Meningitis: Causes, Symptoms and Treatment

Meningitis: Causes, Symptoms and Treatment

Edited by Matthew Martin

AMERICAN
MEDICAL PUBLISHERS
www.americanmedicalpublishers.com

American Medical Publishers,
41 Flatbush Avenue,
1st Floor, New York,
NY 11217, USA

Visit us on the World Wide Web at:
www.americanmedicalpublishers.com

ISBN: 978-1-63927-303-4

Cataloging-in-Publication Data

Meningitis : causes, symptoms and treatment / edited by Matthew Martin.
p. cm.
Includes bibliographical references and index.
ISBN 978-1-63927-303-4
1. Meningitis. 2. Meningitis--Etiology. 3. Meningitis--Treatment.
4. Central nervous system--Diseases--Treatment. I. Martin, Matthew.

RC376 .M46 2022

616.82--dc23

Table of Contents

Preface

Every book is a source of knowledge and this one is no exception. The idea that led to the conceptualization of this book was the fact that the world is advancing rapidly; which makes it crucial to document the progress in every field. I am aware that a lot of data is already available, yet, there is a lot more to learn. Hence, I accepted the responsibility of editing this book and contributing my knowledge to the community.

Meningitis is the inflammation of the protective membranes which cover the brain and the spinal cord. The person affected with meningitis often experiences fever, neck-stiffness, headache, vomiting, sensitivity to light or loud noises and altered consciousness. Viruses, bacteria and other microorganisms are the primary causes of this disease. In some cases, meningitis may be life-threatening due to the proximity of inflammation to the brain and spinal cord. A sample of cerebrospinal fluid is collected from the spinal cord by a lumbar puncture for diagnosis of meningitis. A few forms of meningitis can be prevented through vaccination and antibiotics. Its treatment depends on the cause of meningitis. Bacterial meningitis is treated with intravenous antibiotics, fungal meningitis can be treated with antifungal agents and viral meningitis is treated with intravenous antiviral medications. This book contains some path-breaking studies on meningitis. It presents researches and studies performed by experts across the globe. This book, with its detailed analyses and data, will prove immensely beneficial to professionals and students involved in this area at various levels.

While editing this book, I had multiple visions for it. Then I finally narrowed down to make every chapter a sole standing text explaining a particular topic, so that they can be used independently. However, the umbrella subject sinews them into a common theme. This makes the book a unique platform of knowledge.

I would like to give the major credit of this book to the experts from every corner of the world, who took the time to share their expertise with us. Also, I owe the completion of this book to the never-ending support of my family, who supported me throughout the project.

Editor

1

Human meningitis due to *Streptococcus suis* in Lomé, Togo

Mireille Prince-David[1,2], Mounerou Salou[1,2], Corinne Marois-Créhan[3,4], Komi Assogba[5], Céline Plainvert[6,7], Koffi A. Balogou[5], Claire Poyart[6,7,8] and Asmaa Tazi[6,7,8*]

Abstract

Background: *Streptococcus suis* is a zoonotic pathogen which represents the leading cause of meningitis in Southeast Asia and an emerging pathogen in the Western world, the main risk factor for infection being contact with pigs. In Africa, the prevalence of *S. suis* infections in swine and humans is largely unrecognized, with only one recent report of a limited case series.

Case presentation: We describe a human case of meningitis due to *S. suis* in a 32-year-old man living in Togo. The patient had no particular medical history and no risk factors for immunodeficiency but reported regular contact with pork products. Using specific immunological and molecular methods, we characterized the isolate as *S. suis* serotype 2, ST1, one the most prevalent and virulent clone worldwide. The outcome was favorable after one week of adapted antibiotic therapy but the patient was left with severe hearing disorders.

Conclusions: This work highlights the emergence of this pathogen in Africa and reinforces the need for accurate epidemiological and surveillance studies of *S. suis* infections and for educating clinicians and exposed groups in non-endemic countries.

Keywords: Case report, *Streptococcus suis*, Meningitis, Zoonosis, Neurologic sequelae, Capsular serotype

Background

Streptococcus suis is an emerging zoonotic pathogen in Europe, North-America and South-America [1, 2]. This encapsulated gram-positive coccus is responsible for meningitis, bacteremia, and pneumonia in swine and is mainly associated with meningitis and endocarditis in humans. Incidence is highly correlated to contact with pigs and eating of undercooked pork products, habits which are common in Southeast Asia where *S. suis* is endemic and represents the leading cause of meningitis in adults [1, 2]. In the Western world, rates of *S. suis* infection are low and the vast majority of the cases involves highly-exposed groups such as abattoir workers and pig breeders [1]. Mortality rate reaches approx. 3 % and neurologic sequelae in case of meningitis are frequent (60 %), making the global burden of *S. suis* infections in endemic countries significant [2]. We report, according to the CARE guidelines, a human case of meningitis due to *S. suis* in Africa where the prevalence of this bacterium in swine and humans is largely unrecognized.

Case presentation

A 32-year-old man working as a carpenter in Lomé, Togo, was admitted in August 2015 to the University Hospital Campus of Lomé for a 3 day history of severe headaches, vomiting, fever, and intense agitation (Table 1). He had no particular medical history and no risk factors for immunodeficiency. At admission, the body temperature was of 36.4 °C, and the general state was acceptable, with a correct conservation of consciousness. The neurological examination did not show any sign of motor or sensitive defect, of cranial nerve dysfunction or cerebellar symptoms. There was no hearing or skin abnormalities, no obvious neck stiffness, and the rest of the clinical examination was normal. Acute meningeal hemorrhage was evocated as the initial diagnosis. Cranial computed tomography could not be performed and a symptomatic treatment associating antalgic, antipyretic, and anticonvulsant medication was

* Correspondence: asmaa.tazi@cch.aphp.fr
[6]Service de Bactériologie, Hôpitaux Universitaires Paris Centre, site Cochin, 75679 Paris cedex 14, France
[7]Centre National de Référence des Streptocoques, Hôpital Cochin, 75679 Paris cedex 14, France
Full list of author information is available at the end of the article

Table 1 Case-patient timeline

	Presenting concerns	Physical examination	Evaluations	Diagnosis	Interventions-Treatments
Day of admission	32-year-old man, carpenter in Lomé No particular medical history 3-day history of headaches, agitation, vomiting, fever	Body temperature: 36.4 °C Neurological examination: normal Clinical examination: normal	Cranial computed tomography: not performed	Acute meningeal hemorrhage	Symptomatic treatment
Day 2	Persisting symptoms Fever	Neck stiffness Kernig and Brudzinski signs positive	Lumbar puncture: turbid CSF[a] CSF analysis: -WBC[a]: 2,800/mm3 (65 % lymphocytes,35 % neutrophils) - Protein: 1.8 g/L - Glucose: 0.47 g/L (plasma 1.41 g/L; ratio = 0.33) - Gram stain: negative	Bacterial meningitis	Wide-spectrum antibiotic therapy: ceftriaxone, ofloxacin, metronidazole
Day 3	Vertigo Tinnitus		CSF culture positive: catalase negative, gram-positive cocci in chains		Adapted antibiotic therapy: ampicillin, gentamicin Corticoid therapy
Day 4	Patient reported working as a pork butcher every weekend		Bacterial identification: *Streptococcus suis* Audiogram: severe hearing loss in l eft and right ears (80 dB)	Bacterial meningitis due to *S. suis* with neurological complications	
Month 9	Tinnitus		Audiogram: severe hearing loss in left and right ears (80 dB)	Neurological sequelae of the meningitis	

[a]*CSF* cerebrospinal fluid, *WBC* white blood cells

initiated. At the second day of admission, the patient was febrile, agitated, and still suffered from severe headaches and vomiting. The neck had become stiff, and Kernig and Brudzinski signs were positive. The meningeal signs led to the realization of a lumbar puncture, which yielded a turbid cerebrospinal fluid (CSF) concluding to the diagnosis of bacterial meningitis. An empiric intravenous antibiotic treatment associating ceftriaxone (2 g, 2×/d for 24 h then 1 g, 2×/d), ofloxacin (200 mg, 3×/d), and metronidazole (500 mg, 2×/d) was started.

CSF analysis showed 2,800 leukocytes/mm^3 (65 % lymphocytes and 35 % neutrophils), a protein concentration of 1.8 g/L, and a glucose concentration of 0.47 g/L (2.6 mmol/L) with a plasma glucose concentration of 1.41 g/L (7.8 mmol/L; ratio = 0.33). Gram staining did not reveal any microorganism. Blood and CSF cultures, after 48 h and 24 h of incubation, respectively, grew small beta-hemolytic colonies on horse blood agar plates. The bacteria were catalase negative, gram-positive cocci, in chains or in pairs. They were identified as *S. suis* (score 2.56) by MALDI-TOF (Matrix Assisted Laser Desorption Ionisation Time Of Flight) spectrometry (BrukerTM) and as *S. suis* serotype 1 (97 % probability) by VITEK 2 Gram-positive card system (bioMérieux, Marcy l'Etoile, France). Slide agglutination with type-specific hyperimmune serum and specific multiplex PCR identified the isolate as *S. suis* serotype 2, indicating a serotype misidentification by the automated card system, and concluding, together with Multi-Locus Sequence Typing [3–5], to an infection due to *S. suis* serotype 2, Sequence-Type (ST) 1, one of the most virulent and frequently isolated clone all over the world [1, 6]. Antimicrobial drug-susceptibility testing performed according to the European Committee on Antimicrobial Susceptibility Testing (EUCAST) recommendations characterized the strain as susceptible to penicillin (Minimum inhibitory concentration (MIC) < =0.25 mg/L), erythromycin, clindamycin, levofloxacin, and linezolid and resistant to tetracycline.

After *S. suis* was identified, the patient reported working as a pork butcher every week-end. The patient did not have any sign or symptoms of endocarditis, and the antibiotic treatment was replaced by ampicillin (2 g, 3×/d) and gentamicin (80 mg, 2×/d) for 7 days. While the patient was receiving treatment for 1 day, vertigo and tinnitus developed, for which he received adjunctive corticoid therapy and the treatment was completed with no particular adverse events. Hearing disorders, especially hearing loss, are the most common sequelae of *S. suis* infections and affect more than 50 % of patients who survive meningitis [2]. In that case, hearing disorders evolved into severe hearing loss in the left and right ears (80 dB), and the patient was still suffering from tinnitus 9 months after the diagnosis. One year later, tinnitus had disappeared and the patient's auditory function had improved from severe to moderate hearing loss.

Conclusions

Data for circulation and epidemiology of *S. suis* in Africa remain extremely scarce. This is the second report of a human *S. suis* meningitis in Togo, which, together with a recently published limited case-series [7], highlights the emergence of this zoonotic pathogen in Africa. Nevertheless, swine industry and pork products consumption, although extremely low compared to other continents, are steadily increasing [8], which might lead to a significant rise of *S. suis* infections in the future. Besides, *S. suis* infections are not limited to adult cases but also affect children [7], and specific attention should be paid to this other potential high-risk group. This case-report, for which clinical data, microbiological findings, and outcome were similar to those reported elsewhere [1, 2], emphasizes the need for educating both clinicians and exposed groups about *S. suis* infections and their severity in non-endemic countries. Particularly, accurate epidemiological and surveillance studies appear essential to assess the global burden of *S. suis* infections in swine and humans in Africa.

Abbreviation

CSF: Cerebrospinal fluid

Acknowledgements

Not applicable.

Funding

This work was not supported by any specific funding.

Authors' contributions

MPD and MS analyzed the patient's microbiological data. CMC, CPl, CPo and AT performed and analyzed the molecular characterization of the bacterial isolate. KA and KAB analysed and interpreted the patient data regarding the neurological disease. MS, KA and AT were major contributors in writing the manuscript. All authors reviewed and approved the final manuscript.

Competing interests

The authors declare that they have no competing interests.

Consent for publication

The case-patient gave his written consent to publish.

Author details

[1]Centre de Biologie Moléculaire et d'Immunologie, Université de Lomé, BP 101, Lomé, Togo. [2]Service de Microbiologie, Centre Hospitalier Universitaire Sylvanus Olympio, Tokoin Hôpital, BP 57, Lomé, Togo. [3]Agence nationale de sécurité sanitaire de l'alimentation, de l'environnement et du travail, 22440 Ploufragan, France. [4]Université Bretagne Loire, 22440 Ploufragan, France. [5]Service de Neurologie, Centre Hospitalier Universitaire Campus, BP 30284, Lomé, Togo. [6]Service de Bactériologie, Hôpitaux Universitaires Paris Centre, site Cochin, 75679 Paris cedex 14, France. [7]Centre National de Référence des Streptocoques, Hôpital Cochin, 75679 Paris cedex 14, France. [8]Université Paris Descartes, 75006 Paris, France.

References

1. Huong VTL, Ha N, Huy NT, Horby P, Nghia HDT, Thiem VD, et al. Epidemiology, Clinical Manifestations, and Outcomes of *Streptococcus suis* Infection in Humans. Emerg Infect Dis. 2014;20:1105–14.
2. Van Samkar A, Brouwer MC, Schultsz C, Van der Ende A, Van de Beek D. *Streptococcus suis* Meningitis: A Systematic Review and Meta-analysis. PLoS Negl Trop Dis. 2015;9:e0004191.
3. Marois C, Bougeard S, Gottschalk M, Kobisch M. Multiplex PCR assay for detection of *Streptococcus suis* species and serotypes 2 and 1/2 in tonsils of live and dead pigs. J Clin Microbiol. 2004;42:3169–75.
4. King SJ, Leigh JA, Heath PJ, Luque I, Tarradas C, Dowson CG, et al. Development of a multilocus sequence typing scheme for the pig pathogen *Streptococcus suis*: identification of virulent clones and potential capsular serotype exchange. J Clin Microbiol. 2002;40:3671–80.
5. Gottschalk M, Higgins R, Jacques M, Mittal KR, Henrichsen J. Description of 14 new capsular types of *Streptococcus suis*. J Clin Microbiol. 1989;27:2633–6.
6. Schultsz C, Jansen E, Keijzers W, Rothkamp A, Duim B, Wagenaar JA, et al. Differences in the population structure of invasive Streptococcus suis strains isolated from pigs and from humans in The Netherlands. PLoS ONE. 2012;7, e33854.
7. Tall H, Njanpop-Lafourcade B-M, Mounkoro D, Tidjani L, Agbenoko K, Alassani I, et al. Identification of *Streptococcus suis* Meningitis through Population-Based Surveillance, Togo, 2010–2014. Emerg Infect Dis. 2016;22:1262–4.
8. Food and Agriculture Organization of the United Nations, Statistics Division. http://faostat3.fao.org. Accessed 16 Aug 2016.

2

The diagnostic value of cerebrospinal fluid lactate for post-neurosurgical bacterial meningitis

Xiong Xiao[†], Yang Zhang[†], Liwei Zhang, Peng Kang and Nan Ji[*]

Abstract

Background: Bacterial meningitis is not rare in post-neurosurgical patients. If patients are not treated promptly, the mortality rate can reach 20 to 50 %. The concentration of cerebrospinal fluid (CSF) lactate has been reported to be helpful in the diagnosis of bacterial meningitis; however, no systematic evaluations have investigated CSF from a postoperative perspective. In this study, we performed a systematic evaluation and meta-analysis of the efficacy of using CSF lactate concentrations in the diagnosis of post-neurosurgical bacterial meningitis.

Method: We retrieved studies that investigated the diagnostic value of CSF lactate for the diagnosis of post-neurosurgical bacterial meningitis by searching PubMed, EBSCO, the Cochrane Library and ClinicalTrials.gov. All these databases were searched from inception to November 2015. We used Quality Assessment of Diagnostic Accuracy Studies (QUADAS), a tool for the quality assessment of diagnostic accuracy, to evaluate the quality of the included studies. The Meta-DiSc 1.4 and Review Manager 5.3 software programs were used to analyze the included studies. Forest plots and summary receiver operating characteristics (SROC) curves were also drawn.

Results: Five studies, involving a total of 404 post-neurosurgical patients, were selected from 1,672 articles according to the inclusion criteria. The quality of the five included studies was assessed using QUADAS, and the related results are presented in tables. The meta-analysis revealed the following diagnostic values regarding CSF lactate for post-neurosurgical bacterial meningitis: a pooled sensitivity of 0.92 (95 % CI 0.85–0.96), a pooled specificity of 0.88 (95 % CI 0.84–0.92 with significant heterogeneity), a diagnostic odds ratio of 83.09 (95 % CI 36.83–187.46), an area under the curve (AUC_{SROC}) of 0.9601, an SE(AUC) of 0.0122, a Q* of 0.9046 and an SE(Q*) of 0.0179.

Conclusion: The meta-analysis indicated that the CSF lactate concentration has relatively high sensitivity and specificity for the diagnosis of post-neurosurgical bacterial meningitis and thus has relatively good efficacy.

Keywords: Cerebrospinal fluid lactate, Post-neurosurgical bacterial meningitis, Diagnostic value, Meta-analysis

Background

Bacterial meningitis is not rare in post-neurosurgical patients and has an incidence of approximately 0.3 to 1.5 % [1]. However, the observed incidence in clinical practice is higher than this number. Clinical manifestations such as fever, signs of meningeal irritation and an altered mental status lack specificity and sensitivity [2]. Furthermore, the intraoperative aseptic inflammatory response induced by blood, bone chips, sloughing tissue, and surgical implants as well as the widespread postoperative administration of prophylactic antibiotics increase the difficulty of diagnosing postoperative bacterial meningitis via routine cerebrospinal fluid (CSF) analysis and CSF culture [2–5]. The delayed administration of antibiotics and corticosteroids, as well as the unnecessary administration of these agents, can result in impaired treatment effects [2, 6]. If patients with bacterial meningitis are not treated promptly, the mortality rate can reach 20 to 50 % [6]. Therefore, early and accurate diagnosis is critical for postoperative bacterial meningitis [7].

Previous studies have found that the CSF lactate concentration is associated with bacterial meningitis. The evaluation of CSF lactate levels is relatively efficient in

* Correspondence: neurochina@gmail.com
[†]Equal contributors
Department of Neurosurgery/China National Clinical Research Center for Neurological Diseases, Beijing Tiantan Hospital, Capital Medical University, 6 Tian Tan Xi Li, Beijing 100050, China

distinguishing between bacterial meningitis and aseptic meningitis [8–11] and is superior to routine CSF analysis [10]. However, post-neurosurgical patients were excluded from Huy's study [10], and Sakushima did not perform a stratified analysis of the diagnostic value of CSF lactate in postoperative bacterial meningitis [11]. Recent studies have indicated that CSF lactate shows a certain degree of diagnostic accuracy for differentiating between postoperative bacterial meningitis and aseptic meningitis [12]; however, no systematic evaluations have investigated this aspect.

The CSF lactate exam is simple, objective and affordable [6]. The exam is not affected by blood contamination of the CSF [13, 14]. Many researchers also reported that the CSF lactate concentration was not related to the neutrophil count [6, 15, 16]. The test can be performed at bedside, and the results can be received within 15 min. Additionally, a rapid decrease in the CSF lactate level following antibiotic treatment could suggest a relatively good prognosis. Therefore, CSF lactate may play a significant role in the diagnosis of post-neurosurgical bacterial meningitis. This study performed a systematic evaluation and meta-analysis of the efficacy of CSF lactate concentration in diagnosing post-neurosurgical bacterial meningitis.

Methods

Review of ethics committee

This study is a meta-analysis based on published data from previous studies. Hence, no review by an ethics committee needed.

Standard of systematic reviews

This study is designed and performed according to the "Transparent reporting of systematic reviews and meta-analyses" (PRISMA) guidelines.

Inclusion and exclusion criteria

This analysis included studies that were published in international journals and investigated the CSF lactate concentration in the diagnosis of post-neurosurgical bacterial meningitis.

The inclusion/exclusion criteria were as follows: (1) The study's objectives included an evaluation of the diagnostic value of the CSF lactate concentration in post-neurosurgical bacterial meningitis. (2) The study subjects were patients who underwent neurosurgery. Studies irrelevant to neurosurgery, studies on patients who did not undergo neurosurgery, and animal studies were excluded from this analysis. (3) The studies used etiological methods as basic diagnostic tools, which means that a Gram stain or bacterial culture of CSF was considered the basis of the gold diagnostic standard for postoperative bacterial meningitis. (4) A diagnostic test fourfold table was included in the studies or could be indirectly obtained by calculations utilizing the data provided in the studies. (5) The studies were published in English.

Measured parameters

The indexes included sensitivity, specificity, positive likelihood ratio (LR+), negative likelihood ratio (LR-), diagnostic odds ratio (DOR), area under the curve (AUC) of the summary receiver operating characteristics (SROC) curve, and Q^* (Q^* is the intersection point on the SROC curve where the sensitivity equals specificity).

Literature retrieval, collection, and screening

We searched PubMed, EBSCO, Cochrane and ClinicalTrials.gov. All the databases were searched from inception to November 2015. ("Lactate" OR "lactic acid") AND "meningitis" were used as search terms in both PubMed and EBSCO. To avoid ignoring valuable studies, "Lactate" OR "lactic acid" were used to search studies in ClinicalTrials.gov and the Cochrane library.

Studies were selected from the results of the database search. The title and abstract were read first. For each study that could offer a valuable contribution to this analysis and that could not be excluded based on reading only the title and abstract, the full text of the study was directly assessed. If the original text could not be directly accessed, we acquired the full text by contacting the study authors, performing repeated retrievals, searching Google Scholar, or other legal methods.

According to the above study inclusion and exclusion criteria, two investigators (Xiong Xiao and Yang Zhang) performed the literature search and independently acquired and read the studies to exclude articles that were confirmed to hold no useful information for this analysis. The two investigators crosschecked the results of the literature search, discussed the search results and constructed a table for the included studies. A PRISMA flow diagram was drawn (Fig. 1).

Quality assessment of studies

We evaluated the study quality using the Quality Assessment of Diagnostic Accuracy Studies (QUADAS) method, which contains 14 items for study assessment. Three criteria, "Yes" (satisfies this criterion), "No" (does not satisfy this criterion or was not mentioned) and "unclear" (criterion partially satisfied or cannot obtain sufficient information from the study), were applied to identify the causes of study bias and variations.

Data extraction

Two investigators independently performed the data extraction, which was consistent. We extracted parameters such as the first author's name, the publication year, the location of the study, the type of study and the cut-off value of each included study. If the study presented data regarding the number of true positives, number of false positives, number of true negatives, number of false negatives, sensitivity, or specificity, we recalculated these data to ensure correctness. Otherwise, we derived these data according to the related numbers in the included article. All the extracted data were double-checked to avoid errors.

Statistical analysis

1) We first assessed the heterogeneity of the studies: if the heterogeneity $I^2 > 50$ % and $P < 0.05$, heterogeneity was considered to be significant; otherwise, heterogeneity was not significant. When the heterogeneity was significant, a Spearman correlation coefficient was computed between the logit of sensitivity and the logit of (1 – specificity) to assess the threshold effect. 2) A pooled model analysis was chosen according to the results of the heterogeneity assessment. A random effects model was selected if there was significant heterogeneity; otherwise, a fixed effects model was used. 3) The Review Manager 5.2 (Cochrane Editorial Unit, London, UK) and Meta-DiSc 1.4 (Clinical Biostatistics Unit, Ramon y Cajal Hospital, Madrid, Spain) software programs were used for analysis. Forest plots and SROC cures were plotted. The pooled sensitivity, pooled specificity, pooled positive likelihood ratio (LR+), pooled negative likelihood ratio (LR-), pooled diagnostic odds ratio (DOR) and AUC were computed using the software indicated above. Additionally, a Begg's funnel plot was generated using STATA 12 (StataCorp LP, College Station, TX, USA) to show potential publication bias.

Results

Search results

After excluding overlapping literature, 1,672 studies were retrieved (Fig. 1), among which 523 studies were obtained from PubMed; 190 studies came from EBSCO; 130 studies were obtained from the Cochrane library; and 829 came from ClinicalTrials.gov. We finally included 5 studies in this analysis according to the above inclusion and exclusion criteria, all of which were published in English and involved a total of 404 post-neurosurgical patients. The publication year of these studies ranged from 1999 to 2014. Among the 5 included studies, 3 were prospective, while the other 2 were retrospective. The cutoff values for CSF lactate ranged from 3.45 mmol/L to 5.4 mmol/L (4.41 ± 0.85 mmol/L). The gold standards of these 5 studies are also shown. One study used only CSF bacterial culture or Gram staining to diagnose post-neurosurgical bacterial meningitis, while the other 4 studies employed diagnostic methods including CSF white blood cells (WBC), the CSF neutrophil percentage, or CSF glucose levels (Table 1). The data from fourfold tables for diagnostic tests were extracted from the studies and prepared for the subsequent analysis (Fig. 2).

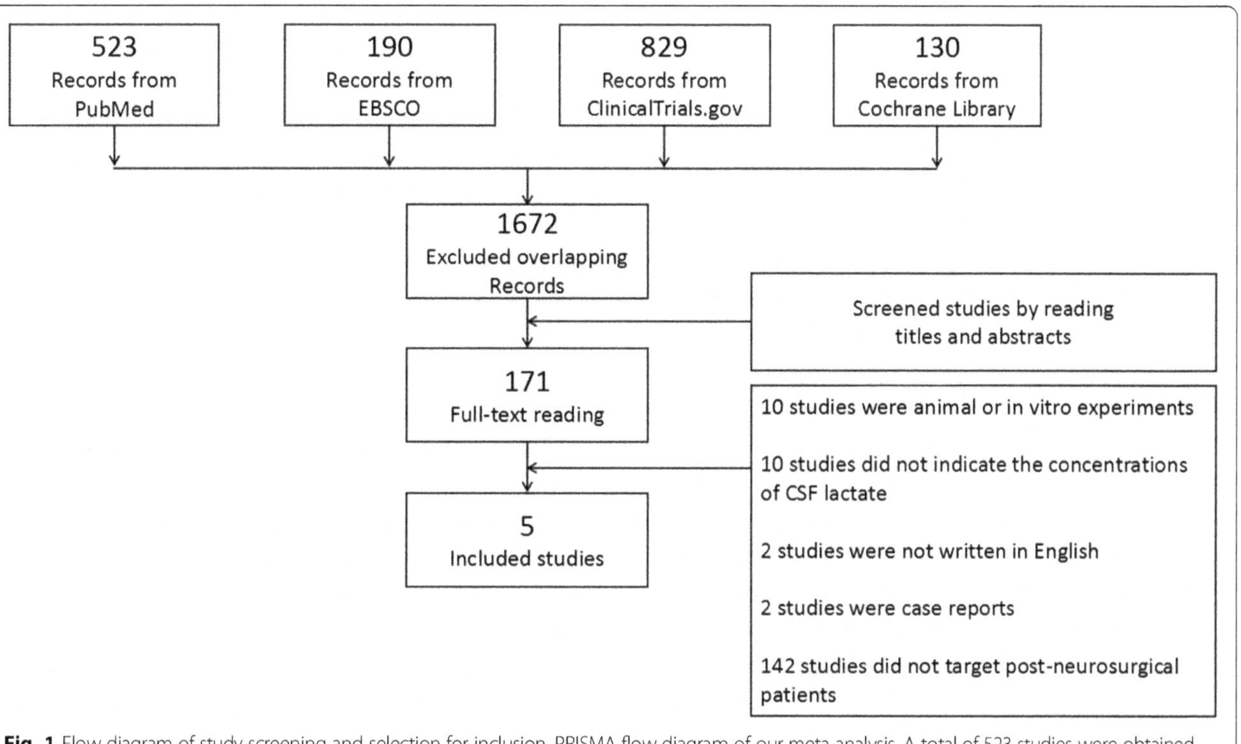

Fig. 1 Flow diagram of study screening and selection for inclusion. PRISMA flow diagram of our meta-analysis. A total of 523 studies were obtained from PubMed, 190 studies from EBSCO, 130 studies from the Cochrane library, and 829 from ClinicalTrials.gov. After excluding overlapping literature, 1,672 studies were retrieved. We finally included 5 studies in this analysis according to the above inclusion and exclusion criteria

Table 1 Studies included in this meta-analysis

Authors	Publication year	Type of study	Cut-off value (mmol/L)	Gold standard
Leib et al. [6]	1999	Retrospective	4.0	1) or 2) or 3): 1) positive bacterial CSF culture and CSF WBC > 2.5×10^8/L 2) CSF WBC > 1×10^9/L and neutrophils >50 % 3) CSF WBC > 2.5×10^8/L and neutrophils >50 % in patients treated with steroids or antibiotics at the time of LP
Tavares et al. [25]	2006	Prospective	5.4	positive bacterial CSF culture or Gram stain
Grille et al. [21]	2012	Prospective	5.2	1) or 2): 1) positive bacterial CSF culture or Gram stain 2) negative bacterial CSF culture or Gram stain and CSF WBC > 1×10^9/L (>50 % neutrophils) in patients treated with antibiotics at the time of lumbar puncture
Maskin et al. [22]	2013	Prospective	4.0	1) or 2): 1) positive bacterial CSF culture or Gram stain and CSF WBC ≥ 1×10^5/L or (CSF glucose <40 mg/dL or CSF glucose/blood glucose <0.4) 2) CSF WBC ≥ 2.5×10^5/L and CSF glucose/blood glucose <0.5 if patients received antibiotics 24 h prior to CSF sampling
Li et al. [18]	2014	Retrospective	3.45	[a] All of the below: 1) clinical symptoms 2) positive bacterial CSF culture or Gram stain 3) CSF WBC count ≥1×10^9/L and polykaryocyte percentage ≥75 % 4) CSF glucose <2.5 mmol/L or CSF glucose/blood glucose <0.4.

[a] Patients who did not meet these criteria with a CSF WBC count <5×10^8/L were classified into the non-PNBM group

We evaluated the quality of the included studies using the QUADAS tool, the results are presented in Table 2.

Analysis results

Forest plots were drawn according to the results of the meta-analysis using the Review Manager 5.2 software (Fig. 2). A Begg's funnel plot was drawn using STATA 12 (Fig. 3) to assess publication bias. All of the dots were within the 95 % CI with a symmetrical distribution in an approximate funnel shape.

It can be seen from the analysis that the heterogeneity of the 5 studies (I2) was 79.5 %, ($P = 0.0006$). This heterogeneity was significant. The Spearman correlation coefficient between the logit of sensitivity and the logit of (1 – specificity) was 0.462 ($P = 0.434$), indicating that there was no obvious threshold effect in the estimates of accuracy. Therefore, the random effects model was chosen for the pooled analysis. Meta-DiSc 1.4 was used to select the random effects model for the pooled analysis. The results were as follows: the pooled sensitivity was 0.92 (95 % CI 0.85–0.96), the pooled specificity was 0.88 (95 % CI 0.84–0.92 with significant heterogeneity), the pooled LR+ was 7.70 (95 % CI 3.94–15.05 with significant heterogeneity), the pooled LR- was 0.11 (95 % CI 0.06–0.19), the pooled DOR was 83.09 (95 % CI 36.83–187.46), the AUC of the SROC curve was 0.9601 and the Q* was 0.9046 (Figs. 4 and 5).

Discussion

When performing this systematic review and meta-analysis, we found only a few diagnostic studies on post-neurosurgical intracranial infection, and two of these were retrospective studies. Few high-quality clinical trials or prospective studies have been conducted. The diagnosis and treatment of intracranial infection has become a critical and urgent problem in neurosurgery. Thus, it is necessary to conduct related clinical research to develop highly specific, sensitive, convenient, fast and affordable early diagnostic indexes. Additionally, scientific and systematic evaluations of the diagnostic efficacy of these indexes should be performed. This work has great

Study	TP	FP	FN	TN	Sensitivity (95% CI)	Specificity (95% CI)
1.Leib 1999	23	1	3	46	0.88 [0.70, 0.98]	0.98 [0.89, 1.00]
2.Tavares 2006	6	2	1	19	0.86 [0.42, 1.00]	0.90 [0.70, 0.99]
3.Grille 2012	13	0	1	32	0.93 [0.66, 1.00]	1.00 [0.89, 1.00]
4.Maskin 2013	32	10	1	36	0.97 [0.84, 1.00]	0.78 [0.64, 0.89]
5.Li 2014	45	20	5	108	0.90 [0.78, 0.97]	0.84 [0.77, 0.90]

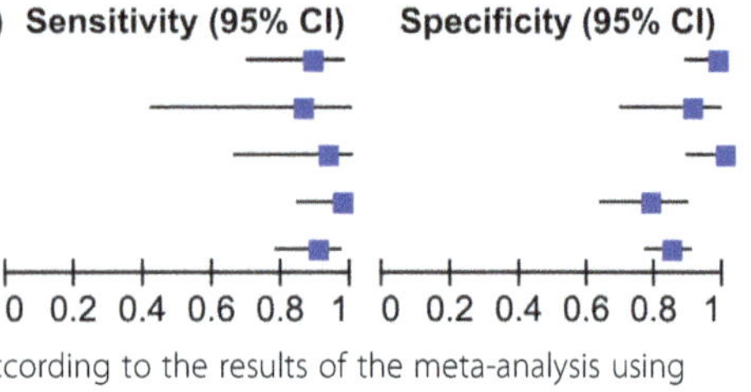

Fig. 2 Forest plot drawn using data from the included studies. Forest plots were drawn according to the results of the meta-analysis using Review Manager 5.2 software. The data extracted from the 5 included studies are shown. TP: true positive; FP: false positive; FN: false negative; TN: true negative

Table 2 Quality assessment of the included studies according to QUADAS

	1	2	3	4	5	6	7	8	9	10	11	12	13	14
Leib 1999 [6]	Yes	Yes	Unclear	Yes	Yes	Yes	Yes	Yes	Yes	Unclear	Yes	Yes	No	No
Tavares 2006 [25]	Yes	Yes	Unclear	Yes	Yes	Yes	Yes	Yes	Yes	Unclear	Unclear	Yes	No	No
Grille 2012 [21]	Yes	Yes	Unclear	Yes	Yes	Yes	Yes	Yes	Yes	Unclear	Unclear	Yes	No	No
Maskin 2013 [22]	Yes	Yes	Unclear	Yes	Yes	Yes	Yes	Yes	Yes	Unclear	Unclear	Yes	No	No
Li 2014 [18]	Yes	Yes	Unclear	Yes	Yes	Yes	Yes	Yes	Yes	Unclear	Unclear	Yes	No	No

significance for the early diagnosis and treatment of post-neurosurgical bacterial meningitis.

According to our results, the CSF lactate exam shows relatively good efficacy. Moreover, this test is fast, simple, objective, and affordable and can be widely applied in hospitals.

Several factors may affect the results of this meta-analysis: 1) A small number of studies, only 5, were included. Moreover, two of these were retrospective studies. The number of study subjects was relatively small (only 404 patients). 2) It was difficult to standardize the CSF lactate measurement exam methods among the 5 studies. 3) Two of the included studies defined the cutoff value before analysis; however, the other three generated the value based on the highest sensitivity and specificity of the ROC curve. The cutoff values in the studies ranged from 3.45 mmol/L to 5.4 mmol/L. Although the Spearman correlation between the logit of sensitivity and the logit of (1 – specificity) showed that there was no obvious threshold effect, the situation would be improved if more studies using same cutoff value were available. 4) Of the 5 included studies, only 1 used etiological examination as the gold standard for diagnosis; the other 4 studies included patients with clinically confirmed diagnoses, which means that the patients had a negative etiology test result but presented with significant clinical symptoms and signs and that their cerebrospinal cell analysis exhibited significantly abnormal results.

Additionally, we found that the CSF lactate cutoff value was defined before the analysis in 2 studies; however, in the others, it was defined based on the best value according to the ROC curve. To determine whether this difference was responsible for the heterogeneity of the studies, we used Meta-DiSc 1.4 to run a Meta-Regression. The results indicated that this difference did not cause the observed heterogeneity ($P = 0.3141$). To further analyze the sources of heterogeneity, we ran a subgroup analysis based on the type, publication year, sample size, and diagnostic method of the studies and whether the cutoff values were defined before analysis. It was found that dividing the studies into two groups based on whether the publication year was before 2013 reduced the heterogeneity in each subgroup. The pooled diagnostic values in the subgroup with earlier publication dates were as follows: sensitivity, 0.894 (95 % CI: 0.769–0.965); specificity, 0.970 (95 % CI: 0.915–0.994); LR+, 21.442 (95 % CI: 5.330–86.101); LR-, 0.120 (95 % CI: 0.054–0.263); DOR, 207.71 (95 % CI:

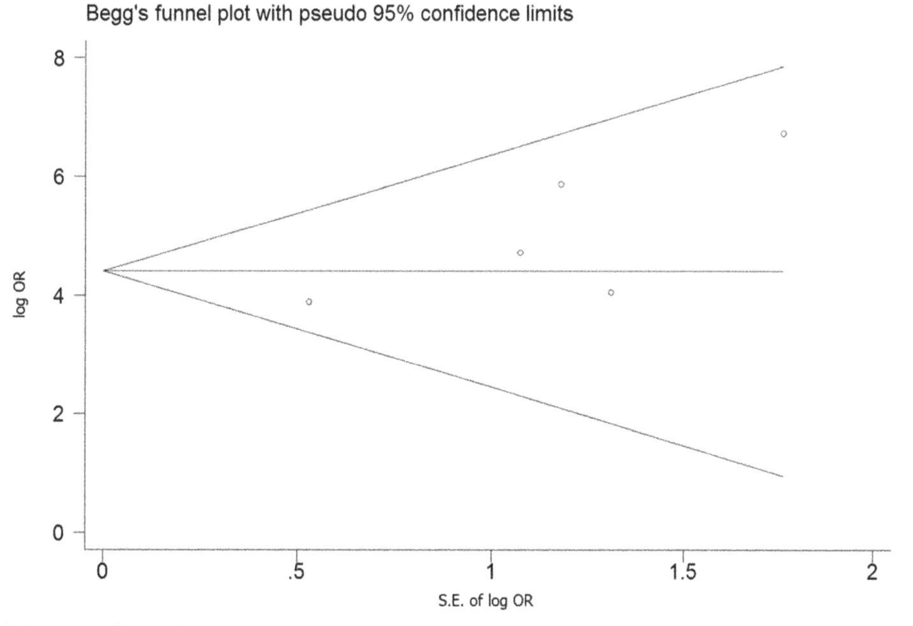

Fig. 3 Begg's funnel plot. Begg's funnel plot was drawn using STATA 12. Each circle means that a study included. OR: odd ratio; S.E.: standard error

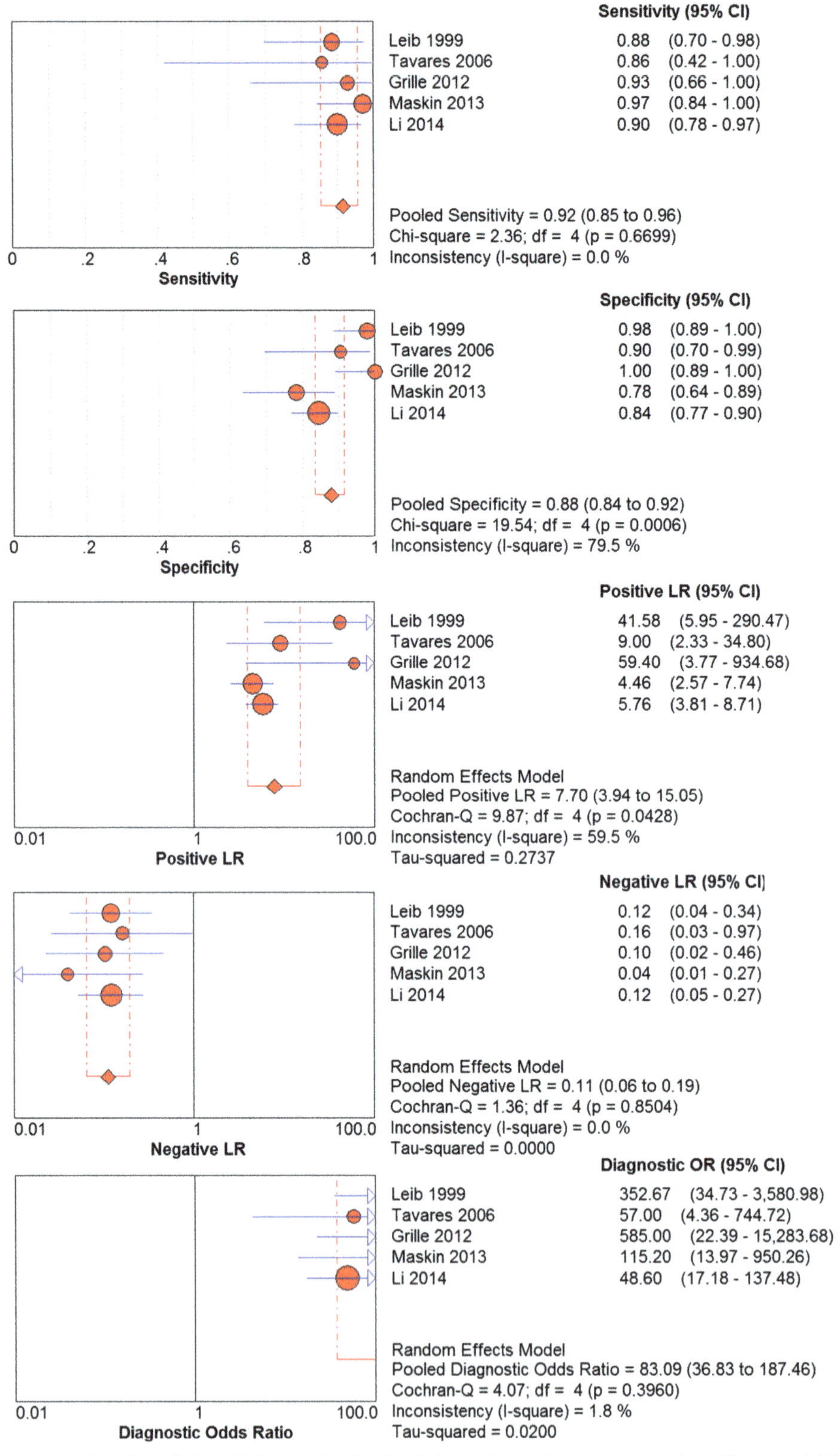

Fig. 4 Results from the pooled analysis of the included studies. Results of the pooled analysis using a random effects model. The sensitivity, specificity, positive LR, negative LR, and diagnostic OR of all of the included studies were pooled. The pooled sensitivity was 0.92 (95 % CI 0.85–0.96); the pooled specificity was 0.88 (95 % CI 0.84–0.92, with significant heterogeneity); and the diagnostic OR was 83.09 (95 % CI 36.83–187.46). LR: likelihood ratio

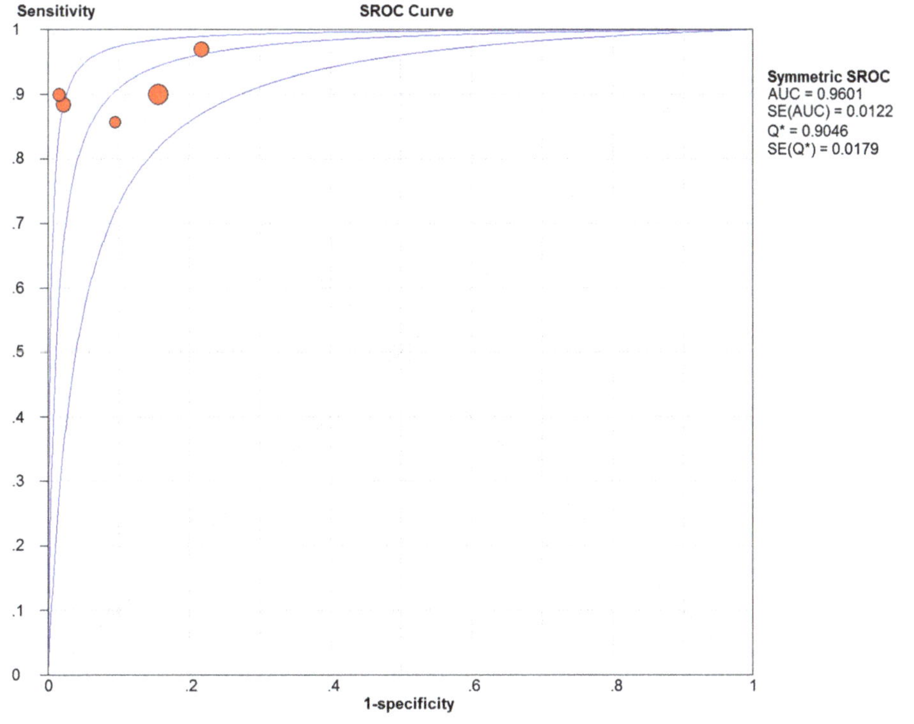

Fig. 5 SROC Curve. SROC curves were plotted. Each red point represent an included study. The AUC of the SROC curve was 0.9601, and the Q* was 0.9046. SROC: summary receiver operating characteristic; AUC: area under curve; Q*: the point on the SROC where sensitivity equals specificity

45.321–951.99); AUCSROC, 0.9795; Q*, 0.9363. The pooled diagnostic values in the subgroups with later publication dates were as follows: sensitivity, 0.928 (95 % CI: 0.849–0.973); specificity, 0.828 (95 % CI: 0.763–0.881); LR+, 5.255 (95 % CI: 3.775–7.313); LR-, 0.095 (95 % CI: 0.040–0.231); DOR, 57.528 (95 % CI: 22.636–146.21); AUCSROC, 0.9469; Q*, 0.8864.

Although positive CSF culture or Gram stain results are the most direct evidence of infection, the percentages of the positive results are low for a variety of reasons, including the low volume, contamination of the CSF sample, time constraints and antibiotic drug administration [17, 18]. This makes the "gold standard" less sensitive and specific, leading to low diagnostic efficacy. It is possible to misdiagnose many patients with postoperative infections when using only the etiological exam to confirm diagnosis. This would result in higher mortality and study bias. Additionally, the CSF culture requires several days to generate a result, which is sometimes too long to wait for treatment. Etiological examinations in addition to CSF cytology and biochemical examinations are widely used to achieve better efficacy. However, there is no specific criterion for the threshold values of the involved items. In other words, there is no other gold standard. As Li reported, the widely used criteria for diagnosing post-neurosurgery bacterial meningitis include those proposed by the Centers for Disease Control and Prevention [19], the Massachusetts General Hospital [20], the Infectious Diseases Society of America and the Beijing Tiantan Hospital [18]. Four of the 5 studies that we included also used standards that differed from those of other studies. However, the evidence indicating whether the patients were suffering from post-neurosurgical meningitis was objective. Regardless of the criterion, meeting the established standard meant a greater chance that the post-neurosurgical meningitis diagnosis was correct. Moreover, the studies we included compared the CSF lactate levels of patients whose diagnoses were etiologically confirmed with those whose diagnoses were clinically confirmed (i.e., those with negative etiological diagnoses but with the presence of significant clinical manifestations and abnormal CSF levels); there was no statistically significant difference between these patients [6, 21, 22].

New techniques, such as polymerase chain reaction (PCR), can improve diagnostic sensitivity; however, these techniques are usually unavailable to most hospitals or laboratories. New diagnostic markers, such as PCT, sCD163 and CRP, have also been reported [18, 23, 24]. Furthermore, some researchers tested the efficacy of combinations of markers and obtained optimistic results [18]. However, most studies concerning these markers are retrospective or have small sample sizes.

Neurosurgery involves the management of many types of diseases. It may not be appropriate to treat these diseases equally and to put all of the post-operative conditions into a single category ("post-neurosurgical") when investigating post-operative infections. The operative procedures vary according to differences in disease type, lesion location, patient condition and other factors. In the design period, we attempted to search for articles on "post-craniotomy meningitis" because we believed that the infections in patients who received craniotomies would differ from those in patients who did not undergo craniotomy. However, the article retrieval results were not optimistic.

This meta-analysis summarized the studies targeting the diagnostic efficacy of CFS lactate in post-neurosurgical bacterial meningitis and reached a relevant conclusion. However, more high-quality, large-scale, prospective studies are required to obtain a more thorough understanding of and better biomarkers or indicators for post-neurosurgical meningitis.

Conclusion

This meta-analysis investigated the diagnostic value of CSF lactate for post-neurosurgical bacterial meningitis. We included 5 studies on a total of 404 post-neurosurgical patients to obtain pooled data. The results indicate that the CSF lactate concentration shows a relatively high sensitivity and specificity in the diagnosis of post-neurosurgical bacterial meningitis and thus has relatively good efficacy. However, additional precise, accurate and convincing data from prospective studies and from those with large samples is necessary.

Abbreviations

CSF: Cerebrospinal fluid; QUADAS: Quality assessment of diagnostic accuracy studies; SROC: Summary receiver operating characteristics; LR+: Positive likelihood ratio; LR-: Negative likelihood ratio; OR: Odds ratio; S.E.: Standard error; WBC: White blood cells

Acknowledgements

We acknowledge all of the work upon which this analysis was based, regardless of whether that work was included in the analysis.

Funding

This work was supported by grants from the Beijing Tiantan Hospital Funds for Young Scholars project (#2014-YQN-YS-26), the National Key Technology Research and Development Program of the Ministry of Science and Technology of China (2013BAI09B03, 2015BAI12B04) and the Beijing Talents Fund (2014000021469G257).

Authors' contributions

All the authors participated in the study conception and design. XX and YZ acquired the data. XX and YZ analyzed and interpreted the data. XX, YZ, PK and NJ drafted the manuscript. All the authors critically revised the article. All the authors reviewed the submitted version of the manuscript. LZ approved the final version of the manuscript on behalf of the authors. XX and YZ performed the statistical analysis. NJ provided administrative/technical/material support and supervised the study. All authors read and approved the final manuscript.

Competing interests

The authors declare that they have no competing interests.

Consent for publication

Not applicable.

Statement

This manuscript has not been previously published in whole or in part or submitted elsewhere for review.

References

1. Blomstedt GC. Infections in neurosurgery: a retrospective study of 1143 patients and 1517 operations. Acta Neurochir. 1985;78(3–4):81–90.
2. Ross D, Rosegay H, Pons V. Differentiation of aseptic and bacterial meningitis in postoperative neurosurgical patients. J Neurosurg. 1988;69(5):669–74. doi:10.3171/jns.1988.69.5.0669.
3. Kaufman BA, Tunkel AR, Pryor JC, Dacey Jr RG. Meningitis in the neurosurgical patient. Infect Dis Clin N Am. 1990;4(4):677–701.
4. Carmel PW, Greif LK. The aseptic meningitis syndrome: a complication of posterior fossa surgery. Pediatr Neurosurg. 1993;19(5):276–80.
5. Wang KW, Chang WN, Huang CR, Tsai NW, Tsui HW, Wang HC, et al. Post-neurosurgical nosocomial bacterial meningitis in adults: microbiology, clinical features, and outcomes. J clin neurosci. 2005;12(6):647–50. doi:10.1016/j.jocn.2004.09.017.
6. Leib SL, Boscacci R, Gratzl O, Zimmerli W. Predictive value of cerebrospinal fluid (CSF) lactate level versus CSF/blood glucose ratio for the diagnosis of bacterial meningitis following neurosurgery. Clin infect dis. 1999;29(1):69–74. doi:10.1086/520184.
7. Kumar A, Roberts D, Wood KE, Light B, Parrillo JE, Sharma S, et al. Duration of hypotension before initiation of effective antimicrobial therapy is the critical determinant of survival in human septic shock. Crit Care Med. 2006;34(6):1589–96. doi:10.1097/01.CCM.0000217961.75225.E9.
8. Genton B, Berger JP. Cerebrospinal fluid lactate in 78 cases of adult meningitis. Intensive Care Med. 1990;16(3):196–200.
9. Pavese P, Francois P, Lafond JL, Kayemba Kay SS, Bosson JL. Assay of lactic acid in the cerebrospinal fluid for the diagnosis of bacterial meningitis. Strategies for the choice of discriminatory threshold. Presse Med. 1997;26(12):551–4.
10. Huy NT, Thao NT, Diep DT, Kikuchi M, Zamora J, Hirayama K. Cerebrospinal fluid lactate concentration to distinguish bacterial from aseptic meningitis: a systemic review and meta-analysis. Crit Care. 2010;14(6):R240. doi:10.1186/cc9395.
11. Sakushima K, Hayashino Y, Kawaguchi T, Jackson JL, Fukuhara S. Diagnostic accuracy of cerebrospinal fluid lactate for differentiating bacterial meningitis from aseptic meningitis: a meta-analysis. J infect. 2011;62(4):255–62. doi:10.1016/j.jinf.2011.02.010.
12. van de Beek D, Drake JM, Tunkel AR. Nosocomial bacterial meningitis. N Engl J Med. 2010;362(2):146–54. doi:10.1056/NEJMra0804573.
13. Begovac J, Bace A, Soldo I, Lehpamer B. Lactate and glucose in cerebrospinal fluid heavily contaminated with blood. Acta medica Croatica. 1991;45(4–5):341–5.
14. Cameron PD, Boyce JM, Ansari BM. Cerebrospinal fluid lactate in meningitis and meningococcaemia. J infect. 1993;26(3):245–52.
15. Bland RD, Lister RC, Ries JP. Cerebrospinal fluid lactic acid level and pH in meningitis. Aids in differential diagnosis. Am J Dis Child. 1974;128(2):151–6.
16. Jordan GW, Statland B, Halsted C. CSF lactate in diseases of the CNS. Arch Intern Med. 1983;143(1):85–7.
17. Simon TD, Pope CE, Browd SR, Ojemann JG, Riva-Cambrin J, Mayer-Hamblett N, et al. Evaluation of microbial bacterial and fungal diversity in cerebrospinal fluid shunt infection. PLoS One. 2014;9(1):e83229. doi:10.1371/journal.pone.0083229.
18. Li Y, Zhang G, Ma R, Du Y, Zhang L, Li F, et al. The diagnostic value of cerebrospinal fluids procalcitonin and lactate for the differential diagnosis of post-neurosurgical bacterial meningitis and aseptic meningitis. Clin Biochem. 2015;48(1–2):50–4. doi:10.1016/j.clinbiochem.2014.10.007.
19. Korinek AM, Baugnon T, Golmard JL, van Effenterre R, Coriat P, Puybasset L. Risk factors for adult nosocomial meningitis after craniotomy: role of

antibiotic prophylaxis. Neurosurgery. 2006;59(1):126–33. doi:10.1227/01.NEU.0000220477.47323.92. discussion –33.
20. Durand ML, Calderwood SB, Weber DJ, Miller SI, Southwick FS, Caviness Jr VS, et al. Acute bacterial meningitis in adults. A review of 493 episodes. N Engl J Med. 1993;328(1):21–8. doi:10.1056/NEJM199301073280104.
21. Grille P, Torres J, Porcires F, Bagnulo H. Value of cerebrospinal fluid lactate for the diagnosis of bacterial meningitis in postoperative neurosurgical patients. Neurocirugia. 2012;23(4):131–5. doi:10.1016/j.neucir.2011.11.005.
22. Maskin LP, Capparelli F, Mora A, Hlavnicka A, Orellana N, Diaz MF, et al. Cerebrospinal fluid lactate in post-neurosurgical bacterial meningitis diagnosis. Clin Neurol Neurosurg. 2013;115(9):1820–5. doi:10.1016/j.clineuro.2013.05.034.
23. Knudsen TB, Larsen K, Kristiansen TB, Moller HJ, Tvede M, Eugen-Olsen J, et al. Diagnostic value of soluble CD163 serum levels in patients suspected of meningitis: comparison with CRP and procalcitonin. Scand J Infect Dis. 2007; 39(6–7):542–53. doi:10.1080/00365540601113685.
24. Shimetani N, Shimetani K, Mori M. Levels of three inflammation markers, C-reactive protein, serum amyloid A protein and procalcitonin, in the serum and cerebrospinal fluid of patients with meningitis. Scand J Clin Lab Invest. 2001;61(7):567–74.
25. Tavares WM, Machado AG, Matushita H, Plese JP. CSF markers for diagnosis of bacterial meningitis in neurosurgical postoperative patients. Arq Neuropsiquiatr. 2006;64(3A):592–5. doi:10.1590/S0004-282X2006000400012.

3

Clinical presentations, diagnosis, mortality and prognostic markers of tuberculous meningitis in Vietnamese children

Nguyen Duc Bang[1,2], Maxine Caws[1,3,4], Thai Thanh Truc[1], Tran Ngoc Duong[2], Nguyen Huy Dung[2], Dang Thi Minh Ha[1,2], Guy E. Thwaites[1,4], Doortje Heemskerk[1,4], Joel Tarning[4,5], Laura Merson[1,4], Pham Van Toi[1,4], Jeremy J. Farrar[1,4], Marcel Wolbers[1,4], Thomas Pouplin[1,4,5] and Jeremy N. Day[1,4*]

Abstract

Background: Tuberculous meningitis in adults is well characterized in Vietnam, but there are no data on the disease in children. We present a prospective descriptive study of Vietnamese children with TBM to define the presentation, course and characteristics associated with poor outcome.

Methods: A prospective descriptive study of 100 consecutively admitted children with TBM at Pham Ngoc Thach Hospital, Ho Chi Minh City. Cox and logistic regression were used to identify factors associated with risk of death and a combined endpoint of death or disability at treatment completion.

Results: The study enrolled from October 2009 to March 2011. Median age was 32.5 months; sex distribution was equal. Median duration of symptoms was 18.5 days and time from admission to treatment initiation was 11 days. Fifteen of 100 children died, 4 were lost to follow-up, and 27/81 (33 %) of survivors had intermediate or severe disability upon treatment completion. Microbiological confirmation of disease was made in 6 %. Baseline characteristics associated with death included convulsions (HR 3.46, 95CI 1.19–10.13, $p = 0.02$), decreased consciousness (HR 22.9, 95CI 3.01–174.3, $p < 0.001$), focal neurological deficits (HR 15.7, 95CI 1.67–2075, $p = 0.01$), Blantyre Coma Score (HR 3.75, 95CI 0.99–14.2, $p < 0.001$) and CSF protein, lactate and glucose levels. Neck stiffness, MRC grade (children aged >5 years) and hydrocephalus were also associated with the combined endpoint of death or disability.

Conclusions: Tuberculous meningitis in Vietnamese children has significant mortality and morbidity. There is significant delay in diagnosis; interventions that increase the speed of diagnosis and treatment initiation are likely to improve outcomes.

Keywords: Tuberculous meningitis, Children, Vietnam, Mycobacterium, Survival

* Correspondence: jday@oucru.org
[1]Oxford University Clinical Research Unit, Wellcome Trust Major Overseas Programme, 764 Vo Van Kiet, Quan 5, Ho Chi Minh City, Vietnam
[4]Centre for Tropical Medicine and Global Health, Nuffield Department of Medicine Research Building, University of Oxford, Old Road campus, Roosevelt Drive, Oxford, UK
Full list of author information is available at the end of the article

Background

Tuberculosis (TB) is an important cause of childhood morbidity - recent estimates of the number of children developing TB each year range from 500 000 to 1 million, significantly higher than previously estimated by the WHO [1, 2]. There may be 50 million children latently infected [3]. 5 % of disease occurs in HIV co-infected children, although this is higher in sub-Saharan Africa [3]. Despite this high burden, in TB as in many other diseases, children are a neglected group - the vast majority of data used to guide management are derived from adult patients.

Tuberculous meningitis (TBM) is the most severe form of tuberculosis, with high rates of disability and death [4]. Children are more likely than adults to develop disseminated TB and TB meningitis following infection [5]. This risk is greatest for infants and children under 2 years of age, probably due to the immaturity of the immune system [6]. The challenges of TBM diagnosis and management are exacerbated in children. Initial symptoms in infants are non-specific, it is difficult to obtain diagnostic samples and more invasive sampling methods are needed, and the diagnostics samples obtained generally proffer extremely low yields of mycobacteria [7, 8]. Death from TBM is strongly associated with delays in diagnosis and treatment both in children and adults [9–12]. It is striking that there has never been a randomized controlled trial of anti-tuberculosis drugs in children with TBM [13].

Vietnam is classified as having a high burden of TB, with a prevalence in the order of 145 per 100 000 of the population as a whole [14]. Tuberculous meningitis in adults is well characterized in Vietnam, and these data have been key in developing treatment guidelines, but there are no data on the disease in children [11, 15–17]. In accordance with historic WHO policy, the Vietnamese National TB Programme has focused on the systematic notification of smear positive cases of TB. However, the majority of pediatric TB cases are smear negative, and subsequently limited data are available on pediatric TB in Vietnam. In line with WHO policy revisions, Vietnam has recently implemented disaggregated data collection for pediatric TB. Improving outcomes in children is dependent upon a better understanding of the epidemiology of childhood TB, and early diagnosis and instigation of effective treatment.

Methods

Study aim

This study aimed to describe the current practice in the management of Vietnamese children with TBM, the presenting clinical features and predictors of poor outcome (death and neurological disability), in order to define the challenges in management and prioritise research.

Study design

A prospective descriptive study of 100 consecutive cases of TBM in children (aged ≤15 years).

Setting and participants

The study was conducted at Pham Ngoc Thach Hospital (PNT), Ho Chi Minh City (HCMC). PNT is the tertiary referral centre for tuberculosis in the south of Vietnam, serving 40 million people. All children diagnosed or suspected of having TBM in HCMC and the surrounding provinces are referred here. Approximately 500 inpatient cases of pediatric TB are treated each year; around 20 % have meningitis.

Entry criteria

All patients aged ≤15 years presenting to Pham Ngoc Thach Hospital with a clinical syndrome consistent with TBM (meaning one or more of: fever, headache, neck stiffness, vomiting, confusion, coma, convulsions, cranial nerve palsies, hemiplegia or paraplegia) and considered to have tuberculous meningitis by their attending physician (i.e. meriting anti-TB therapy) were eligible to enter the study. TBM was classified as "definite", "probable" or "possible", as follows:

Definite TBM: acid-fast bacilli (AFB) seen or cultured from cerebrospinal fluid (CSF).
Probable TBM: Clinical syndrome consistent with TBM, and one or more of the following criteria: suspected active pulmonary tuberculosis on chest radiography, AFB found in any specimen other than the CSF, brain imaging consistent with TBM, or clinical evidence of other extrapulmonary tuberculosis.
Possible TBM: Clinical syndrome consistent with TBM and at least 4 of the following: past medical history of tuberculosis, predominance of lymphocytes in the CSF, illness of ≥6 days in duration, CSF: blood glucose ratio <0.5, altered consciousness, yellow CSF, and focal neurological signs.

Patient assessment

All patients had clinical assessments by the dedicated study team at study entry, 2 weeks, 1, 2, 3 and 8 months.

Lumbar puncture

All patients underwent lumbar puncture either at the referring centre or on admission to PNT hospital. Lumbar puncture was repeated at days 30 and 90 following study entry/treatment initiation. Cerebrospinal fluid (CSF) investigations included cell count, glucose, protein, lactate, Gram's stain, and India ink test, and culture for fungi and pyogenic bacteria. CSF Ziehl-Neelsen smear and culture were not available at referring centres. When patients were referred from other centres, lumbar puncture was only repeated at baseline if felt to be clinically indicated by the attending physician. The GeneXpert test was not available at the time the study took place.

Other investigations

All children had haematology and biochemistry investigations according to standard of care in the hospital. Sputum was examined for acid fast bacteria (AFB) when available; gastric washings for AFB were done at the discretion of the attending physician. All patients had HIV testing - counselling and HIV testing were available for the parents of children diagnosed with HIV. All patients had a chest radiograph performed at study entry. 40 patients were entered into a descriptive radiological substudy and underwent cranial Magnetic Resonance Imaging (MRI) at study entry, on day 60 and day 270. Other imaging was performed at the discretion of the attending physician.

Classification of severity

All patients were graded for severity at study entry. For children older than 5 years severity was graded according to a modified United Kingdom Medical Research Council criteria based on Glasgow Coma Score: Grade I had a Glasgow coma score (GCS) of 15/15 with no focal neurological signs, grade II either had a GCS 11–14 or GCS 15 with focal neurological signs, Grade III had a GCS of ≤ 10.

For children less than 5 years of age severity of TBM was graded according to the Blantyre Coma Score. Patients with grade I disease had a Blantyre coma score of 4–5 with no focal neurological signs; patients with grade II disease had a Blantyre coma score of 2–3 or a score of 4–5 with focal neurological signs; and grade III had a Blantyre coma score ≤1.

Treatment and follow-up

Anti-tuberculosis treatment was according to Vietnamese treatment guidelines, which at the time were consistent with the 2006 WHO guidelines. Patients received oral isoniazid (5 mg/kg), rifampicin (10 mg/kg), pyrazinamide (25 mg/kg), ethambutol 15 mg/kg and intramuscular streptomycin (15 mg/kg) for 2 months, followed by oral isoniazid, rifampicin, pyrazinamide and ethambutol for 1 month and oral isoniazid, rifampicin, and ethambutol at the same doses for 5 months [2HRZES/1HRZE/5HRE]. Streptomycin was not used for HIV-infected patients. Patients with MRC grades II and III and BCS grades II and III disease received adjuvant dexamethasone for the first six weeks; patients with MRC grade I and BCS grade I received adjuvant dexamethasone for 4 weeks as per Vietnamese guidelines [11]. All patients were reviewed daily by the study team while in-patients, at days 30, 60 and 90, and on completion of treatment after 8 months. DOT was used to secure and monitor treatment adherence, and drugs were administered via nasogastric tube to unconscious children.

Assessment of outcome

We were interested in two outcomes: survival, and a combined endpoint of neurological disability or death. Disability status was assessed at the end of 8 months of treatment with the use of the two simple questions ("Does the child require help from anybody for everyday activities [e.g., eating, drinking, washing, brushing teeth, and going to the toilet]?" and "Has the illness left the child with any other problems?") and the modified Rankin scale (scores range from 0 [no symptoms at all] to 6 [death]) and was classified as good (i.e., no disability), intermediate, severe, or death, as described elsewhere [11]. For children under 5 years, the response was determined by the study clinician in relation to the expected functioning in normal children of the same age.

Study size

The study was designed as a prospective descriptive study to include all patients less than or equal to 15 years of age presenting with suspected TBM to Pham Ngoc Thach Hospital. Approximately 100 such patients are admitted each year, and we planned to recruit 100 consecutively admitted patients.

Statistical analysis

The raw data was imported into a secure anonymised in-house data management system (CliRes). Between group comparisons of baseline characteristics were based on the Wilcoxon rank sum test and Fisher's exact test for continuous and categorical variables, respectively. Mortality at 8 months was estimated with the Kaplan-Meier method. Univariate Cox regression was used to identify significant factors influencing time to death. Factors relating to the probability of a combined endpoint of neurological sequelae (intermediate or severe disability) or death were determined using univariate logistic regression and the Firth correction was applied in case of separation [18]. Multivariable regression models were not fitted due to the relatively low number of events and large number of factors of interest. All analyses were performed using R software version 2.9.1 [19].

Results

Demographic and clinical characteristics

Enrollment was conducted between October 2009 and March 2011. During this period 133 children were admitted to PNT hospital with suspected TBM. Twelve children declined to join the study and 21 were not recruited because they were already receiving treatment.

Follow-up completed in December 2011. The median duration from first hospital admission to making the diagnosis of TBM (and instigation of treatment) was 11 days (range 1–74 days).

Baseline characteristics and outcomes for the cohort are shown in Table 1.

Fifty-six percent ($n = 56/100$) of patients were male. The majority of children (67 %) were less than 5 years old (median age 32.5 months, range 2 to 180 months). Four of 96 children tested were HIV infected (4 %); 5 % ($n = 5/96$) were hepatitis B surface antigen positive. Concomitant extra-pulmonary TB was common, seen in 42 patients (36 pulmonary, 4 pulmonary with peripheral lymphadenitis, 1 pulmonary disease with pleural involvement, and 1 pulmonary disease with concomitant TB arthritis. A family history of TB was reported for 27 patients (27 %); one patient had a previous history of TB.

Table 1 Baseline characteristics and outcomes of 100 childhood TBM patients

Symptoms and signs	Number affected (%)		Median duration in days (range)
Fever	96/97 (99 %)		23; (6–96)
Vomiting	76/100 (76 %)		13; (1–96)
Weight loss	59/98 (60 %)		15.5; (7–90)
Confusion	15/100 (15 %)		10.4; (2–30)
Unconsciousness	27/100 (27 %)		5.3; (1–16)
Headache[a]	49/55 (89 %)		21; (4–66)
Fits	39/100 (39 %)		8.5; (1–35)
Neck stiffness	75/100 (75 %)		
Hemiparesis/ Hemiplegia	20/98 (20 %)		
Paraparesis/ paraplegia	6/98 (6 %)		
Monoplegia	4/98 (4 %)		
Quadriplegia	2/98 (2 %)		
II nerve involvement	3/98 (3 %)		
III nerve palsy	4/98 (4 %)		
VI nerve palsy	20/98 (20 %)		
VII nerve palsy	7/98 (7 %)		
Anemia (Hb < 11 g/dL)	46/99 (46 %)		
HIV infection	4/96 (4 %)		
HBV infection	5/96 (5 %)		
MRC Grades >5 years (33)	I: 16 (48 %)	II: 11 (33 %)	III: 6 (18 %)
Blantyre < 5 years (67)	4–5: 43 (64 %)	2–3: 12 (18 %)	0–1: 12 (18 %)
Deaths	15/100 (15 %)		
Sequelae			
Severe	6/81 (7 %)		
Intermediate	21/81 (26 %)		

[a]Unable to ascertain in 44 due to the age of the child; headache was not assessed for one additional subject

Fever, vomiting and nuchal rigidity were the most frequently elicited symptoms. Seizures were common reported in 39 cases. Headaches occurred in at least 49 (49 %) cases - in 44 cases (44 %) the presence of headache was uncertain because the child was too young to describe the symptom. Of 33 (33 %) children ≥ 5 years of age, 16 (48 %) had MRC grade I disease, 11 (33 %) grade II disease, and 6 (18 %) grade III disease. The remaining 67 children under 5 years were graded using the Blantyre coma score (BCS): BCS I (4–5): 43 (64 %), BCS II (2–3): 12 (18 %) and BCS III (0–1): 12 (18 %) (Table 1). Focal neurological signs were frequent occurring in 58 %, most commonly VIth cranial nerve palsies (22 %), followed by hemiplegia (20 %), VIIth cranial nerve palsy 7 %, paraplegia 6 %, monoparesis 4 %, IIIrd cranial nerve palsy 4 %, optic nerve atrophy 3 %, and quadriparesis 2 %. Four patients (4 %) were lost to follow up after 3 months of treatment.

Cerebrospinal fluid results

Lumbar puncture was performed on all patients ($n = 100$) at referring hospitals; 22 (22 %) children had repeat lumbar puncture at PNT. All CSF was analyzed for protein, lactate and glucose concentrations, and for cell count and differentials (Table 2). The median white cell count was 202 cells/uL. 92 of 95 (97 %) patients had lymphocyte predominance (>50 %). The mean CSF:blood glucose ratio was 0.25 (range 0.07 to 0.69; 7 of 100 patients had ratios >0.5). 77 patients had CSF lactate measured; the median was 5.3 mmol/L (10th and 90th centiles 2.36 and 8.8 mmol/L respectively). All but 8 patients had elevated CSF protein concentrations (median 1.2 g/L, upper limit of the normal range 0.4 g/L).

Microbiology results

None of 22 CSF samples taken at PNT were AFB smear positive, However, *M. tuberculosis* was cultured from 6 of these samples. Smears of sputum and gastric aspirates were positive for AFB in only 2 (7 %) of 29 patients and 5 (7 %) of 67 patients, respectively. Drug susceptibility testing was not performed.

TBM classification

Six cases met the definition of definite TBM. Sixty-six cases fulfilled the case definition of probable TBM: seven had positive AFB smears and/or *M. tuberculosis* cultured from sputum or gastric aspirate; 33 had abnormal chest X-rays consistent with TB and an abnormal brain imaging, and 26 cases had an abnormal CT or MRI brain imaging consistent with TBM.

Table 2 Baseline characteristics of possible TBM and definite/probable TBM

Variables	Possible TBM ($n = 28$)	Definite/Probable TBM ($n = 72$)	P-value for comparison
Age[a] (months)	24.5 (2–165)	36.5 (2–180)	0.09
Male (%)	18/28 (64 %)	38/72 (53 %)	0.03
Fever	28/28 (100 %)	71/72 (99 %)	0.99
Symptom duration[a] (days)	16 (6–60)	19.5 (6–96)	0.172
Vomiting	20/28 (71 %)	56/72 (78 %)	0.50
Altered sensorium	6/28 (21 %)	36/72 (50 %)	0.01
Fits	9/28 (32 %)	30/72 (40 %)	0.38
Neck stiffness	17/28 (61 %)	58/72 (81 %)	0.04
Motor deficit	4/25 (16 %)	28/60 (47 %)	0.01
Cranial nerve palsy	9/28 (32 %)	18/72 (25 %)	0.91
HIV infection	1/28 (4 %)	3/72 (4 %)	0.99
HBV infection	2/28 (7 %)	3/72 (4 %)	0.86
Family TB history	7/28 (25 %)	19/72 (26 %)	0.89
Death	2/27 [b] (7 %)	13/69 (19 %) [c]	0.28
Permanent sequelae	2/25 (8 %)	25/56 (45 %)	0.002
CSF WCC[a] (cells/uL)	144 (4–780)	150 (1–802)	0.37
CSF Lymph[a] (cells/uL)	80 (40–100)	80 % (50–100)	0.44
CSF Protein[a] (g/L)	0.8 (0.2–5)	1.3 (0.1–4.8)	0.08
CSF Lactate[a] (mmol/L)	4.3 (1.4–8.8)	5.6 (1.21–19.2)	0.08
CSF: Blood Glucose ratio[a]	0.30 (0.09–0.61)	0.25 (0.07–0.69)	0.51

[a] Values are medians/ranges
[b] 1 lost to follow-up
[c] 3 lost to follow-up

The remaining 28 cases fulfilled the definition of possible TBM, with clinical features and CSF biochemistry consistent with the diagnosis. The differences in baseline characteristics and outcome between definite/probable and possible cases are illustrated in Table 2. There were statistically significant lower rates of altered sensorium, neck stiffness and motor deficits at baseline, and a reduced risk of neurological sequelae in possible cases, suggesting that these patients may have had less severe disease.

Imaging findings

All children had chest X-ray examinations at admission: 42 % (42/100) had abnormalities consistent with TB (14 % mediastinal lymphadenopathy 14 %, consolidation 11 %, miliary pattern 9 %, nodules 6 %, cavity 1 % and atelectasis 1 %).

Forty-three patients underwent cranial MRI before beginning treatment (42 with contrast enhancement). Findings are shown in Table 3.

Abnormalities were frequent, detected in 86 % of patients: 62 % (26/42) had basal meningeal enhancement, 44 % (19/43) hydrocephalus, 30 % (13/43) infarctions and 14 % (6/42) tuberculomas. 35 of these 43 patients had repeat cranial MRI scans performed 60 days post randomization: 37 % (13/35) had basal meningeal enhancement, 29 % (10/35) hydrocephalus, 34 % (12/35) infarctions and 29 % (10/35) tuberculomas.

Death and sequelae

Fifteen patients died by 8 months (Kaplan-Meier estimate of mortality 15.7 %, 95CI: 9.56–24.3 %, 4 patients lost to follow-up). Eight (53 %) deaths occurred within the first 6 days of treatment; 14 within 45 days of diagnosis. At the end of treatment, six of 81 surviving patients (7.4 %) were classified with severe disability and 21/81 (26 %) were classified with intermediate disability (Table 1).

Baseline predictors associated with increased risk of death or neurological sequelae are shown in Table 4.

More severe BCS was predictive of increased risk of death, as were history of coma, fits, focal neurological deficits and CSF levels of protein, lactate and glucose. The study did not detect a statistically significant association between risk of death and MRC score but this may be due to the low number of children in the study aged ≥5 years. However, there was a consistent increase in the hazard of death as MRC grade worsened. Hydrocephalus, neck stiffness and MRC grade at baseline were associated with an increased risk of the combined endpoint of neurological sequelae or death ($p = 0.01$). Neither brain infarctions nor

Table 3 Baseline brain MRI scan results for 43 patients

Finding	Absolute frequency (%)
Any abnormality	37/43 (86 %)
Meningeal enhancement	26/42 (62 %)
Basal	25 (60 %)
Sylvian Fissure	16 (37 %)
Suprasellar cistern	4 (9 %)
Hydrocephalus	19/43 (44 %)
Tuberculoma	6/42 (14 %)
Infarction	13/43 (30 %)
Basal Ganglia	8/43 (19 %)
Cerebral cortex	3/43 (7 %)
Internal capsule	1/43 (2 %)
Brain stem	1/43 (2 %)

basal meningeal enhancement identified on brain imaging were associated with mortality or the combined endpoint.

Two patients developed drug induced liver injury (DILI) according to the classification of antituberculosis drug-induced hepatotoxicity based on the WHO Adverse Drug Reaction Terminology [20]. This occurred at 2 and 4 weeks following treatment initiation. Neither case was infected with Hepatitis B or C virus. In both cases, PZA was discontinued completely and INH and RIF were reintroduced successfully. Both patients survived.

Uniform case definition for tuberculous meningitis

After this study was designed and recruited, a consensus document was published suggesting criteria to standardize the categorization of TB meningitis as possible, probable or definite, in order to allow comparison of different populations in intervention trials [21]. The criteria are based upon the expert opinion of a number of international experts. We reclassified our patients according to these new criteria, and this resulted in 18 cases moving from the 'probable' diagnosis to the new 'possible' category, and 8 cases moving from our 'possible' category to the new 'probable' category. Following re-categoristaion, male sex was no longer statistically significantly differently distributed between possible and probable/definite cases; altered sensorium, neck stiffness, motor deficit and permanent sequelae remained significantly more common amongst probable and definite cases. Cranial nerve palsies and death became significantly more associated with probable and definite cases.

Discussion

This study demonstrates the challenges in delivering effective treatment for TBM in children in Vietnam. First, TBM is associated with considerable mortality and morbidity, with a risk of death at the end of treatment of 15 %, and 33 % of survivors having intermediate or severe disability. These figures are similar to those reported from other studies in children, and to the rates of death and disability seen in HIV uninfected adults with TBM in Vietnam, but while in adult disease considerable progress has been made and large studies are on-going, childhood TBM remains a neglected area [11, 13, 22–29]. Treatment guidelines for children are largely derived from studies in adults, and although efforts are underway to develop pediatric formulations in appropriate ratios, at the present time dosing schedules are limited by adult fixed dose combination tablets. Randomised controlled trials and pharmacokinetic studies of novel dosing strategies and agents in children are needed to ensure treatment is optimized.

Secondly, the timely instigation of treatment in TBM remains a significant challenge, even in countries such as Vietnam where the burden of TB is high and the diagnosis is at the forefront of clinicians' minds. In this study, the median time from presentation to treatment was 19 days, and 50 % of deaths occurred within the first 6 days of treatment. Earlier instigation of treatment may be able to prevent these deaths. Delays in diagnosis and treatment are likely explained by 3 main factors. First, poverty is a barrier to accessing health care. Since the study Vietnam has made important progress in rolling out free access to healthcare for children under the age of 6 years; however, this is beyond the means of many countries where the TB burden is highest. Secondly, TBM presents in a non-specific manner and it is rare to confirm the diagnosis microbiologically even in high resource settings. In this study, a definitive diagnosis was made in only 6 % of cases. This is partly explained because only 22 % (22/100) of patients had a CSF smear and culture, although the study is representative of real world practice. Of note, no patients were CSF smear positive. Most papers report finding AFB in fewer than 20 % of TBM patients [30]. Improving laboratory training and infrastructure, and improving access to WHO endorsed technologies such as the GeneXpert, would potentially reduce this delay but will not alter the fact that clinical specimens from children are limited both by their volume and their paucibacillary nature [31]. An adequate volume of CSF significantly affects the likelihood of confirming the diagnosis [32] and appropriate sampling for TB at other sites should be performed. Moreover, while TB diagnostic tests remain poorly sensitive, increasing the capacity to identify and exclude other central nervous system pathogens is key in giving clinicians the confidence to instigate treatment in a timely manner and will reduce unnecessary prescription of lengthy TB regimens. Of note, an approach that has shown promise in South African children with TBM, which resulted in a doubling of diagnostic sensitivity, is

Table 4 Univariate analysis of potential predictors of mortality and neurological sequelae in patients with tuberculous meningitis

Characteristic	Time to death ($N = 100$)			Neurological sequelae or death ($N = 96$)		
	Death/No at risk	HR (95 % CI)	*P*	Events/No at risk	OR (95 % CI)	*P*
Sex						
[a]Male	10/56 (17.9 %)	0.61	0.36	23/54 (42.6 %)	1.11	0.80
Female	5/44 (11.4 %)	(0.21–1.78)		19/42 (45.2 %)	(0.49–2.52)	
Age						
[a]<5 years	11/67 (16.5 %)	0.70	0.54	30/64 (46.9 %)	0.68	0.38
≥5 years	4/33 (12.1 %)	(0.22–2.20)		12/32 (37.5 %)	(0.28–1.61)	
Duration of symptoms $N = 89$		1.00	0.4	–	1.01	0.43
(per +1 day)		(0.98–1.01)			(0.98–1.04)	
Neck stiffness						
[a]No	1/25 (4.0 %)	5.15	0.11	5/24 (20.8 %)	4.02	0.01
Yes	14/75 (18.7 %)	(0.68–39.16)		37/72 (51.4 %)	(1.44–13.18)	
HIV co-infection						
[a]No	13/92 (14.1 %)	1.85	0.55	39/88 (44.3 %)	0.42	0.43
Yes	1/4 (25.0 %)	(0.24–14.17)		1/4 (25.0 %)	(0.02–3.42)	
BCS Grade						
age <5 years						
[a]BI	0/43 (0 %)	1.00	<0.001	10/40 (25.0 %)	1.00	<0.001
BII	3/12 (25.0 %)	27.96 [b]		9/12 (75.0 %)	9.00	
		(2.71–3760)			(2.21–47.06)	
BIII	8/12 (67.0 %)	94.64 [b]		11/12 (91.7 %)	33.00	
		(11.71–12,260)			(5.44–643.12)	
TBM grade						
(age ≥ 5 years)						
[a]I	1/16 (6.3 %)	1.00	0.28	2/15 (13.3 %)	1.00	0.01
II	1/11 (9.1 %)	1.41		5/11 (45.5 %)	5.41	
		(0.09–22.5)			(0.81–36)	
III	2/6 (33.3 %)	6.26		5/6 (83.3 %)	32.5	
		(0.57–69.2)			(2.4–443)	
Convulsions						
[a]No	5/61 (8.2 %)	3.46	0.02	20/59 (33.9 %)	2.86	0.01
Yes	10/39 (25.6 %)	(1.18–10.13)		22/37 (59.5 %)	(1.24–6.81)	
Decreased level of consciousness						
[a]No	1/58 (1.7 %)	22.9	<0.001	10/54 (18.5 %)	14.08	<0.001
Yes	14/42 (33.3 %)	(3.01–174.3)		32/42 (76.2 %)	(5.46–39.85)	
Focal neurological deficits						
[a]No	0/53 (0 %)	15.66	0.01	6/50 (12.0 %)	15.4	<0.001
Yes	4/32 (12.5 %)	(1.67–2075)		21/31 (67.7 %)	(5.22–51.96)	
Extra meningeal TB						
[a]No	6/51 (11.8 %)	2.3	0.11	19/57 (33.3 %)	2.87	0.01
Yes	9/30 (30.0 %)	(0.82–6.45)		23/39 (59.0 %)	(1.25–6.80)	
TB culture						
[a]Negative	2/14 (14.3 %)	2.72	0.33	4/16 (25.0 %)	4.50	0.16

Table 4 Univariate analysis of potential predictors of mortality and neurological sequelae in patients with tuberculous meningitis *(Continued)*

Positive	2/3 (66.7 %)	(0.38–19.4)		3/5 (60.0 %)	(0.56–45.4)	
Hydrocephalus[c]						
[a]No	2/31 (6.5 %)	3.46	0.10	6/31 (19.4 %)	9.72	<0.001
Yes	6/30 (20.0 %)	(0.70–17.16)		21/30 (70.0 %)	(2.97–32)	
Cranial nerve palsy						
No	14/70 (20.0 %)	5.42	0.10	29/70 (41.4 %)	0.71	0.45
Yes	1/26 (3.8 %)	(0.71–42.2)		13/26 (50.0 %)	(0.29–1.75)	
CSF Protein	*N* = 99	1.74	0.002	*N* = 94	1.65	0.01
(per + 1 g/L)		(1.22–2.49)			(1.14–2.51)	
CSF Lactate	*N* = 77	1.14	0.04	*N* = 73	1.20	0.03
(per + 1 mmol/L)		(1.01–1.29)			(1.01–1.47)	
CSF Glucose	*N* = 100	0.45	0.05	*N* = 96	0.65	0.10
(per + 1 mmol/L)		(0.20–0.98)			(0.38–1.08)	

[a]Baseline category. HR and OR give comparisons to the baseline category. *P*-value is an overall likelihood ratio test for the significance of the factor
[b]Model fitted by logistic regression with Firth correction
[c]hydrocephalus diagnosed by MRI brain (43 patients or CT brain 19 patients)

the use of more than one nucleic acid amplification test on CSF [33]. However, the investigators still found a combination of microscopy and culture to be most effective. We have found GeneXPert and CSF smear to have similar sensitivities of in adult patients; the challenge for Vietnam remains in obtaining significant volumes of CSF from infants and balancing the risk of investigation with the benefits of a definitive diagnosis [31]. The early identification of drug resistance is likely to be an important factor in improving outcomes. A South African study found that drug resistance was associated with delays in instigation of effective treatment, and that multidrug resistance was associated with worse outcomes [34]. In this study isoniazid mono-resistance was not clearly associated with worse outcomes [34]. However, this mimics the experience in adult patients – initial small studies failed to show a deleterious effect of isoniazid mono-resistance on outcome, but later larger datasets demonstrated that indeed such resistance is disadvantageous [35, 36].

Thirdly, TB treatment is onerous, both in regards to side effects and duration, which may lead to reluctance to start empirical treatment where the risk and consequences of disease are perceived to be low. However, *M. tuberculosis* has been reported to be a more frequent cause of meningitis than pyogenic organisms in South Africa – given that 50 % of deaths are occurring within the first week of treatment a case could be made for early empirical TB treatment in such centres [37]. Few data exist on the optimal duration of treatment for TBM. Drugs such as the fluoroquinolones, which have good tolerability and excellent CSF penetration, potentially offer more effective and palatable treatment regimens, but are relatively untested in children [38]. Randomized controlled trials in children specifically designed to improve TB treatment by 1) identifying shorter equally effective courses and 2) new treatment combinations, may go some way to addressing this issue, although recent trials in adult patients have had mixed results [39–42]. The effective dose of rifampicin appears to be key in improving outcomes. Such regimes would enable a move towards an empirical therapeutic approach similar to that used in acute bacterial meningitis to be employed in high burden settings.

Finally, it is reassuring that drug induced liver injury necessitating treatment interruption was rare and not associated with a poor outcome in this study, affecting just 2 % of the patients. Our study is small and thus our estimates are somewhat imprecise. However, the rate is considerably lower than the 13 % quoted for DILI in adults, supporting the concept that higher doses could be used in children, as advocated in the recent WHO guidelines. [2, 43–45].

Our study had some limitations. It was limited by its small size, and thus estimates around the rates of death and other sequelae lack precision, although findings are generally in keeping with other series [13]. Secondly, we used all-cause mortality. However, 50 % of all deaths occurred within 1 week of treatment initiation, and the rates of co-morbidities (such as HIV) were low, meaning that it is reasonable to assume that all deaths were either a direct consequence of TB or a result of its sequelae. Thirdly, children were only followed up until the end of treatment, and we may have missed later deaths and relapse. The main limitation is the low rate of microbiological confirmation of tuberculosis. This is consistent with other studies in children and represents the very real practical difficulties of managing these children. It is possible that some of these cases, particularly those meeting the 'possible' case definition, may have had some other pathology. However, when the possible cases are excluded, then the mortality and morbidity rate rises further underlying the need to improve diagnostics and treatment for this devastating disease.

Our study was designed and completed before the publication of the universal case definition (UCD) for TBM was published and thus we present our results as originally intended, with a secondary analysis using this classification [21]. The UCD is based upon a non-linear scoring system derived from expert opinion, and has been shown to misclassify 14 % of cases of culture proven TBM as possible TBM in children in a South African study [46]. This underlines the danger of using this research tool as a diagnostic aid, particularly where microbiological diagnostic facilities are poorly developed. Moreover, it is not yet clear that the UCD achieves that which it set out to achieve – i.e allowing robust comparison of patients across diverse study groups according to the UCD defined likelihood of there being definite, probable or possible TBM. As an illustration, a study from South Africa found that patients with 'possible' versus other 'probable/definite' TBM had significant differences in CSF protein concentrations and CSF/serum glucose concentrations. This difference was not apparent in our children, suggesting that our 'possible' cases may be more likely to actually have TBM than possible cases from South African series [47]. There is a need to develop more robust data-driven classification systems, and given the number of patients enrolled into intervention trials in the last 15 years this should be feasible [11, 15, 38, 48].

Conclusions

Tuberculous meningitis in children carries significant morbidity and mortality in Vietnam. A particular challenge is in reducing the time to diagnosis, and institution of effective treatment. However, improving outcomes will also require the development of treatment regimens tailored to children. Given the recent disappointing results of fluoroquinolone boosted treatment regimens in adults with TBM, randomized controlled trials of boosted rifampicin dosing would seem the most important strategy to develop.

Abbreviations

AFB: Acid fast bacilli; BCS: Blantyre coma score; CSF: Cerebrospinal fluid; DILI: Drug induced liver injury; DOT: Directly observed treatment; E: Ethambutol; GCS: Glasgow coma score; H: Isoniazid; HCMC: Ho Chi Minh City; HIV: Human immunodeficiency virus; INH: Isoniazid; MRC: Medical Research Council; MRI: Magnetic Resonance Imaging; PNT: Pham Ngoc Thach Hospital; PZA: Pyrazinamide; R: Rifampicin; RIF: Rifampicin; S: Streptomycin; TB: Tuberculosis; TB: Tuberculosis; TBM: Tuberculous meningitis; UK: United Kingdom; WHO: Word Health Organisation; Z: Isoniazid

Acknowledgements

We thank the study participants, their parents, and the ward, administrative and laboratory staff of PNT, and the funders for making this study possible.

Funding

Funded by the Wellcome Trust UK. JND is a Wellcome Trust Intermediate Fellow Grant No WT097147MA.

Authors' contributions

JND, TP, NDB and JF designed the study; NDB, JND, TND, NHD, PVT, DTMH, MC, LM and TP generated the data; NDB, JND, TTT and MW analysed the results; JND wrote the first draft of the manuscript; all authors reviewed and edited the manuscript. All authors read and approved the final manuscript.

Competing interests

The authors declare that they have no competing interests.

Author details

[1]Oxford University Clinical Research Unit, Wellcome Trust Major Overseas Programme, 764 Vo Van Kiet, Quan 5, Ho Chi Minh City, Vietnam. [2]Pham Ngoc Thach Hospital, 120 Hung Vuong, Quan 5, Ho Chi Minh City, Vietnam. [3]Department of Clinical Sciences, Liverpool School of Tropical Medicine, Pembroke Place, L3 5QA Liverpool, UK. [4]Centre for Tropical Medicine and Global Health, Nuffield Department of Medicine Research Building, University of Oxford, Old Road campus, Roosevelt Drive, Oxford, UK. [5]Mahidol-Oxford Tropical Medicine Research Unit, Faculty of Tropical Medicine, 420/6 Ratchawithi Rd., Bangkok, Thailand.

References

1. Cruz AT, Starke JR. What's in a number? Accurate estimates of childhood tuberculosis. The Lancet Global Health. 2014;2(8):e432–3.
2. WHO. Guidance for national tuberculosis programmes on the management of tuberculosis in children second edition. 2nd ed. Geneva: WHO; 2014.
3. Dodd PJ, Gardiner E, Coghlan R, Seddon JA. Burden of childhood tuberculosis in 22 high-burden countries: a mathematical modelling study. The Lancet Global Health. 2014;2(8):e453–9.
4. Thwaites GE, van Toorn R, Schoeman J. Tuberculous meningitis: more questions, still too few answers. Lancet Neurol. 2013;12(10):999–1010.
5. Beyers N, Gie RP, Schaaf HS, Van Zyl S, Talent JM, Nel ED, Donald PR. A prospective evaluation of children under the age of 5 years living in the same household as adults with recently diagnosed pulmonary tuberculosis. Int J Tuberc Lung Dis. 1997;1(1):38–43.
6. Marais BJ, Gie RP, Schaaf HS, Hesseling AC, Obihara CC, Starke JJ, Enarson DA, Donald PR, Beyers N. The natural history of childhood intra-thoracic tuberculosis: a critical review of literature from the pre-chemotherapy era. Int J Tuberc Lung Dis. 2004;8(4):392–402.
7. Kent SJ, Crowe SM, Yung A, Lucas CR, Mijch AM. Tuberculous meningitis: a 30-year review. Clin Infect Dis. 1993;17(6):987–94.
8. Cuevas LE, Browning R, Bossuyt P, Casenghi M, Cotton MF, Cruz AT, Dodd LE, Drobniewski F, Gale M, Graham SM, et al. Evaluation of tuberculosis diagnostics in children: 2. Methodological issues for conducting and reporting research evaluations of tuberculosis diagnostics for intrathoracic tuberculosis in children. Consensus from an expert panel. J Infect Dis. 2012; 205 Suppl 2:S209–15.
9. Ertekin V, Alp H, Altinkaynak S, Selimoglu MA. Tuberculous meningitis in Turkish children: an evaluation of 38 cases. Trop Doct. 2005;35(3):183–4.

10. Mihailidou E, Goutaki M, Nanou A, Tsiatsiou O, Kavaliotis J. Tuberculous meningitis in Greek children. Scand J Infect Dis. 2012;44(5):337–43.
11. Thwaites GE, Nguyen DB, Nguyen HD, Hoang TQ, Do TT, Nguyen TC, Nguyen QH, Nguyen TT, Nguyen NH, Nguyen TN, et al. Dexamethasone for the treatment of tuberculous meningitis in adolescents and adults. N Engl J Med. 2004;351(17):1741–51.
12. The Lancet N. Tuberculosis of the CNS remains a lethal threat. Lancet Neurol. 2011;10(5):395.
13. Chiang SS, Khan FA, Milstein MB, Tolman AW, Benedetti A, Starke JR, Becerra MC. Treatment outcomes of childhood tuberculous meningitis: a systematic review and meta-analysis. Lancet Infect Dis. 2014;14(10):947–57.
14. Hoa NB, Sy DN, Nhung NV, Tiemersma EW, Borgdorff MW, Cobelens FG. National survey of tuberculosis prevalence in Viet Nam. Bull World Health Organ. 2010;88(4):273–80.
15. Torok ME, Yen NT, Chau TT, Mai NT, Phu NH, Mai PP, Dung NT, Chau NV, Bang ND, Tien NA, et al. Timing of initiation of antiretroviral therapy in human immunodeficiency virus (HIV)–associated tuberculous meningitis. Clin Infect Dis. 2011;52(11):1374–83.
16. Heemskerk D, Day J, Chau TTH, Dung NH, Yen NTB, Bang ND, Merson L, Olliaro P, Pouplin T, Caws M, et al. Intensified treatment with high dose Rifampicin and Levofloxacin compared to standard treatment for adult patients with Tuberculous Meningitis (TBM-IT): protocol for a randomized controlled trial. Trials. 2011;12:25.
17. Torok ME, Chau TT, Mai PP, Phong ND, Dung NT, Chuong LV, Lee SJ, Caws M, de Jong MD, Hien TT, et al. Clinical and microbiological features of HIV-associated tuberculous meningitis in Vietnamese adults. PLoS One. 2008; 3(3):e1772.
18. Heinze G, Schemper M. A solution to the problem of separation in logistic regression. Stat Med. 2002;21(16):2409–19.
19. R: A language and environment for statistical computing. [http://www.R-project.org]. Accessed 13 Oct 2016.
20. Tostmann A, Boeree MJ, Aarnoutse RE, de Lange WC, van der Ven AJ, Dekhuijzen R. Antituberculosis drug-induced hepatotoxicity: concise up-to-date review. J Gastroenterol Hepatol. 2008;23(2):192–202.
21. Marais S, Thwaites G, Schoeman JF, Torok ME, Misra UK, Prasad K, Donald PR, Wilkinson RJ, Marais BJ. Tuberculous meningitis: a uniform case definition for use in clinical research. Lancet Infect Dis. 2010;10(11):803–12.
22. Farinha NJ, Razali KA, Holzel H, Morgan G, Novelli VM. Tuberculosis of the central nervous system in children: a 20-year survey. J Infect. 2000;41(1):61–8.
23. Yaramis A, Gurkan F, Elevli M, Soker M, Haspolat K, Kirbas G, Tas MA. Central nervous system tuberculosis in children: a review of 214 cases. Pediatrics. 1998;102(5):E49.
24. Paganini H, Gonzalez F, Santander C, Casimir L, Berberian G, Rosanova MT. Tuberculous meningitis in children: clinical features and outcome in 40 cases. Scand J Infect Dis. 2000;32(1):41–5.
25. Girgis NI, Sultan Y, Farid Z, Mansour MM, Erian MW, Hanna LS, Mateczun AJ. Tuberculosis meningitis, Abbassia Fever Hospital-Naval Medical Research Unit No. 3-Cairo, Egypt, from 1976 to 1996. Am J Trop Med Hyg. 1998;58(1):28–34.
26. Doerr CA, Starke JR, Ong LT. Clinical and public health aspects of tuberculous meningitis in children. J Pediatr. 1995;127(1):27–33.
27. Delage G, Dusseault M. Tuberculous meningitis in children: a retrospective study of 79 patients, with an analysis of prognostic factors. Can Med Assoc J. 1979;120(3):305–9.
28. Kumar R, Dwivedi A, Kumar P, Kohli N. Tuberculous meningitis in BCG vaccinated and unvaccinated children. J Neurol Neurosurg Psychiatry. 2005; 76(11):1550–4.
29. van Well GT, Paes BF, Terwee CB, Springer P, Roord JJ, Donald PR, van Furth AM, Schoeman JF. Twenty years of pediatric tuberculous meningitis: a retrospective cohort study in the western cape of South Africa. Pediatrics. 2009;123(1):e1–8.
30. Garg RK. Tuberculosis of the central nervous system. Postgrad Med J. 1999; 75(881):133–40.
31. Nhu NT, Heemskerk D, Thu do DA, Chau TT, Mai NT, Nghia HD, Loc PP, Ha DT, Merson L, Thinh TT, et al. Evaluation of GeneXpert MTB/RIF for diagnosis of tuberculous meningitis. J Clin Microbiol. 2014;52(1):226–33.
32. Thwaites GE, Chau TT, Farrar JJ. Improving the bacteriological diagnosis of tuberculous meningitis. J Clin Microbiol. 2004;42(1):378–9.
33. Solomons RS, Visser DH, Friedrich SO, Diacon AH, Hoek KG, Marais BJ, Schoeman JF, van Furth AM. Improved diagnosis of childhood tuberculous meningitis using more than one nucleic acid amplification test. Int J Tuberc Lung Dis. 2015;19(1):74–80.
34. Seddon JA, Visser DH, Bartens M, Jordaan AM, Victor TC, van Furth AM, Schoeman JF, Schaaf HS. Impact of drug resistance on clinical outcome in children with tuberculous meningitis. Pediatr Infect Dis J. 2012;31(7):711–6.
35. Tho DQ, Torok ME, Yen NT, Bang ND, Lan NT, Kiet VS, van Vinh CN, Dung NH, Day J, Farrar J, et al. Influence of antituberculosis drug resistance and Mycobacterium tuberculosis lineage on outcome in HIV-associated tuberculous meningitis. Antimicrob Agents Chemother. 2012;56(6):3074–9.
36. Thwaites GE, Lan NT, Dung NH, Quy HT, Oanh DT, Thoa NT, Hien NQ, Thuc NT, Hai NN, Bang ND, et al. Effect of antituberculosis drug resistance on response to treatment and outcome in adults with tuberculous meningitis. J Infect Dis. 2005;192(1):79–88.
37. Wolzak NK, Cooke ML, Orth H, van Toorn R. The changing profile of pediatric meningitis at a referral centre in Cape Town, South Africa. J Trop Pediatr. 2012;58(6):491–5.
38. Thwaites GE, Bhavnani SM, Chau TT, Hammel JP, Torok ME, Van Wart SA, Mai PP, Reynolds DK, Caws M, Dung NT, et al. Randomized pharmacokinetic and pharmacodynamic comparison of fluoroquinolones for tuberculous meningitis. Antimicrob Agents Chemother. 2011;55(7):3244–53.
39. Alvarez-Uria G, Midde M, Pakam R, Naik PK. Initial antituberculous regimen with better drug penetration into cerebrospinal fluid reduces mortality in HIV infected patients with tuberculous meningitis: data from an HIV observational cohort study. Tuberc Res Treat. 2013;2013:242604.
40. Ruslami R, Ganiem AR, Dian S, Apriani L, Achmad TH, van der Ven AJ, Borm G, Aarnoutse RE, van Crevel R. Intensified regimen containing rifampicin and moxifloxacin for tuberculous meningitis: an open-label, randomised controlled phase 2 trial. Lancet Infect Dis. 2013;13(1):27–35.
41. Te Brake L, Dian S, Ganiem AR, Ruesen C, Burger D, Donders R, Ruslami R, van Crevel R, Aarnoutse R. Pharmacokinetic/pharmacodynamic analysis of an intensified regimen containing rifampicin and moxifloxacin for tuberculous meningitis. Int J Antimicrob Agents. 2015;45(5):496–503.
42. Heemskerk AD, Bang ND, Mai NT, Chau TT, Phu NH, Loc PP, Chau NV, Hien TT, Dung NH, Lan NT, et al. Intensified antituberculosis therapy in adults with tuberculous meningitis. N Engl J Med. 2016;374(2):124–34.
43. Baghaei P, Tabarsi P, Chitsaz E, Saleh M, Marjani M, Shemirani S, Pooramiri MV, Kazempour M, Farnia P, Fahimi F, et al. Incidence, clinical and epidemiological risk factors, and outcome of drug-induced hepatitis due to antituberculous agents in new tuberculosis cases. Am J Ther. 2010;17(1):17–22.
44. Tariq S, Khan TS, Malik S, Anwar MS, Rashid A. Frequency of anti-tuberculous therapy-induced hepatotoxicity in patients and their outcome. J Ayub Med Coll Abbottabad. 2009;21(4):50–2.
45. Altman C, Biour M, Grange JD. Hepatic toxicity of antitubercular agents. Role of different drugs. 199 cases. Presse Med. 1993;22(26):1212–6.
46. Solomons RS, Wessels M, Visser DH, Donald PR, Marais BJ, Schoeman JF, van Furth AM. Uniform research case definition criteria differentiate tuberculous and bacterial meningitis in children. Clin Infect Dis. 2014;59(11):1574–8.
47. Solomons RS, Visser DH, Donald PR, Marais BJ, Schoeman JF, van Furth AM. The diagnostic value of cerebrospinal fluid chemistry results in childhood tuberculous meningitis. Childs Nerv Syst. 2015;31(8):1335–40.
48. Heemskerk AD, Bang ND, Mai NT, Chau TT, Phu NH, Loc PP, Chau NV, Hien TT, Dung NH, Lan NT, et al. Intensified antituberculosis therapy in adults with tuberculous meningitis. N Engl J Med. 2016;374(2):124–34.

4

Role of matrix metalloproteinase –9 in progression of tuberculous meningitis: a pilot study in patients at different stages of the disease

S. Majeed[1], P. Singh[2], N. Sharma[3] and S. Sharma[1*]

Abstract

Background: TBM (Tuberculous meningitis) is severe form of tuberculosis causing death of one third of the affected individuals or leaving two-third of the survivors disabled. MMP-9 (Matrix metalloproteinase-9) is produced by the central nervous system in a variety of inflammatory conditions and has a role in the breakdown of extracellular matrix and blood–brain barrier.

Methods: In this study, the levels of MMP-9 and its inhibitor, TIMP-1 (tissue inhibitor of metalloproteinases-1), were screened using zymography and reverse zymography in cerebrospinal fluid and serum of tuberculous meningitis patients at different stages of the disease. Further, role of MMP-9 as therapeutic target was studied in C6 glioma cells infected with *Mycobacterium tuberculosis* $H_{37}R_V$. Cells were treated with dexamethasone or SB-3CT (specific inhibitor of MMP-9) in combination with conventional antitubercular drugs.

Results: MMP-9 levels in patients were increased as the disease progressed to advanced stages. The infection led to increased MMP-9 levels in C6 glioma cells and specific inhibition of MMP-9 by SB-3CT augmented bacillary clearance when used along with antitubercular drugs.

Conclusion: MMP-9 plays a prominent role in progression of tuberculous meningitis from initial to advanced stages. Increased levels of MMP-9 during advancement of the disease leads to degeneration of nervous tissue and blood brain barrier disruption. Hence, MMP-9 can be considered as a therapeutic target for efficient management of TBM and can be explored to inhibit further progression of the disease if used at an early stage.

Keywords: Antitubercular drugs, Inflammation, *Mycobacterium tuberculosis*, Matrixmetalloproteinase-9, SB-3CT, Tissue inhibitor of metalloproteinase-1, Tuberculous meningitis

Background

Tuberculous meningitis is the highest mortality causing form of tuberculosis, one third of the patients die and more than half of survivors are left disabled after contracting the disease [1, 2]. Severe clinical manifestations of tuberculous meningitis occur due to robust inflammatory response generated in the brain against pathogenic bacilli [3]. During this process, microglial cells are activated to secrete proteases which have ability to degrade extracellular matrix and cause tissue destruction [4, 5]. Among these proteases, MMPs seem to have prominent role in tissue destruction. MMPs are endopeptidases which degrade all the components of the extracellular matrix and thus have potential to disrupt blood brain barrier and cause CNS damage [5]. Tuberculosis infection elicits the production of MMP-9 by direct interaction between cell wall components of bacilli, human monocytes and macrophages.[6] The higher increase of MMP-9 in pleural effusions of tuberculous meningitis patients than in patients with malignant pleural disease also signifies the role of MMP-9 in tuberculous infections and vice versa [7]. Besides, the synergistic effects of

* Correspondence: sadhnabiochem@gmail.com
[1]Department of Biochemistry, Postgraduate Institute of Medical Education & Research, Chandigarh 160012, India
Full list of author information is available at the end of the article

MMP-9 and Mycobacteria on each other, specific MMP-9 substrates type IV collagen and laminin, constitute essential structural components of the blood brain barrier reflecting its importance in tissue damage. The possibility of using MMP-9 inhibition as therapeutic target can be considered for preventing progression of disease to advanced stages and control disabilities. Currently corticosteroids like dexamethasone or prednisolone are usually given along with conventional antitubercular drugs to combat the inflammatory tissue degradation which nonspecifically inhibits MMP 9 as well [8, 9]. Specific inhibitor of MMP-9, SB-3CT has come forth with desirable properties of crossing blood brain barrier and therapeutic effects for treating neurological diseases due to inflammation [10]. This inhibitor has been studied for ischemia of immature brain and found to work efficiently; showing its utility in pediatric cases [11]. In this study, role of MMP-9 has been evaluated in progression of TBM. The levels of MMP-9 at different stage of the disease were compared to evaluate if any correlation exists between the worsening prognosis and MMP-9 levels. Though the inflammatory tissue destruction amplifies as the disease progresses from stage I to stage III, no study is available on the exact contribution of these MMPs in advancement of the disease. Effect of specific inhibition of MMP-9 on clearing the bacterial burden were further evaluated in C6 glioma cells infected with *Mycobacterium tuberculosis* $H_{37}R_v$.

Methods: availability of data and material section

Ethical considerations

The plan of work was approved by Institutional Ethics Committee (IEC) of Postgraduate Institute of Medical education and Research, Chandigarh, and sample collection was done according to the ethical guidelines. CSF and blood samples were used after written consent from the patients or their attendants in case of unconscious or confused patients. The written consent was recorded in patient proforma approved by Institutional Ethical Committee.

Chemicals and consumables

Isoniazid, Rifampicin, Pyrazinamide, Dexamethasone, MMP-9 standard, MMP-9 inhibitor (SB-3CT) and gelatin were obtained from Sigma (St. Louis USA). OADC (Oleic albumin dextrose catalase) enrichment and 7H11 agar were obtained from Difco-Becton-Dickinson (USA), FBS (fetal bovine serum) and MEM (minimum essential medium) were obtained from Invitrogen Corporation (Gibco), New York, USA. Acrylamide, bisacrylamide, ammonium persulphate and other reagents used were of molecular grade. Ultrapure water was used throughout the study.

Mycobacterial culture and cell lines

Mycobacterium tuberculosis $H_{37}R_v$ (NCTC7416) was originally obtained from National Collection of Type Culture (NCTC) London, UK. Bacteria were grown in sterile Sautons's medium and maintained in sterile lowenstein-jensen medium. Cultures were grown under shaking conditions at 180 rpm, 37 °C.

Cell lines

C6 glioma and HT1080 cell lines were purchased from National Centre for Cell Science, Pune. C6 glioma cells were grown in MEM supplemented with 10% FBS, HT1080 cells were also grown in MEM supplemented with 10 mM sodium pyruvate and 10% FBS, grown at 37 °C in a humidified incubator under 5% $C0_2$ and 95% air. Cells were maintained as frozen aliquots of 10% DMSO in FBS at −80 °C. Conditioned media containing gelatinases was obtained by growing HT-1080 cells initially in MEM supplemented with 10% FBS and then in serum-free MEM for 24 h.

Study design, site and population

Study subjects included patients with TBM attending Neurology, Emergency or Internal medicine departments at PGIMER, Chandigarh, India. Patients above 12 years of age and of either sex were included in the study. Patients infected with HIV or suffering from any other infectious disease in addition to TBM were excluded from the study. The plan of work was approved by Institutional Ethics Committee of Postgraduate Institute of Medical Education and Research, Chandigarh and sampling was carried out according to the ethical guidelines. CSF and blood samples were used after written consent from the patients or their attendants in case of unconscious or confused patients. Samples were taken during treatment of patients. The written consent was recorded in patient proforma, which was approved by Institutional Ethical Committee. Performa was used to collect the demographic and clinical information, including age, sex, HIV status, duration, regimen, tests and examinations of previous treatment, etc. Ninety-one patients with clinical symptoms of TBM and 16 control subjects were included in the study. The selection of patients was based on the criteria defined by Mahadevan et al. [12] i.e. fever over a period of week, high protein sugar ratio in cerebrospinal fluid, imaging studies of head showing exudates, hydrocephalus, infarcts, cranial nerve palsies, response to antitubercular drug therapy and final confirmation of tuberculous meningitis by the clinician attending the patient. According to the guidelines of British Medical Research Council (MRC), the patients were categorized into three stages I, II and III as per the symptoms shown by the patients. Stage I included conscious and rational patients with no signs of focal or neurological deficits or neck stiffness, Stage II patients were conscious but confused had focal signs such as cranial nerve palsies or hemiparesis. Patients in stage III were comatose or delirious with or without dense neurological deficit. Controls subjects were those having non inflammatory disease. CSF and blood samples were obtained from patients in different stages of TBM (10 patients with stage I, 42 with stage II, 39 with stage III) and 16 control subjects. CSF sample was obtained by lumbar puncture during their hospitalization and blood sample (5 ml) was drawn in sterile tube and processed for serum separation. CSF and serum samples were sterile filtered and immediately frozen at −80 °C till assayed for MMP-9 and TIMP-1 levels.

Gelatin-substrate zymography

MMP-9 levels in CSF and serum were monitored by gelatin zymography using 8% polyacrylamide gels containing 0.3% SDS and gelatin (1 mg/ml) [13]. Undiluted CSF and serum (1:100 dilutions) was mixed with zymography buffer [50 mM Tris–HCl, 10% glycerol, 2% SDS and 0.01%bromophenol blue]. Samples were loaded and run at 20 mA for 20 min and then at 30 mA for 60 min. Equal amount of each sample was used for analysis. Authentic MMP-9 standard was also run as control. Gels were agitated in 2.5% TritonX-100 and washed in 50 mM Tris–HCl buffer, pH 7.5 containing 200 mM NaCl. Thereafter, gels were incubated overnight at 37 °C in renaturing buffer (50 mM Tris–HCl buffer, pH 7.5 containing 200 mM NaCl, 5 mM $CaCl_2$, 0.02% (w/v) brij-35, and 0.01% sodium azide. Finally, gels were stained with Comassie G blue and or silver stained to obtain the bands. Intensities of gelatinolytic bands corresponding to MMP-9 were measured by software analysis [13, 14] The densitometric intensities of known concentrations of MMP-9 standard were plotted to obtain standard curve from which MMP-9 concentrations in patient samples was determined.

Reverse zymography

TIMP-1 in CSF and serum samples was analyzed by reverse zymography. 15% polyacrylamide gels with gelatin and gelatinases copolymerized into the matrix were prepared. Gelatinases were obtained from serum free media of HT1080 fibrosarcoma cell line. Samples were mixed with zymography buffer and run for electrophoresis. Gels were agitated in 2.5% TritonX-100, washed in 50 mM Tris–HCl buffer, and incubated overnight in renaturation buffer for action of gelatin and gelatinases. During the activation step, gelatinases present in gel digest the gelatin but only in areas where TIMPs are absent. Upon staining, the levels were monitored as blue bands of undigested gelatin on a clear gelatinolytic background [15].

Effect of MMP-9 inhibition on C6 glioma cells infected with *Mycobacterium tuberculosis*

C6 glioma cells were plated in 24 well plates and infected with *Mycobacterium tuberculosis* $H_{37}R_V$ in ratio of 10 bacilli per cell. After 90 min., the cells were washed extensively to remove extracellular bacteria. Cells were divided into seven groups Group I: uninfected cells, Group II: cells infected with *Mycobacterium tuberculosis* $H_{37}R_V$, Group III: infected cells treated with dexamethasone, Group IV: infected cells treated with MMP-9 inhibitor (SB- 3CT), Group V: infected cells treated with antitubercular drugs, Group VI: infected cells treated with antitubercular drugs along with dexamethasone, Group VII: infected cells treated with antitubercular drugs along with SB-3CT. Concentration of drugs, dexamethasone and SB-3CT used was as described [16–18]. After 5 days of treatment, cells were lysed with 0.1% SDS. Mixture of extra cellular media and cell lysate was processed for CFU enumeration and MMP-9 analysis.

Statistical analysis

Comparison of MMP-9 levels amongst patients in different stages of TBM was performed using Kruskal-Wallis test. If the overall test was significant ($p < 0.05$) the Mann–Whitney test was applied to compare control subjects with stage I, II, III patients; stage I patients with stage II, III patients and stage II patients with stage III patients. All the comparisons were based on mean rank.

Results

Levels of MMP-9 and TIMP-1 in CSF of patients with advanced stages of TBM

TBM patients selected for the study were grouped into stage I, II and III as per details given in Table 1. The amount of MMP-9 in CSF samples was quantified by comparing their densitomertic values with those of known concentration of MMP-9 standard. CSF zymography revealed that MMP-9 levels increased with advanced stages of TBM (Fig. 1a). MMP-9 levels were 0.62 ± 0.40 ng/ml for controls, 9.0 ± 0.87 ng/ml for stage I, 12.0 ± 1.34 ng/ml for stage II and 16.86 ± 2.7 ng/ml for stage III tuberculous meningitis patients (Fig. 1b and c). MMP-9 levels showed significant increase in samples of stage III patients as compared to stage I and stage II. TIMP-1 was detectable in

Table 1 Demography data of the subjects included in the study Patients in advanced stages of the disease showed higher protein and lower glucose content in their CSF

	No. of individuals	Average age (years)	Male: Female	CSF Protein (mg/ml)	CSF glucose (mg/ml)
Stage 1	10	36.75±14.1	6:4	121.7±21.5	32.3±6.5
Stage 11	42	34.66±15.5	24:18	135±44.5	31.8±16.3
Stage III	39	53.6±10.5	23:16	245±89.2	25.72±7.9
Control	16	35.93±8.3	10:6	21.2±6.5	63.88±11.3

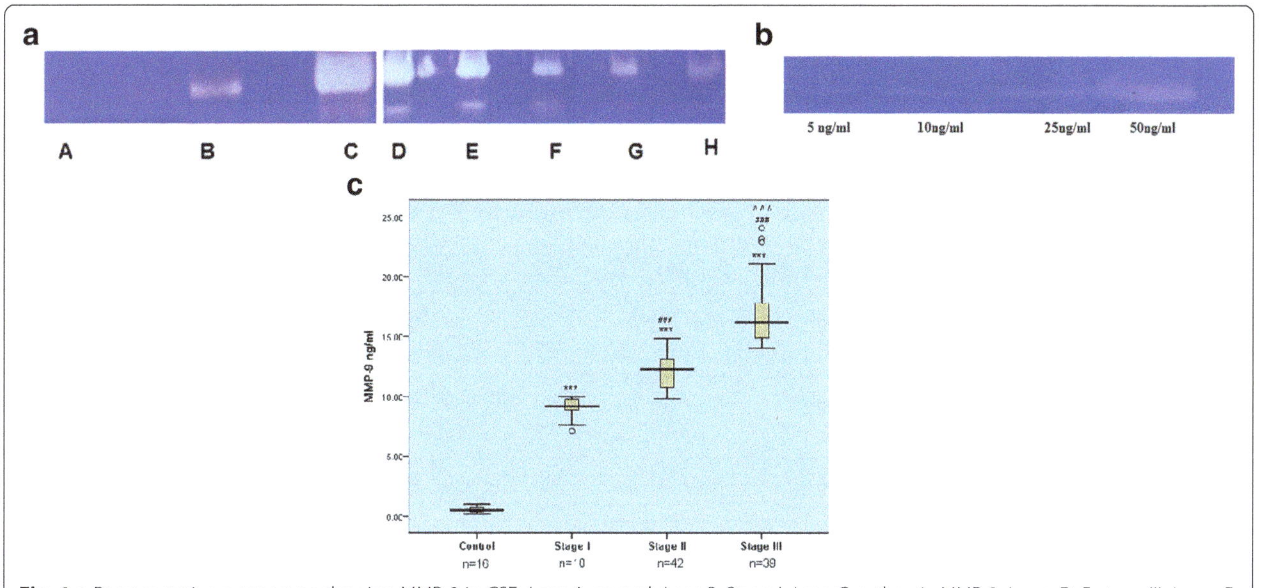

Fig. 1 a Representative zymograms showing MMP-9 in CSF: *Lane A:* control, *Lane B:* Stage I, *Lane C:* authentic MMP-9, *Lanes D, E:* stage III; *Lanes F, G, H:* stage II. Equal amount of sample was loaded in each lane (**b**) Zymogram of known concentrations of standard MMP-9 (**c**) Box plot showing MMP-9 levels in CSF of patients in different stages of tuberculous meningitis***$p < 0.001$ compared to control, ### $p < 0.001$ compared to stage I and control, ^^^ $p < 0.001$ compared to stage II

stage I TBM patients only. Out of 10 stage I patients, it was detected in only 3 patients. However, TIMP-1 was detected in all control samples but no sample from stage II or III patients showed the presence of TIMP-1 (Fig. 2).

Levels of MMP-9 and TIMP-1 in serum samples of patients with advanced stages of TBM

Increase in MMP-9 levels with advancement of the disease was observed in serum samples hence confirming the results obtained with CSF (Fig. 3a). Densitometric analysis revealed MMP-9 levels of 5.67 ± 2.45 ng/ml for controls, 830.66 ± 83.07 ng/ml for stage I, 1202.55 ± 136.81 ng/ml for stage II and 1679 ± 277.4 ng/ml for stage III TBM patients (Fig. 3b). TIMP-1 was not detected in serum sample of any subject.

Evaluation of MMP-9 as therapeutic target using SB-3CT (MMP-9 inhibitor) and dexamethasone in C6 glioma cells infected with *Mycobacterium tuberculosis* $H_{37}R_v$

Levels of MMP-9 were increased in *Mycobacterium tuberculosis* infected C6 cells as compared to the uninfected cells (Fig. 4a). Ex vivo study can mimic the in vivo model of *Mycobacterium tuberculosis* infection where MMP-9 levels are known to be elevated due to infection. After confirming the elevation of MMP-9 levels in infected cells, the effect of MMP-9 inhibitor (SB-3CT) and dexamethasone was monitored in the infected C6 glioma cells. Levels of MMP-9 were reduced to greater extent after treatment with either SB-3CT or dexamethasone (Fig. 4b). Levels of MMP-9 remained unaffected when treated with antitubercular drugs alone (Fig. 4c.) and were markedly reduced when drugs were given along with dexamethasone or SB-3CT, (Fig. 4d). Cells treated with only SB-3CT or dexamethasone did not show decrease in CFUs. Interestingly, cells when treated with antitubercular drugs along with dexamethasone or SB-3CT, showed almost undetectable CFUs after 5 days of treatment (Fig. 5).

Discussion

In this study, MMP-9 in CSF as well as serum was increased with progression of disease from stage I to III. Though increased levels of MMP-9 in TBM has been

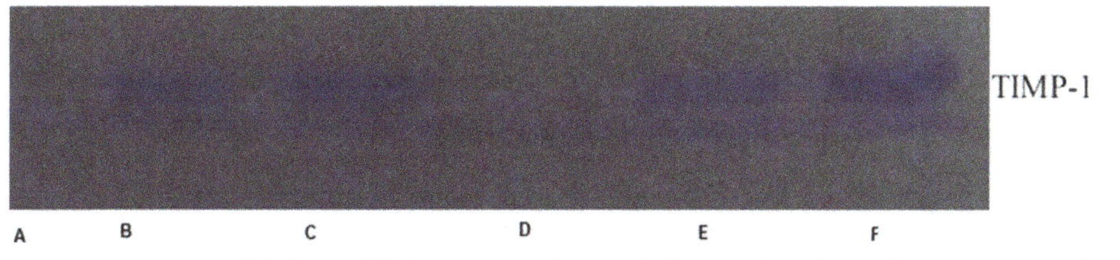

Fig. 2 Representative reverse zymogram of TIMP-1 in CSF: *Lanes A:* stage II; *Lanes B, C:* stage I; *Lane D,* stageIII; *Lanes E, F:* control subjects. Equal amount of sample was loaded in each lane

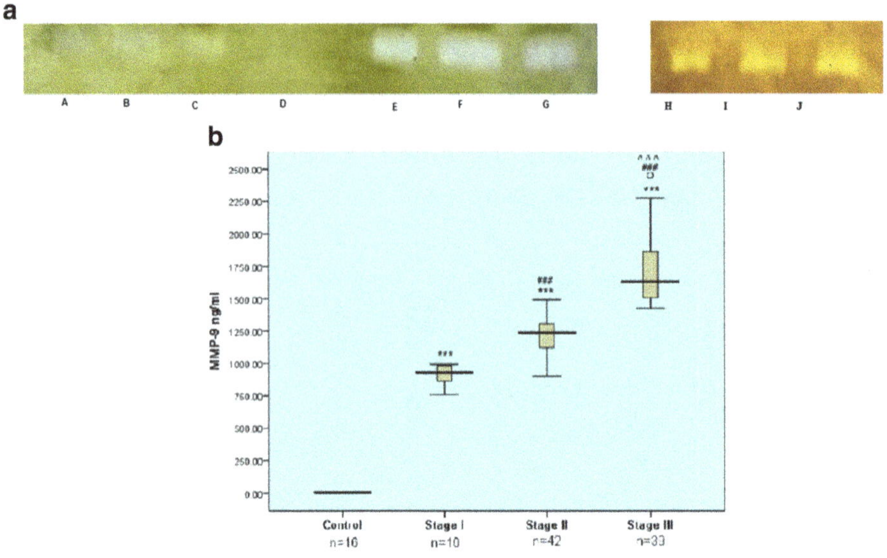

Fig. 3 Representative zymogram of MMP-9 in serum samples of tuberculous meningitis patients. **a** *Lanes A, B, C:* stage I; *Lane D:* control subject; *Lanes H, I, J:* stage II. **b** Box plot showing MMP-9 levels in serum of patients in different stages of TBM ***$p < 0.001$ compared to control, ### $p < 0.001$ compared to stage I and control, ^^^ $p < 0.001$ compared to stage II

reported earlier [13, 19] this study compared the concomitant increase in MMP-9 levels with progression of the disease from earlier to its advanced stages. It was found that MMP-9 levels were significantly increased as disease progressed from stage I to II and significant increase was seen as the disease progressed to stage III. Other low MW gelatinase was also detected which is predicted to be MMP-2 based on its position on the gel. The concomitant increase of this gelatinase was also found with the advancement of the disease but increment in MMP-9 levels was significantly higher (Fig. 6a and b). Association of MMP-9 has been observed in necrotic meningeal vessels in TBM. CSF concentrations of MMP-9 has been correlated with involvement of brain ischaemia in TBM [20]. MMP-9 levels could not be detected in control samples while the low MW gelatinase was detected in these samples demonstrating that it is constitutively expressed. TIMP-1 levels in CSF samples were decreased with advancement of the disease and were undetectable in serum samples. Thus overall ratio of MMP-9/TIMP-1 was found to be increased leading to matrix degrading phenotype. Studies have found generation of matrix-degrading phenotype in tuberculosis and implicate MMP-9 as key mediator in tuberculosis pathology [21]. Other studies have reported uncontrolled rise of MMP-9 in CNS TB due to insignificant levels of

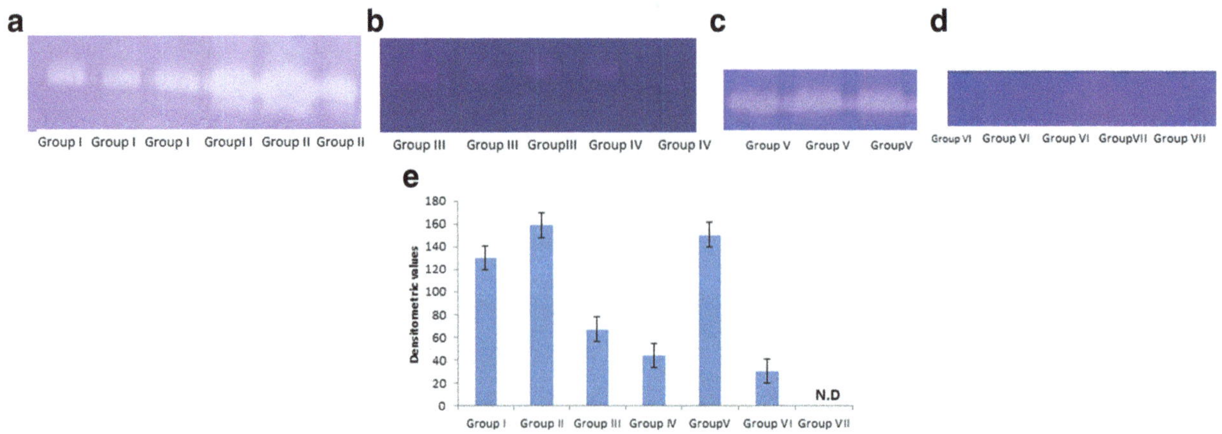

Fig. 4 Zymograms of MMP-9 levels in C6 cells (**a**) *Group I:* uninfected and *Group II:* infected cells (**b**) *Group III:* dexamethasone treated and *Group IV:* SB-3CT treated cells (**c**) Group V:treated with antitubercular drugs only (**d**) *Group VI:* treatment with antitubercular drugs along with dexamethasone and *Group VII:* treatment with antitubercular drugs along with SB-3CT (**e**) Graphical representation of Densitometric units corresponding to MMP-9 bands in different treatment groups of C6 Glioma Cells

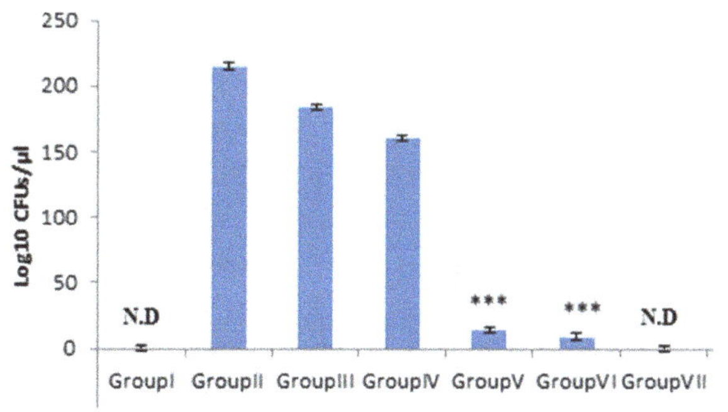

Fig. 5 Log_{10} CFUs of *Mycobacterium tuberculosis* $H_{37}R_v$ infected C6 glioma cells after 5 days of treatment. *Group I:* uninfected cells, *Group II:* Untreated C6 cells infected with *Mycobacterium tuberculosis* $H_{37}R_v$,*Group III:* Infected C6 cells treated with Dexamethasone, *Group IV:* Infected C6 cells treated with SB-3CT, *Group V:* Infected C6 cells treated with antitubercular drugs (Isoniazid + Rifampicin + Pyrazinamide) *Group VI:* Infected cells treated with antitubercular drugs along with dexamethasone, *Group VII:* Infected cells treated with antitubercular drugs along with SB-3CT. Values are mean ± SD of cells processed in triplicate. *** $p < 0.001$, respect to *Group II*

TIMP-1 in comparison to MMP-9 which results in matrix degrading phenotype [22]. Role of *Mycobacterium tuberculosis* infections in elevating MMP-9 levels has also been documented [23]. Thus TBM seems to have dual relation with MMP-9. MMP-9 is involved in inflammatory response to disease and on the other hand *Mycobacterium tuberculosis* is involved in increasing MMP-9 levels. The data supporting the inflammatory as well as pathological role of MMP-9 in tuberculosis reveals the possibility of its prominent therapeutic role. This pilot study demonstrates the apparent role of MMP-9 in TBM pathology. Further, *Mycobacterium tuberculosis* infection enhanced levels of MMP-9 in C6 glioma cells as explained in earlier studies [24] wherein, conditioned media from *Mycobacterium tuberculosis* infected monocytes induced MMP-9 secretion from astrocytes. MMP-9 inhibitor SB-3CT and dexamethasone was used to inhibit *Mycobacterium tuberculosis* induced MMP-9 in C6 glioma cells. MMP-9 levels were decreased in cells treated with SB-3CT or dexamethasone. These results are in agreement with earlier studies [25]. Levels of MMP-9 were not apparently affected with antitubercular drugs only indicating that antitubercular drugs are not involved in reducing inflammation in tuberculous meningitis patients which explains the lifelong neurological defects even after bacillary clearance. When drugs were used along with SB-3CT or dexamethasone, the MMP-9 levels were decreased to almost undetectable levels. CFU counts were significantly decreased upon treatment with antitubercular drugs. Bacillary counts were further decreased when SB-3CT or dexamethasone was used along with antitubercular drugs. No report about combined effects of antitubercular drugs with SB-3CT is available in the literature. MMP-9 seems to be a promising molecule to resolve the destructive outcome of TBM; however, further studies are required to assign therapeutic significance to MMP-9 inhibition for better management of TBM.

Conclusions

The present work suggested important role of MMP-9 in tissue destruction during TBM and its progression to the advanced stages. Specific inhibition of MMP-9 can be beneficial approach to overcome the limitations of corticosteroids with equivalent benefits for treatment of the disease.

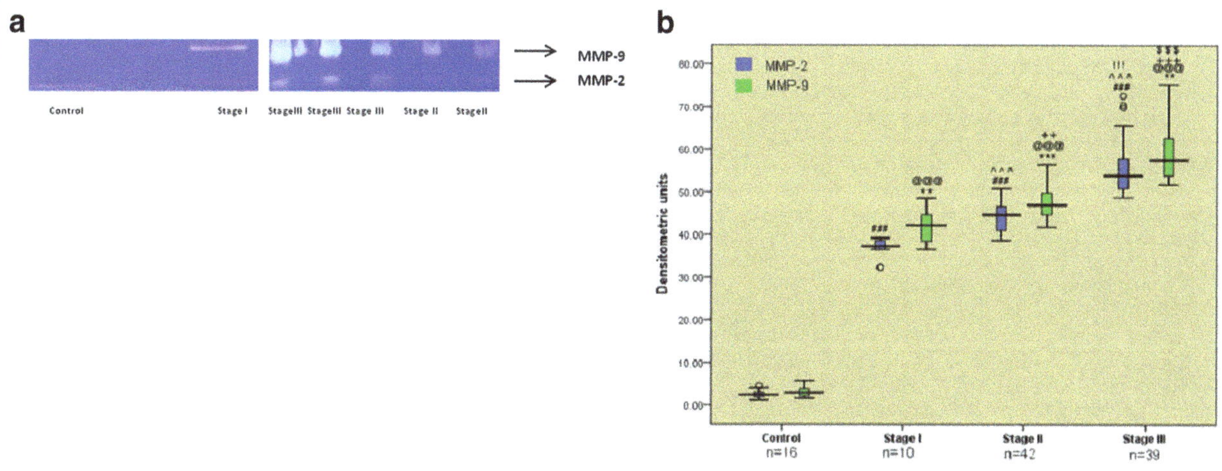

Fig. 6 **a** Representative zymograms showing Low MW gelatinase in different stages of TBM. **b** Box plot showing comparison of densitometric values and low MW gelatinase in samples of control subjects and TBM patients

Abbreviations

CNS: Central nervous system; CSF: Cerebrospinal fluid; MMP-9: Matrix metalloproteinase-9; TBM: Tuberculous meningitis; TIMP-1: Tissue inhibitor of metalloproteinase-1

Funding

No specific funding was available for this study. During the period of study S. Majeed received research fellowship from Indian Council of Medical Research, New Delhi.

Authors' contributions

SM was involved in design of the study; experimentation, analysis and interpretation of data and preparation of the manuscript; critical revision of the manuscript for important intellectual content. PS and NS were involved in the diagnosis and confirmation of tuberculous meningitis patients at different stages of the disease and analysis of the data. Corresponding author was responsible for study concept design; analysis, interpretation and integrity of the data, preparation of the manuscript and reviewed the manuscript for intellectual content. All authors read and approved the final manuscript.

Competing interests

The authors declare that they have no competing interests.

Consent for publication

Not applicable.

Author details

[1]Department of Biochemistry, Postgraduate Institute of Medical Education & Research, Chandigarh 160012, India. [2]Department of Neurology, Postgraduate Institute of Medical Education & Research, Chandigarh 160012, India. [3]Department of Internal Medicine, Postgraduate Institute of Medical Education & Research, Chandigarh 160012, India.

References

1. Thwaites G, Hien T, Thwaites G, Hien T. Tuberculous meningitis: many questions, too few answers. The Lancet Neurology. 2005;4(3):160-170
2. Isabel B. S. RHP. Pathogenesis and Immune Response in Tuberculous Meningitis. J Med Sci. 2014;21(1):4-10.
3. Thwaites GE, Simmons CP, Than Ha Quyen N, Thi Hong Chau T, Phuong Mai P, Thi Dung N, Hoan Phu N, White NP, Tinh Hien T, Farrar JJ. Pathophysiology and prognosis in vietnamese adults with tuberculous meningitis. J Infect Dis. 2003;188(8):1105–15.
4. Rivera-Marrero CA, Schuyler W, Roser S, Ritzenthaler JD, Newburn SA, Roman J. M. Tuberculosis induction of matrix metalloproteinase-9: the role of mannose and receptor-mediated mechanisms. Am J Physiol Lung Cell Mol Physiol. 2002;282(3):L546–55.
5. Spanos JP, Hsu NJ, Jacobs M. Microglia are crucial regulators of neuro-immunity during central nervous system tuberculosis. Front Cell Neurosci. 2015;9:182.
6. Chang JCWA, Tchou-Wong KM, Moskowitz N, Zhang Y, Rom WN. Effect of mycobacterium tuberculosis and its components on macrophages and the release of matrix metalloproteinases. Thorax. 1996;51:306–11.
7. Sheen P, O'Kane CM, Chaudhary K, Tovar M, Santillan C, Sosa J, Caviedes L, Gilman RH, Stamp G, Friedland JS, et al. High mmp-9 activity characterises pleural tuberculosis correlating with granuloma formation. Eur Respir J. 2009;33(1):134–41.
8. Li YT, Shen F, Bai JY, Cheng GF. Inhibition of dexamethasone, indomethacin and resveratrol on matrix metalloproteinase-9 and the mechanism of inhibition. Yao Xue Xue Bao. 2003;38(7):501–4.
9. Russell RE, Culpitt SV, DeMatos C, Donnelly L, Smith M, Wiggins J, et al. Release and activity of matrix metalloproteinase-9 and tissue inhibitor of metalloproteinase-1 by alveolar macrophages from patients with chronic obstructive pulmonary disease. Am J Respir Cell Mol Biol. 2002;26(5):602–9.
10. Cui J, Chen S, Zhang C, Meng F, Wu W, Hu R, Hadass O, Lehmidi T, Blair GJ, Lee M, Chang M, Mobashery S, Sun GY, Gu Z. Inhibition of mmp-9 by a selective gelatinase inhibitor protects neurovasculature from embolic focal cerebral ischemia. Mol Neurodegener. 2012;7:21.
11. Ranasinghe HS, Scheepens A, Sirimanne E, Mitchell MD, Williams CE, Fraser M. Inhibition of mmp-9 activity following hypoxic ischemia in the developing brain using a highly specific inhibitor. Dev Neurosci. 2012;34(5):417–27.
12. Mahadevan BMS, Tiroumourougane V, Narahsiman R. Tuberculin reactivity in tuberculous meningitis. Indian J Pediatr. 2005;72:213–5.
13. Matsuura EUF, Hashiguchi T, Fujimoto N, Okada Y, et al. Marked increase of matrix metalloproteinase 9 in cerebrospinal fluid of patients with fungal or tuberculous meningoencephalitis. J Neurol Sci. 2000;173:45–52.
14. DE Kleiner SW. Quantitative zymography: detection of picogram quantities of gelatinases. Anal Biochem. 1994;218:325–9.
15. Oliver GWLJ, Stevenson WG, Kleiner DE. Quantitative reverse zymography: analysis of picogram amounts of metalloproteinase inhibitors using gelatinase a and b reverse zymograms. Anal Biochem. 1997;244:161–6.
16. Chanwong S, Maneekarn N, Makonkawkeyoon L, Makonkawkeyoon S. Intracellular growth and drug susceptibility of mycobacterium tuberculosis in macrophages. Tuberculosis (Edinb). 2007;87(2):130–3.
17. Lin CW, Shen SC, Hou WC, Yang LY, Chen YC. Heme oxygenase-1 inhibits breast cancer invasion via suppressing the expression of matrix metalloproteinase-9. Mol Cancer Ther. 2008;7(5):1195–206.
18. Schierloh P, Yokobori N, Aleman M, Landoni V, Geffner L, Musella RM, et al. Mycobacterium tuberculosis-induced gamma interferon production by natural killer cells requires cross talk with antigen-presenting cells involving toll-like receptors 2 and 4 and the mannose receptor in tuberculous pleurisy. Infect Immun. 2007;75(11):5325–37.
19. Lee KY, Kim EH, Yang WS, Ryu H, Cho SN, Lee BI, Heo JH. Persistent increase of matrix metalloproteinases in cerebrospinal fluid of tuberculous meningitis. J Neurol Sci. 2004;220(1–2):73–8.
20. Lammie GHR, Schoeman JF, Donald PR. Tuberculous cerebrovascular disease. J Infect. 2009;59:155–66.
21. Elkington PT, Friedland JS, GCAU. Matrix metalloproteinases in tuberculosis. Eur Respir J. 2011;38:456–64.
22. Yu AE, Hewitt RE, Kleiner DE, Stetler-Stevenson WG. Molecular regulation of cellular invasion–role of gelatinase a and timp-2. Biochem Cell Biol. 1996;74(6):823–31.
23. Harris JE, Green JA, Elkington PT, Friedland JS. Monocytes infected with mycobacterium tuberculosis regulate map kinase-dependent astrocyte mmp-9 secretion. J Leukoc Biol. 2007;81(2):548–56.
24. Harris JE, Nuttall RK, Elkington PT, Green JA, Horncastle DE. Monocyte-astrocyte networks regulate tuberculosis in vitro and in vivo and secretion in central nervous system matrix metalloproteinase gene expression. J Immunol. 2007; 178:1199–207.
25. Harkness KA, Adamson P, Sussman JD, Davies-Jones GAB, Greenwood J, Woodroofe MN. Dexamethasone regulation of matrix metalloproteinase expression in cns vascular endothelium. Brain. 2000;123(4):698–709.

5

Paradoxical reaction in tuberculous meningitis: presentation, predictors and impact on prognosis

Anurag Kumar Singh[1†], Hardeep Singh Malhotra[1†], Ravindra Kumar Garg[1*†], Amita Jain[2], Neeraj Kumar[1], Neera Kohli[3], Rajesh Verma[1] and Praveen Kumar Sharma[1]

Abstract

Background: Awareness about paradoxical reactions in tuberculous meningitis is crucial as a paradoxical reaction may lead to certain wrong conclusions (for example, an erroneous diagnosis, and a possibility of treatment failure, mycobacterial drug-resistance, drug toxicity, or presence of a malignancy). The present study was planned to evaluate the incidence and predictive factors of paradoxical reactions in light of clinical, cerebrospinal fluid, and neuroimaging characteristics.

Methods: In this prospective cohort study, consecutive patients fulfilling the International Consensus criteria of tuberculous meningitis were included. Patients were subjected to clinical evaluation, cerebrospinal fluid evaluation, and neuroimaging. Patients were treated with anti-tuberculosis drugs along with corticosteroids. Patients were regularly followed up at 3 monthly intervals. At each follow up patients were evaluated clinically and repeat cerebrospinal fluid analysis was performed along with repeat neuroimaging. Disability assessment was done using Barthel index.

Results: We enrolled 141 patients of tuberculous meningitis. Approximately one-third of patients (44/141; 31.2 %) developed a paradoxical reaction. Twenty-seven patients developed hydrocephalus, 26 developed tuberculomas, 12 developed optochiasmatic arachnoiditis and 4 patients had spinal arachnoiditis. In 41 patients (out of 44) cerebrospinal fluid paradoxically worsened (increase in cells and/or protein); 2 demonstrated a decrease in cells with polymorph predominance while in one it was normal. In 3 patients, paradoxical cerebrospinal fluid changes were not associated with neuroimaging changes. On multivariate analysis, predictors of paradoxical reaction were female gender ($p = 0.013$), HIV positivity ($p = 0.01$) and a shorter duration of illness ($p = 0.049$). Development of paradoxical reactions did not predict the disability status of the patients.

Conclusions: Paradoxical reaction occurs in approximately one-third of patients with tuberculous meningitis. Female gender, concomitant HIV infection, and a shorter duration of illness were significant predictors. Paradoxical reactions did not adversely affect the outcome.

Keywords: Tuberculoma, Optochiasmatic arachnoiditis, Hydrocephalus, Cerebrospinal fluid, Immune reconstitution inflammatory syndrome

* Correspondence: garg50@yahoo.com
†Equal contributors
[1]Department of Neurology, King George Medical University, Uttar Pradesh, Lucknow PIN-226003, India
Full list of author information is available at the end of the article

Background

Paradoxical reaction, in patients with tuberculous meningitis, is characterized by either worsening of pre-existing tuberculous lesions or the appearance of new tuberculous lesions in patients who show initial improvement following anti-tuberculosis treatment. The clinical or radiological deterioration associated with such a reaction may fallaciously suggest either a drug resistant state or treatment failure, and might even prompt to look for an alternative diagnosis [1–3]. The manifestations of paradoxical reaction, that have been described, are mostly derived from case reports and small case series. These include a variety of clinical manifestations and neuroimaging abnormalities, along with an altered cerebrospinal fluid picture. Cerebrospinal fluid changes may include lymphocytic pleocytosis, a change in cellular components in the direction of polymorphonuclear predominance, or an increase in protein levels. Paradoxical reaction does not necessarily represent treatment failure and corticosteroids have been shown to have a beneficial effect [4–6].

In human immunodeficiency virus (HIV)-infected patients, paradoxical reactions are termed as the immune reconstitution inflammatory syndrome (IRIS), which is a condition characterized with worsening of pre-existing infective processes, following treatment with antiretroviral therapy. Tuberculosis-associated immune reconstitution inflammatory syndrome is characterized by worsening of clinical symptoms, signs, and imaging characteristics of tuberculosis subsequent to initiation of antiretroviral therapy after initial improvement with anti-tuberculosis treatment [7, 8].

Most of the current information about paradoxical reaction in tuberculous meningitis is in the form of isolated case reports, small case series, and articles with small number of patients. The exact frequency and spectrum of paradoxical reaction is not precisely known. Its impact on prognosis is also not clear. This prospective follow up study has been planned to answer all these questions.

Methods

This prospective study was conducted in Department of Neurology, King George Medical University Uttar Pradesh, Lucknow. Our institute is a tertiary care hospital serving a population of approximately 100 million. It is situated in an area which is highly endemic for tuberculosis. Formal ethical approval was taken from the Institutional Ethics Committee, King George's Medical University, U.P., India. Written informed consent was obtained from all patients and/or their legal guardians.

Inclusion criteria

All consecutive newly-diagnosed patients of tuberculous meningitis, fulfilling the consensus diagnostic criteria as described by Marais et al., were included. Patients were categorized into definite, probable, or possible tuberculous meningitis groups on the basis of clinical, imaging, and laboratory criteria. The definite cases of tuberculous meningitis had either the presence of acid-fast bacilli in cerebrospinal fluid, or mycobacterium could be cultured from cerebrospinal fluid, or cerebrospinal fluid was positive for mycobacterial nucleic acids by polymerase chain reaction. The probable cases fulfilled the clinical entry criteria plus a total diagnostic score of 10 or more points (when cerebral imaging was not available) or 12 or more points (when cerebral imaging was available) plus exclusion of alternative diagnoses. The possible cases included clinical entry criteria plus a total diagnostic score of 6–9 points (when cerebral imaging was not available) or 6–11 points (when cerebral imaging was available) along with the exclusion of alternative diagnoses [9].

Disease severity

Patients were classified as per British Medical Research Council staging system. Patients with stage-I disease had a Glasgow Coma Scale score of 15 with no focal neurologic signs; patients with stage-II had signs of meningeal irritation with slight or no alteration of sensorium and minor neurological deficit (like cranial nerve palsies) or no deficit (Glasgow coma scale score 11 to14), and patients with stage-III had severe alteration of sensorium, convulsions, focal neurological deficit and involuntary movements (Glasgow coma scale score <10) [10].

Evaluation of patients

All enrolled patients were subjected to detailed clinical, radiological, and laboratory evaluation. Occurrence of systemic tuberculosis, such as involvement of pulmonary system, lymph node, bone, and other organs, were recorded. The work up included complete blood count, peripheral blood smear examination, erythrocyte sedimentation rate, blood urea nitrogen, blood sugar, serum creatinine, serum electrolytes, liver function tests, chest X-ray, and enzyme linked immunosorbent assay for HIV. Cerebrospinal fluid biochemical and microscopic examination, including India ink preparation, were performed. Cerebrospinal fluid sediments were stained, cultured (Lowenstein Jensen media), and tested for drug susceptibility by standard methods. Cerebrospinal fluid specimens were also tested for mycobacterial nucleic acids by polymerase chain reaction. Appropriate patients were also evaluated by performing bacterial screen with culture, cryptococcal latex antigen detection, antinuclear antibody, antineutrophil cytoplasmic antibody screen, hepatitis B and C, and angiotensin converting enzyme level. Patients were subjected to MR imaging of the brain and/or spinal cord using Signa Excite 1.5 Tesla instrument (General Electric Medical Systems, Milwaukee, WI, USA.

Exclusion criteria

Patients with cryptococcal meningitis or any other cause for meningitis were excluded from the study.

Definition of paradoxical reaction

A paradoxical reaction was defined as the worsening of pre-existing tuberculous lesions or the appearance of new tuberculous lesions in patients whose clinical symptoms initially improved and had been on anti-tuberculosis treatment for at least 10 days [2, 3, 11]. For the purpose of the calculation of "time of onset of paradoxical reaction" in the study participants only clinical deteriorations were considered from the time of initiation of anti-tuberculosis treatment; non-symptomatic radiological worsening was defined either at the time of clinical deteriorations or at the pre-defined follow-up visit.

Definition of other neuroimaging findings

Hydrocephalus was defined as ventriculomegaly with Evan's ratio (maximal width of frontal horns/maximal width of inner skull) of more than 30 % and/or size of one or both temporal horns greater than 2 mm. Communicating hydrocephalus was characterized with ventriculomegaly with a dilated fourth ventricle. Meningeal inflammation, on gadolinium-enhanced MRI, was defined as an enhancement of pia-arachnoid mater covering subarachnoid spaces of the sulci and basal cisterns. Exudates were defined as a thick area of enhancement, predominantly in basal cisterns and Sylvian fissure. Optochiasmatic tuberculoma and arachnoiditis were characterized with confluent enhancing lesions involving interpeduncular fossa, pontine cistern, and perimesencephalic and suprasellar cisterns. Spinal arachnoiditis was defined with the presence of enhancement of spinal meninges, and nerve roots, obliteration of the spinal subarachnoid space, cysts and loculations in subarachnoid space, or syrinx formation. Tuberculomas were defined as discrete or coalescing cerebral masses showing nodular or ring shaped enhancement. Infarcts were areas of abnormal signal intensity in a vascular distribution, predominantly in periventricular region. Infarcts appeared hyperintense on T2-weighted images and hypointense on T1-weighted images, with corroborating changes on diffusion-weighted and apparent diffusion coefficient images.

Treatment

All included patients received anti-tuberculosis treatment as per World Health Organization guidelines for the treatment of central nervous system tuberculosis. Patients received 2 months of daily oral isoniazid (5 mg/ kg of body weight; maximum, 300 mg), rifampicin (10 mg/ kg; maximum, 600 mg), pyrazinamide (25 mg/kg; maximum, 2 g/day) and intramuscular streptomycin (20 mg/kg; maximum 1 gm/day), followed by at least 7 months administration of isoniazid and rifampicin [12]. Corticosteroid regimen consisted of intravenous dexamethasone for 4 weeks (0.4 mg/kg body weight per day and then tapered off decreasing 0.1 mg/kg every week) and then oral treatment for 4 weeks, starting at a total of 4 mg per day and decreasing by 1 mg each week [13]. Pyridoxine was given orally 20–40 mg/day to all the patients. In addition, patients received symptomatic treatment as well. Neurosurgical opinion was sought, whenever required.

In HIV-infected patients antiretroviral therapy was administered under supervision of the Nodal antiretroviral therapy unit. Antiretroviral therapy was started as soon as anti-tuberculosis treatment was tolerated (between 2 weeks and 2 months), as per National AIDS Control Organization, Government of India, guidelines [14].

Disability assessment

Disability assessment was done using Barthel index (BI), which is a 20 point scoring system. Assessment of disability included degree of dependence for bowel and bladder, grooming, toilet use, transfer, mobility, dressing, feeding, use of stairs and bathing. For each activity, a score of 0 indicated a complete dependence, and an individual score of 2 or 3 indicated that the patient was able to perform activities independently. A score of ≤ 12 indicated poor functional status and a score of >12 indicated good functional status.

Follow up

Patients were regularly followed up for 9 months. Besides a defined follow up at 3, 6, and 9 months, clinical assessment and cerebrospinal fluid analysis were also done at the time of clinical deterioration. Changes in cerebrospinal fluid parameters (like cells, protein and sugar) were noted. Polymorphonuclear predominance was defined when these constituted >50 % of cells. Repeat neuroimaging were performed after 3 months and 6 months, or at periods of clinical deteriorations. Neuroimaging were looked for any deterioration or new findings. Assessment of disability was done at the end 9 months of follow up. Barthel index >12 was considered as good outcome. Intervening visits mandated by clinical deteriorations generated off-pre-defined visit data which was additionally recorded.

Statistical analysis

Statistical analysis was performed using the Statistical Package for Social Sciences, version 16 for windows (SPSS, Chicago IL, USA). Both univariate and multivariate analysis were done to evaluate the predictors of paradoxical reaction. Univariate analysis was performed by Chi-square test for categorical variables and independent sample "t" test for continuous variables. Odds ratio with 95 % confidence interval were ascertained. For multivariate analysis, binary logistic regression was performed to see the impact of individual predictors of paradoxical reaction. Paired sample "t" test and McNemar tests were used to compare quantitative and qualitative variables before and during development of paradoxical reaction. Kaplan Meier analysis was performed to estimate the event free survival for the outcome with or without baseline paradoxical reaction using the Log Rank test. Statistical significance was defined at a p value of <0.05. All statistical analyses were two-tailed.

Results

Baseline characteristics

We screened 156 consecutive patients of tuberculous meningitis during the study period which ranged from October 2013 to March 2015. Fifteen patients were excluded. Reasons for exclusion of 15 patients have been provided in Fig. 1. Finally, 141 patients were included and evaluated. Majority of our patients 66 (46.8 %), at inclusion, were in stage-II. Thirteen patients were HIV positive. There were 54 (38.3 %) microbiologically-confirmed cases. One patient had multidrug resistant tuberculous meningitis and was included in the non-paradoxical reaction group. In the paradoxical reaction group the mean duration of illness was 42.93 ± 21.58 (median = 38, range 18–107) days while in the non-paradoxical reaction group the mean duration of illness was 52.49 ± 27.54 (median = 45, range 5–180) days (Table 1).

Incidence of paradoxical reaction

In our study, 44 (31.2 %) patients developed some form of paradoxical reaction. In majority (29 patients), paradoxical reactions were noted within 3 months of start of anti-tuberculosis treatment. Mean duration of paradoxical reaction was 82.45 days (16–320 days) (Additional file file 1: Table S1).

Manifestations of paradoxical reaction

Fever, headache, altered sensorium, decreased vision, and seizures were common clinical paradoxical reactions among 44 patients who presented with a paradoxical reaction. Among neuroimaging changes, enhancing basal exudates, a new or enlargement of pre-existing tuberculoma, development of infarcts, and increasing ventriculomegaly were the more frequent paradoxical reactions. Twenty-six (59 %) patients developed either a new (15 patients) or enlargement (11 patients) of pre-existing tuberculoma. Twenty patients demonstrated newly developed hydrocephalus while in 7 cases ventricular size had increased further. Optochiasmatic arachnoiditis was the other common but disabling paradoxical manifestation. Four patients, additionally, had spinal arachnoiditis. In 41 patients, cerebrospinal fluid paradoxically

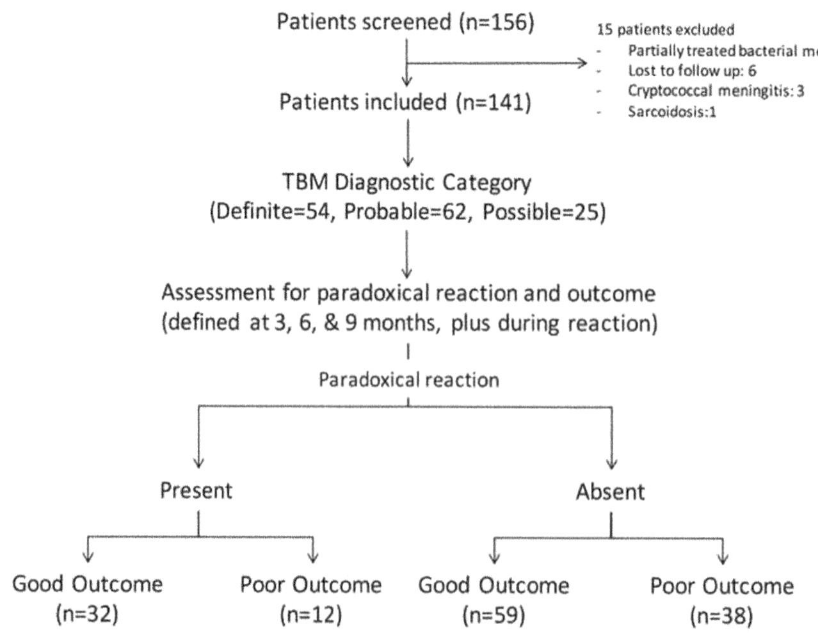

Fig. 1 Flow chart of the study

Table 1 Baseline characteristics, radiological and cerebrospinal fluid parameters, and outcome of patients with tuberculous meningitis

	Total numbers of patients included (*n*=141)	Paradoxical manifestation (*n*=44)	No paradoxical manifestation (*n*=97)
Demographic			
Age (Mean±SD)	29.75±12.79	27.295±10.95	30.866±13.44
Duration of illness (Mean±SD)	49.51±26.13	42.932±21.58	52.495±27.53
Gender (n, %)			
Male	76(53.9 %)	18(40.9 %)	58(59.8 %)
Female	65(46.1 %)	26(59.1 %)	39(40.2)
HIV (n, %)	13(9.2 %)	11(25 %)	2(2.1 %)
Clinical (n, %)			
BMRC stage 1	31(22.0 %)	8(18.2 %)	23(23.7 %)
BMRC stage 2	66(46.8 %)	21(47.7 %	45(46.4 %)
BMRC stage 3	44(31.2 %)	15(34.1 %)	29(29.9 %)
Fever	138(97.8 %)	43(97.7 %)	95(97.9 %)
Headache	131(92.90 %)	39(88.6 %)	92(94.8 %)
Seizure	48(34.0 %)	12(27.3 %)	36(37.1 %)
Altered Sensorium	44(31.2 %)	15(34.1 %)	29(29.9 %)
Decreased vision	35(24.8 %)	10(22.7 %)	25(25.8 %)
Hemiparesis	23(16.3 %)	7(15.9 %)	16(16.5 %)
Paraparesis	12(8.5 %)	2(4.5 %)	10(10.3 %)
Meningeal signs	125(88.7 %)	41(93.2 %)	84(86.6 %)
Lymphadenopathy	13(9.2 %)	10(22.7 %)	3(3.1 %)
Diplopia	59(41.8 %)	17(38.6 %)	42(43.3 %)
Cranial Nerve involvement	80(56.7 %)	27(61.4 %)	53(54.6 %)
Papilloedema	50(62.5 %)	13(29.5 %)	42(43.3 %)
Imaging (n, %)			
Hydrocephalus	53(37.6 %)	13(29.5 %)	40(41.2 %)
Basal Exudates	38(27.0 %)	9(20.5 %)	29(29.9 %)
Tuberculoma	51(36.2 %)	15(34.1 %)	36(37.1 %)
Infarct	25(17.7 %)	7(15.9 %)	18(18.6 %)
Optochiasmatic arachnoiditis	21(14.9 %)	7(15.9 %)	14(14.4 %)
Spinal arachnoiditis	12(8.5 %)	2(4.5 %)	10(10.3 %)
Cerebrospinal fluid			
White blood cells (cells/mL±SD)	189.610±185.66	200.864±121.26	184.505±208.809
Protein mg%	253.704±455.84	188.5382±115.145	283.2649±542.511
Sugar mg%	35.311±18.46	33.620±18.231	36.086±18.61
Neutrophil differential in percentage, mean±SD	17.21±19.250	19.705±21.368	16.072±18.210
Lymphocyte differential in percentage (mean±SD)	83.65±18.02	80.295±21.368	85.175±16.166
AFB smear (n, %)	4(2.8 %)	1(2.27 %)	3(3.09 %)
AFB culture positive (n, %)	21(14.9 %)	11(25 %)	10(10.30 %)
TB PCR-positive (n, %)	50(35.5 %)	22(50 %)	28(28.86 %)

Table 1 Baseline characteristics, radiological and cerebrospinal fluid parameters, and outcome of patients with tuberculous meningitis *(Continued)*

Diagnostic category (n, %)			
Definite	54(38.3 %)	20(45.5 %)	34(35.1 %)
Probable	62(44.0 %)	19(43.2 %)	43(44.3 %)
Possible	25(17.7 %)	5(11.4 %)	20(20.6 %
Disability (n, %)			
Baseline BI(<12)	93(66.0 %)	34(77.3 %)	59(60.8 %)
Baseline BI(>12)	48(34.0 %)	10(22.7 %)	38(39.2 %)
Outcome (n, %)			
Poor (BI<12)	50(35.5 %)	12(27.3 %)	38(39.2 %)
Good (BI>12)	91(64.5 %)	32(72.7 %)	59(60.8 %)

AFB acid fast bacilli, *BMRC* British Medical Research Council, *HIV* human immunodeficiency virus, *BI* Barthel index, *TB PCR* tuberculosis polymerase chain reaction

worsened (increase in cells with or without rise in protein level). Out of the remaining 3, two patients demonstrated a decrease in the cell count but with polymorph predominance (not present at the baseline) while in one the cerebrospinal fluid was normal. In cerebrospinal fluid, major changes observed were increase in protein level and increase in polymorphs. In 3 patients with paradoxical reaction, only cerebrospinal fluid changes (without imaging changes) were noted. Fourteen patients had paradoxical lymphadenopathy while three patients had developed miliary tuberculosis (Fig. 2) (Additional file 1: Table S1). Statistically significant changes from the baseline to the time of development of paradoxical reaction was observed in fever, headache, hydrocephalus, tuberculoma, c-reactive protein, erythrocyte sedimentation rate, and cerebrospinal fluid polymorphs, lymphocytes, and protein (Table 2).

Predictors of paradoxical reaction

On univariate analysis, female gender ($p = 0.037$), HIV positivity ($p = <0.001$), lymphadenopathy ($p = 0.001$) and a shorter duration of illness ($p = 0.028$) were significantly associated with development of paradoxical reaction (Table 3). On multivariate analysis, female gender ($p = 0.013$, OR =2.87, CI 1.24-6.62), HIV positivity ($p = 0.010$, OR = 31.49; CI = 2.31-426.21), and a shorter duration of illness ($p = 0.049$, OR = 0.98 CI = .963-1.00) were found to be statistically significant predictors of paradoxical reaction (Table 4).

Impact on prognosis

Overall, duration of illness, alteration in consciousness, stage-III of tuberculous meningitis, and hydrocephalus predicted poor prognosis among patients with tuberculous meningitis. In the paradoxical group 24 % patients had poor outcome compared to 35.2 % with good outcome, which was statistically not significant (Table 5). We did not observe any significant difference in the proportion of patients having poor disability status after end of follow up. Kaplan-Meier survival statistics did not demonstrate any significant difference in survival between both groups (Fig. 3).

Discussion

In this prospective study approximately one-third of patients with tuberculous meningitis developed paradoxical

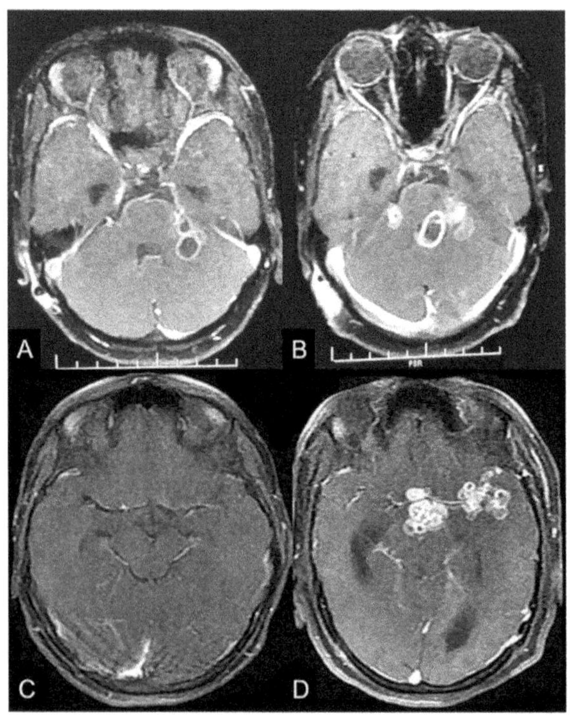

Fig. 2 T1-weighted Gadolinium-enhanced MRI (axial sections) of the brain of a patient with TBM depict the development of additional (paradoxical) tuberculoma (Baseline-**a**, at 5th month-**b**) at the pontocerebellar level. Similar sequence in another patient shows development of paradoxical optochiasmatic arachnoiditis along with multiple tuberculomas (Baseline-**c**, at 3rd month-**d**)

Table 2 Comparative analysis of variables of patients with paradoxical reaction

Variable	At baseline	During pxaradoxical reaction	*P* value
Fever	43	29	*.001*
Headache	39	27	*.008*
Seizure	12	11	1.0
Altered Sensorium	15	12	.664
Decreased vision	10	16	.180
Hemiparesis	7	9	.791
Paraparesis	2	4	.688
Hydrocephalus	13	27	*.009*
Tuberculoma	15	26	*.019*
Basal Exudate	9	12	.648
Optochiasmatic arachnoiditis	7	12	.332
Infarct	7	9	.791
Spinal arachnoiditis	2	4	.688
CRP	19	28	*.004*
ESR	27.818±4.876	33.20±5.889	*.027*
CSF cells	200.864±121.260	210.295±125.761	.058
CSF Polymorph	19.705±21.368	37.84±23.716	*.008*
CSF Lymphocytes	80.295±21.368	62.39±23.398	*.012*
CSF Protein	188.538±115.145	261.355±152.0650	*<.001*
CSF sugar	33.620±43.2566	43.256±17.998	.261

CRP C-reactive protein, *CSF* cerebrospinal fluid, *ESR* Erythrocyte sedimentation rate
Note: Statistically significant *P*-values are depicted in italics

changes. In almost all patients, clinical/imaging paradoxical manifestations accompanied paradoxical cerebrospinal fluid changes. We encountered a variety of manifestations of paradoxical reactions. These paradoxical clinical and neuroimaging manifestations were either aggravated or appeared for the first time during illness, despite of an adequate anti-tuberculosis treatment. Expansion of existing cerebral tuberculomas and appearance of new tuberculomas, hydrocephalus, and optochiasmatic and spinal arachnoiditis, were common paradoxical manifestations.

Paradoxical reactions in these patients result because of an excessive inflammatory response against mycobacterial antigens. Mycobacterial cell wall antigens are present in the affected brain tissues and trigger an exaggerated inflammatory reaction following treatment with anti-tuberculosis drugs. Cheng and colleagues had noted a surge in blood lymphocyte counts accompanied by an increased tuberculin skin reaction during paradoxical response indicating that this immune response is similar to immune restoration syndrome seen in HIV-infected patients. Possibly, due to a paradoxical shift in the cellular components of the cerebrospinal fluid (from lymphocytic predominance to polymorph predominance), neutrophils also play a role in the pathogenesis of paradoxical reaction in patients with tuberculous meningitis. [15] Sütlaş and co-workers followed 61 patients with confirmed or presumed tuberculous meningitis. Patients were categorized into two groups according to the presence of paradoxical response (progressive increase of lymphocytes or increase of polymorphonuclear cells instead of lymphocytes) in cerebrospinal fluid samples. Paradoxical response in the cerebrospinal fluid was seen in 20 patients. New tuberculomas developed more frequently in the group having paradoxical cerebrospinal fluid response. We had similar observations in our study where 41 patients with clinical/imaging paradoxical changes had paradoxical cerebrospinal fluid changes. Interestingly, in two patients where the cells actually decreased, there was a shift towards polymorph predominance. It has been observed that paradoxical cerebrospinal fluid changes occur after several weeks of starting anti-tuberculosis treatment and may not be associated with any clinical or neuroimaging deterioration [16].

We observed that female gender, concomitant HIV infection, and a shorter duration of illness, were significant predictors of paradoxical reactions in patients with tuberculous meningitis. Females exhibit more-robust immune responses to antigenic challenges, like infection and vaccination, in comparison to that in males. Given the fact that immune cells express specific receptors for

Table 3 Predictors of paradoxical reaction on univariate analysis

Characteristic	Paradoxical reaction		*P* value	Odds ratio	95 % Confidence interval	
	Present (*n*=44)	Absent (*n*=97)			Lower bound	Upper bound
Age in years Mean ± SD	27.295 ± 10.958	30.866 ± 13.446	0.125		−1.004	8.145
Duration of illness (days) Mean ± SD	42.932± 21.583	52.495± 27.538	*0.028*		0.276	18.850
Gender (female)	26 (59.1 %)	39 (40.2 %)	*0.037*	2.148	1.04	4.436
HIV positive	11(25 %)	2(2.1 %)	*<0.001*	15.833	3.334	75.184
Fever	43(97.7 %)	95(97.9 %)	0.936	0.905	0.080	10.255
Headache	39(88.6 %)	92(94.8 %)	0.183	0.424	0.116	1.548
Seizure	12(27.3 %)	36(37.1 %)	0.253	0.635	0.291	1.387
Altered Sensorium	15(34.1 %)	29(29.9 %)	0.618	1.213	0.567	2.593
Decreased vision	10(22.7 %)	25(25.8 %)	0.698	0.847	0.366	1.960
Hemiparesis	7(15.9 %)	16(16.5 %)	0.930	0.958	0.363	2.526
Paraparesis	2(4.5 %)	10(10.3 %)	0.341	0.414	0.087	1.976
Meningeal signs	41(93.2 %)	84(86.6 %)	0.253	2.115	0.571	7.837
Lymphadenopathy	10(22.7 %)	3(3.1 %)	*0.001*	9.216	2.393	35.496
Diplopia	17(38.6 %)	42(43.3 %)	0.603	0.825	0.398	1.707
Cranial Nerve involvement	27(61.4 %)	53(54.6 %)	0.455	1.319	0.638	2.727
Papilloedema	13(29.5 %)	42(43.3 %)	0.121	0.549	0.256	1.177
Hydrocephalus	13(29.5 %)	40(41.2 %)	0.184	0.598	0.279	1.282
Basal Exudates	9(20.5 %)	29(29.9 %)	0.242	0.603	0.257	1.413
Tuberculoma	15(34.1 %)	36(37.1 %)	0.729	0.876	0.415	1.850
Infarct	7(15.9 %)	18(18.6 %)	0.703	0.830	0.319	2.161
Optochiasmatic Arachnoiditis	7(15.9 %)	14(14.4 %)	0.820	1.122	0.418	3.008
Spinal cord	2(4.5 %)	10(10.3 %)	0.256	0.414	0.087	1.976
CRP	19(43.2 %)	38(39.2 %)	0.653	1.180	0.573	2.430
Stage 3 TBM	15(34.1 %)	29(29.9 %)	0.618	1.213	0.567	2.593
Baseline BI (<12)	34(77.3 %)	59(60.8 %)	0.056	2.190	0.970	4.944
Definite TBM	20(45.5 %)	34(35.1 %)	0.312	1.544	.748	3.189
Good outcome (BI>12)	32(72.7 %)	59(64.8 %)	0.171	0.582	0.267	1.268
ESR mm in 1 h Mean ± SD	27.818 ± 4.876	27.093 ± 7.593	0.497		−3.194	1.743
CSF Cells/μL Mean ± SD	200.864 ± 121.261	184.505 ± 208.810	0.630		83.265	56.548
CSF protein (mg/dl) Mean ± SD	188.5382 ± 115.145	283.2649 ± 542.511	0.254		−68.924	258.377
CSF sugar (mg/dl) Mean ± SD	33.620 ± 18.231	36.086 ± 18.617	0.465		4.193	9.125

BI Barthel Index, *CRP* C-reactive protein, *CSF* cerebrospinal fluid, *ESR* Erythrocyte sedimentation rate, *HIV* Human Immunodeficiency Virus, *TBM* Tuberculous meningitis
Note: Statistically significant *P*-values are depicted in italics

Table 4 Predictors of paradoxical reaction on multivariate analysis

Characteristic	*P* value	Odds ratio	95 % Confidence interval	
			Lower bound	Upper bound
Duration	*.049*	.981	0.963	1.000
Gender (female)	*.013*	2.873	1.246	6.626
HIV	*.010*	31.407	2.314	426.215
Lymphadenopathy	.813	0.746	0.066	8.465

HIV human immunodeficiency virus
Note: Statistically significant *P*-values are depicted in italics

sex hormones and are responsive to changes in hormone levels, this gender variation might be explained by the modulatory effect of female sex hormones on the immune response towards *Mycobacterium tuberculosis* associated antigens [17, 18].

Patients with disseminated or extrapulmonary disease are considered to have higher bacillary/antigen loads, with a relative immunodeficient response, resulting in an increased risk of both paradoxical reactions and IRIS. Use of bactericidal drugs, such as isoniazid, may cause a massive release of bacterial components and provoke

Table 5 Predictors of disability and outcome on univariate analysis in patients with tuberculous meningitis

Characteristics	BI≤12 (*n*=50)	BI>12 (*n*=91)	*P* value	Odds Ratio	95 % Confidence interval	
					Lower bound	Upper bound
Age	29.320±11.881	29.989±13.322	.768		−3.797	5.135
Duration of illness	42.140±21.204	53.560±27.761	*.013*		2.495	20.345
Gender	22(44 %)	54(59.3 %)	.080	.538	.268	1.082
HIV						
Fever	49(98 %)	89(97.8 %)	.938	1.101	.097	12.453
Headache	44(88 %)	87(95.6 %)	.092	.337	.090	1.257
Seizure	15(30.0 %)	33(36.3 %)	.453	.753	.359	1.580
Altered Sensorium	31(62.0 %)	13(14.3 %)	*<.001*	9.789	4.316	22.206
Decreased vision	16(32.0 %)	19(20.9 %)	.144	1.783	.817	3.891
Hemiparesis	9(18.0 %)	14(15.4 %)	.688	1.207	.482	3.027
Paraparesis	6(12.0 %)	6(6.6 %)	.271	1.932	.588	6.342
Meningeal signs	44(88.0 %)	81(89 %)	.856	.905	.308	2.657
Lymphadenopathy	4(8.0 %)	9(9.9 %)	.711	.792	.231	2.716
Diplopia	19(38.0 %)	40(44.0 %)	.493	.821	.402	1.675
Cranial Nerve involvement	28(56.0 %)	52(57.1 %)	.896	.955	.476	1.914
Papilloedema	18(36.0 %)	37(40.7 %)	.587	.821	.402	1.675
Hydrocephalus	40(80.0 %)	13(14.3 %)	*<.001*	24.0	9.677	59.520
Basal Exudates	12(24.0 %)	26(28.6 %)	.558	.789	.357	1.744
Tuberculoma	22(44.0 %)	29(31.9 %)	.151	1.680	.825	3.422
Infarct	9(18.0 %)	16(17.6 %)	.950	1.029	.418	2.533
Optochiasmatic arachnoiditis	7(14.0 %)	14(15.4 %)	.825	.895	.336	2.388
Spinal arachnoiditis	6(12.0 %)	6(6.6 %)	.271	1.932	.588	6.342
Stage-III TBM	31(62.0 %)	13(14.3 %	*<.001*	9.789	4.316	22.206
Definite TBM	23(46.0 %)	31(34.1 %)	.163			
Paradoxical reaction	12(24.0 %)	32(35.2 %)	.171	.582	.267	1.268
CSF Cells	159.340	206.242	.152		−17.474	111.277
CSF protein	256.772	252.019	.953		−163.99	154.488
CSF sugar	35.112	35.422	.925		−6.153	6.773

CSF cerebrospinal fluid, *HIV* human immunodeficiency virus, *BI* Barthel index, *TBM* tuberculous meningitis
Note: Statistically significant *P*-values are depicted in italics

inflammatory changes that could produce clinical deterioration and imaging changes [19]. Another significant predictor of paradoxical reaction was a shorter duration of illness. Possibly, a large mycobacterial load and subsequent release of mycobacterial antigen following anti-tuberculosis treatment resulted in a higher frequency of paradoxical reactions among patients who developed tuberculous meningitis comparatively rapidly.

A substantial proportion of our HIV-infected patients (11 out of 13 patients) developed paradoxical reactions. Many studies in the past have noted that many patients develop tuberculous meningitis associated IRIS. Manifestations of central nervous system tuberculosis IRIS include meningitis, cerebral parenchymal tuberculoma, brain abscesses, spinal cord complications like myeloradiculopathy, and spinal epidural abscesses [20–22]. In a prospective study, 47 % (16/34) of tuberculous meningitis patients developed tuberculous meningitis-IRIS. At inclusion, tuberculous meningitis-IRIS patients had a higher cerebrospinal fluid neutrophil counts compared with non-tuberculous meningitis-IRIS patients [20]. There is a consensus that antiretroviral therapy should be started early (around 2 weeks) in HIV/tuberculosis co-infected patients. In HIV and tuberculous meningitis co-infected patients, because of a potential risk of tuberculous meningitis associated IRIS, antiretroviral therapy may be delayed; however, there is no consensus on this point [23].

We observed that the development of paradoxical reactions did not adversely affect the outcome of tuberculous meningitis. Several studies in the past had

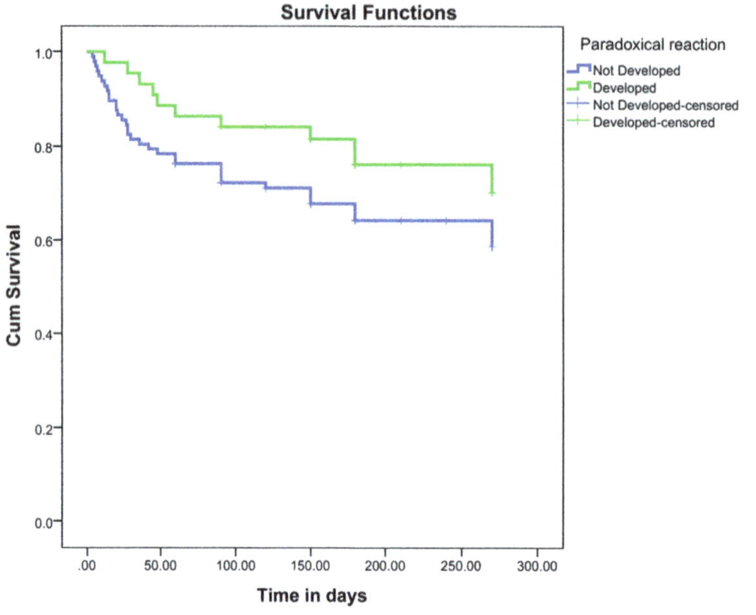

Fig. 3 Kaplan Meyer survival analysis showed no significant difference in the cumulative survival of patients with or without paradoxical reaction (Log rank test: X^2 (1) = 2.198, P = 0.138)

similar observations. Clinical, laboratory, radiological, and outcome data of 14 cases of paradoxical tuberculoma in tuberculous meningitis patients (out of 22 patients who had intracranial tuberculoma) were compared with 41 tuberculous meningitis patients without tuberculomas. The analysis suggested that there was no statistical difference between two groups regarding age, stage of tuberculous meningitis, duration between disease onset and treatment initiation, cerebrospinal fluid protein levels, and in long-term disabilities [24]. Many manifestations of paradoxical reactions like optochiasmatic and spinal arachnoiditis, and a large cerebral tuberculoma are serious conditions associated with severe disabilities, and a potential for death [25]. These conditions warrant urgent treatment with immunomodulatory drugs. High doses of corticosteroids are currently the most preferred treatment. Many other immunomodulatory drugs like, tissue necrosis factor-α antagonists, thalidomide, and interferon– γ have also been used, though sparingly [3].

There were certain limitations of our study. It is difficult to pin-point exactly the timing of onset of a paradoxical reaction clinically. Besides this, the differential diagnosis of a paradoxical reaction may also pose a challenge. A wrong diagnosis, possibility of treatment failure, multidrug-resistance, atypical mycobacterial infection, drug toxicity, or clinical deterioration due to some unrelated cause should always be co-considered. One of our patients with apparent paradoxical reaction later turned out to have multidrug-resistant tuberculosis.

Conclusion

Paradoxical reaction occurs in approximately one-third of patients with tuberculous meningitis. Female gender, concomitant HIV infection, and a shorter duration of illness are significant predictors of such reactions. Duration of illness, alteration in consciousness, stage-III of tuberculous meningitis, and hydrocephalus, predict a poor prognosis in patients with tuberculous meningitis; paradoxical reactions, however, do not seem to affect the outcome adversely.

Abbreviations

AIDS, acquired immune deficiency syndrome; B, barthel index; HIV, human immunodeficiency virus; IRIS, immune reconstitution inflammatory syndrome; MRI, magnetic resonance imaging

Acknowledgement

None.

Funding

Funding was not obtained for this study.

Authors' contributions

AKS: concept of study, execution of study and data analysis and writing the manuscript. HSM: concept of study, execution of study and data analysis and writing the manuscript. RKG: concept of study, execution of study and data analysis and writing the manuscript. AJ: responsible for microbiological studies and manuscript writing. NK: concept of study, execution of study and data analysis and writing the manuscript. NK: responsible for conduct and assessment of Neuroimaging in the study. RV: patient evaluation and manuscript writing. PKS: patient evaluation and manuscript writing. All authors have read and approve of the final version of the manuscript.

Competing interest

On behalf of all authors, the corresponding author states that there is no conflict of interest.

Consent for publish

Not applicable.

Author details

[1]Department of Neurology, King George Medical University, Uttar Pradesh, Lucknow PIN-226003, India. [2]Department of Microbiology, King George Medical University, Uttar Pradesh, Lucknow, India. [3]Department of Radiodiagnosis, King George Medical University, Uttar Pradesh, Lucknow, India.

References

1. Afghani B, Lieberman JM. Paradoxical enlargement or development of intracranial tuberculomas during therapy: case report and review. Clin Infect Dis. 1994;19:1092–9.
2. Nicolls DJ, King M, Holland D, Bala J, del Rio C. Intracranial tuberculomas developing while on therapy for pulmonary tuberculosis. Lancet Infect Dis. 2005;5:795–801.
3. Garg RK, Malhotra HS, Kumar N. Paradoxical reaction in HIV negative tuberculous meningitis. J Neurol Sci. 2014;340:26–36.
4. Garcia-Monco JC, Ferreira E, Gomez-Beldarrain M. The therapeutic paradox in the diagnosis of tuberculous meningitis. Neurology. 2005;65:1991–2.
5. Teoh R, O'Mahony G, Yeung VT. Polymorphonuclear pleocytosis in the cerebrospinal fluid during chemotherapy for tuberculous meningitis. J Neurol. 1986;233:237–41.
6. Kim SH, Kim YS. Immunologic paradox in the diagnosis of tuberculous meningitis. Clin Vaccine Immunol. 2009;16:1847–9.
7. Meintjes G, Lawn SD, Scano F, Maartens G, French MA, Worodria W, Elliott JH, Murdoch D, Wilkinson RJ, Seyler C, John L, van der Loeff MS, Reiss P, Lynen L, Janoff EN, Gilks C, Colebunders R. International Network for the Study of HIV-associated IRIS. Tuberculosis-associated immune reconstitution inflammatory syndrome: case definitions for use in resource-limited settings. Lancet Infect Dis. 2008;8:516–23.
8. Marais S, Meintjes G, Pepper DJ, Dodd LE, Schutz C, Ismail Z, Wilkinson KA, Wilkinson RJ. Frequency, severity, and prediction of tuberculous meningitis immune reconstitution inflammatory syndrome. Clin Infect Dis. 2013;56:450–60.
9. Marais S, Thwaites G, Schoeman JF, et al. Tuberculous meningitis: a uniform case definition for use in clinical research. Lancet Infect Dis. 2010;10:803–12.
10. Council BMR. Streptomycin treatment of tuberculous meningitis. BMJ. 1948;1:582–97.
11. Hawkey CR, Yap T, Pereira J, Moore DA, Davidson RN, Pasvol G, Kon OM, Wall RA, Wilkinson RJ. Characterization and management of paradoxical upgrading reactions in HIV-uninfected patients with lymph node tuberculosis. Clin Infect Dis. 2005;40:1368–71.
12. World Health Organization. Treatment of tuberculosis: guidelines. WHO/HTM/TB/2009.420. 4th ed. World Health Organization; 2012 [http://whqlibdoc.who.int/ publications/2010/9789241547833_eng.pdf; 2010; accessed on 9 January.2016]
13. Thwaites GE, Nguyen DB, Nguyen HD, et al. Dexamethasone for the treatment of tuberculous meningitis in adolescents and adults. N Engl J Med. 2004;351:1741–51.
14. National AIDS Control Organization. National Guidelines on Second-line and Alternative First-line ART For Adults and Adolescents. Department of Health & Family Welfare Government of India New Delhi, India. Downloaded from http://www.naco.gov.in/upload/Policies%20&%20Guidelines/Antiretroviral%20Therapy%20Guidelines%20for%20HIV-Infected%20Adults%20and%20Adolescents.pdf Assessed on January 7, 2016.
15. Cheng VC, Yam WC, Woo PC, Lau SK, Hung IF, Wong SP, et al. Risk factors for development of paradoxical response during antituberculosis therapy in HIV-negative patients. Eur J Clin Microbiol Infect Dis. 2003;22:597–602.
16. Sütlas PN, Unal A, Forta H, Senol S, Kirbas D. Tuberculous meningitis in adults: review of 61 cases. Infection. 2003;31:387–91.
17. Nhamoyebonde S, Leslie A. Biological differences between the sexes and susceptibility to tuberculosis. J Infect Dis. 2014;209 Suppl 3:S100–6.
18. Neyrolles O, Quintana-Murci L. Sexual inequality in tuberculosis. PLoS Med. 2009;6, e1000199.
19. Bell LC, Breen R, Miller RF, Noursadeghi M, Lipman M. Paradoxical reactions and immune reconstitution inflammatory syndrome in tuberculosis. Int J Infect Dis. 2015;32:39–45.
20. Crump JA, Tyrer MJ, Lloyd-Owen SJ, Han LY, Lipman MC, Johnson MA. Miliary tuberculosis with paradoxical expansion of intracranial tuberculomas complicating human immunodeficiency virus infection in a patient receiving highly active antiretroviral therapy. Clin Infect Dis. 1998;26:1008–9.
21. Pepper DJ, Marais S, Maartens G, Rebe K, Morroni C, Rangaka MX, Oni T, Wilkinson RJ, Meintjes G. Neurologic manifestations of paradoxical tuberculosis-associated immune reconstitution inflammatory syndrome: a case series. Clin Infect Dis. 2009;48(11):e96–107.
22. Marais S, Scholtz P, Pepper DJ, Meintjes G, Wilkinson RJ, Candy S. Neuroradiological features of the tuberculosis-associated immune reconstitution inflammatory syndrome. Int J Tuberc Lung Dis. 2010;14:188–96.
23. Lawn SD, Wood R. Poor prognosis of HIV-associated tuberculous meningitis regardless of the timing of antiretroviral therapy. Clin Infect Dis. 2011;52(11):1384–7.
24. Unal A, Sutlas PN. Clinical and radiological features of symptomatic central nervous system tuberculomas. Eur J Neurol. 2005;12:797–804.
25. Sinha MK, Garg RK, Anuradha HK, Agarwal A, Singh MK, Verma R, et al. Vision impairment in tuberculous meningitis: predictors and prognosis. J Neurol Sci. 2010;290:27–32.

6

Increased activity of the complement system in cerebrospinal fluid of the patients with Non-HIV Cryptococcal meningitis

Lei Shen[1†], Jianming Zheng[2†], Yan Wang[3], Mengqi Zhu[2], Haoxiang Zhu[2], Qi Cheng[2] and Qian Li[2*]

Abstract

Backgrounds: Cryptococcal meningitis (CM) has been known to lead to significant morbidity and mortality. The relative contribution of the complement system in protection and pathogenesis during CM remains largely unknown. The purpose of this study was to evaluate the baseline complement component profiles in human cerebrospinal fluid (CSF) and plasma from non-HIV patients with CM, and therefore to provide insights of possible roles of the complement system in CM.

Methods: CSF and blood samples from forty two CM patients not infected with HIV and thirteen non-CM control patients (Ctrl) were retrospectively selected and evaluated from the patients admitted to the hospital with a suspected diagnosis of CM. CSF and blood samples were collected at the admission. Enzyme-linked immunosorbent assay (ELISA) for complement components, cytokine IL-12 and western blot for C3 activation were performed on CSF and plasma samples. The levels of complement C1q, factor B (FB), mannose binding lectin (MBL), C2, C3, C4, C5, C4 binding protein (C4BP), Factor I (FI), Factor H (FH), sC5b-9 in CSF and plasma samples were compared. Pearson's correlation coefficients were calculated on variables between complement components and the levels of total protein in the CSF samples.

Results: Our data demonstrated that the CSF levels of complement components of C1q, FB, MBL as well as complement pathway factors sC5b-9 and complement regulator FH were all elevated in patients with CM as compared to the controls, CSF C3 breakdown products iC3b were found in both CSF and plasma samples of the CM patients. A positive correlation was found between the levels of CSF protein and MBL, C1q or FB.

Conclusions: The activity of the complement system in CSF was increased in non-HIV patients with CM. C1q, MBL and FB are the important participants in the complement activation in CM. The relative contribution of each of the specific complement pathways and complement cascades in protection and inflammation resolution against CM warrant further investigation.

Keywords: Cryptococcal meningitis, Complement, Cryptococcus

* Correspondence: qiannub2000@sina.com
†Equal contributors
[2]Department of Infectious Diseases, Huashan Hospital, Fudan University, Shanghai, China
Full list of author information is available at the end of the article

Background

Cryptococcal meningitis (CM) is one of the most common diseases in HIV patients and other immune-compromised patients [1]. Over 1 million CM cases with 600,000 deaths per year in HIV patients worldwide have been reported [2]. Additionally, non-HIV related CM also contributes a significant mortality and morbidity in the developed world despite advances in antifungal therapy [1]. In China, the main pathogen of cryptococcal infections is *C. neoformans*, resulting in pulmonary cryptococcosis that has a predilection to disseminate to the central nervous system (CNS) leading to life threatening meningoencephalitis [3].

The complement system is well known as a major component of the host innate immune defense system against infection. Activation of the complement system in response to invading pathogens is initiated through the classical (CP), alternative (AP) and lectin (LP) pathways. Activation results in C3 cleavage, releasing anaphylatoxins C3a and C5a, and formation of a membrane attack complex to lyse the target cells. Cleavage of C3 generates the key opsonins, C3b and iC3b. These proteins tag the pathogens for phagocytosis [4]. The complement system has the inhibitory proteins to regulate the location and efficacy of complement activation. Key fluid phase complement regulators include Factor H (FH), Factor I (FI), C4-binding protein (C4BP) and C1 inhibitor (C1INH).

It has been suggested that the complement system is of central importance in host defense against bacterial meningitis. Mice deficient in C1q and C3 demonstrated a decreased survival and enhanced growth of pneumococci in cerebrospinal fluid (CSF) after induction of meningitis [5]. Complement factors C1q, MBL, C3a, iC3b, C5a, sC5b-9 and FH were all elevated in CSF of patients with bacterial meningitis as compared to the controls [6]. Depletion of C3 or elevated C5a levels in CSF of patients with pneumococcal meningitis was associated with poor clinical prognosis [7, 8].

In contrast to bacterial meningitis, most fungal microorganisms cause a chronic instead of an acute or subacute meningitis [9]. Investigations from animal model and human patients have shown the importance of the complement system against cryptococcal infections [10]. Mice lacking hemolytic complement activity in their sera were sensitive to *C.neoformans* [11]. Guinea pigs and mice treated with cobra venom (depletion of C3 to C9) showed reduced ability to clear *C.neoformans* from extraneural sites [12]. *C5*$^{-/-}$ mice were more susceptible to intravenously injected *C.neoformans*, and more easily developed acute, fatal cryptococcal pneumonia [13]. Patients with cryptococcal fungemia showed reduced levels of C3 and FB [14]. Brain sections from patients with CM did not show C3 binding to the pathogen [15]. Moreover, both the classical and alternative complement pathways play a critical role in opsonophagocytosis of *C.neoformans* by neutrophils [16]. In vitro experiments demonstrated that C5a-C5aR signaling guided neutrophils to migrate to *C.neoformans*, resulting in optimal phagocytosis and subsequent killing of the organisms [17]. The complement opsonization is required in the anti-cryptococcal activity of human dendritic cells and macrophages [18, 19]. These data suggest that the major functions of the complement system are to stimulate the chemotaxis of the phagocytic effector cells and enhance the uptake of cryptococcal cells by these phagocytes. Complement functionality can be crucial to fight off and kill invading *Cryptococcus*.

To our knowledge, no study has been reported which examines the complement system activity in CSF and plasma from CM patients. The purpose of this study was to investigate whether the complement system is activated systemically and/or intrathecally during CM. The levels of the complement components in CSF and plasma samples from CM patients were determined and compared with that in the patient control group who were diagnosed with pulmonary cryptococcosis without CNS infection and inflammation involvement.

Methods

Patient selection, clinical sample collection and processing

This study was carried out from November 2014 to December 2015 at Huashan Hospital, Shanghai China. Both lumbar CSF and plasma samples were simultaneously obtained from patients with a suspected CM diagnosis at admission for routine chemistry, cytology and culture analysis. Venous blood was collected from individuals for plasma and routine blood cell and culture analysis. The remaining CSF samples were centrifuged and single use aliquots of these samples were stored at −80 °C.

CM group and patient control group were retrospectively selected from the collected samples. CM group consisted of 42 patients who were ≥18 year old and not infected with HIV with a first episode of CM as diagnosed according to the criteria reported previously [20]. Confirmed cases were patients meeting the laboratory criteria with positive culture of *C. neoformans* or positive India ink smear of CSF. Possible cases were patient with positive cryptococcal antigen titer in undiluted CSF and met at least one of the following criteria : (1) abnormal laboratory tests or an increased open pressure (≥200 mmH_2O) of CSF, (2) abnormalities of cranial imaging (Computerized Tomography or Magnetic Resonance Imaging) which could not be explained by other factors. Cryptococcal antigen in CSF was determined with the Latex-*Cryptococcus* antigen detection system (Immuno-Mycologics) [21].

Control CSF or blood samples were obtained from patients who presented to the hospital with suspicion of CM but subsequently tested negative for CM or any other pathogen in CSF with normal CSF leukocyte count and protein concentration. The control patients were diagnosed as pulmonary cryptococcosis based on histologic presence of the organism in lung biopsy specimens, or positive result of the serum cryptococcal antigen test with radiographic characteristics of pulmonary disease. [22]. The ethical and scientific committee of the College of Medicine, Fudan University approved this study.

ELISA

Human Complement C1q, FB, MBL, C2, C3, C4, C5, C4BP, FH, FI, sC5b-9, and cytokine Interleukin (IL) -12 were measured with commercial ELISA kits (Cusabio Biotech, Wuhan, P.R. China, R&D Systems, Minneapolis, USA, Abcam, Cambridge, UK, QuidelSan Diego, USA). Experiment protocols were followed according to the manufacturer's instructions.

Western blot

For comparison of complement C3 activation in CSF and plasma samples, 20 μl of CSF and 2 μl of plasma samples were loaded on an SDS-PAGE gel. Samples were transferred to polyvinylidene difluoride (PVDF) membranes. The membranes were blocked and then incubated with mouse anti-human C3/C3b/iC3b/C3dg monoclonal antibody (1:1,000, Cedarlane, Ontario, Canada) in TBST (Tris-buffered saline supplemented with Tween 20) containing 5% dry milk at 4 °C overnight. Blots were then washed and incubated with goat anti-mouse IgG (1:15,000, LI-COR Bioscience, Nebraska, USA) diluted in TBST containing 2% dry milk. The membranes were developed with an Odyssey system (Li-COR Bioscience) according to the manufacturer's protocol.

Statistical analysis

Results were graphed and analyzed using Prism 5.0 (GraphPad). Comparisons between the CM and control groups were made using unpaired *t* tests or Mann–Whitney tests (when the variances were significantly different). Nominal data were analyzed with Fisher exact test or Chi χ^2 test. Pearson's correlation coefficients were calculated on the variability between the levels of CSF complement components and CSF total protein. In all cases, a *p* value of <0.05 was set as the measure of significance.

Results

The clinical characteristics of participants

The study groups consisted of 42 CM patients and 13 patients diagnosed with pulmonary cryptococcosis without CNS infection and inflammation served as Ctrl group. As shown in Table 1, there were no significant differences in gender, age, blood routine test, CSF concentration of glucose and chloride between the two groups. However, WBC counts and concentrations of protein in CSF were significantly higher in CM group than that in the Ctrl group.

Complement components in CSF and plasma samples

The CSF concentrations of C1q, MBL and FB of CSF in CM were greatly elevated compared to that in Ctrl, and correlated with CSF protein concentrations

We first examined the concentrations of the complement classical pathway component (C1q), the lectin pathway (MBL) and the alternative pathway (FB) in plasma and CSF samples from CM and Ctrl group. The concentrations of C1q, MBL and FB in CSF samples were significantly higher in CM group than that in Ctrl group (Fig. 1a). The mean CSF concentration of C1q was 1673.14 ng/ml in the CM group, but only 162.72 ng/ml in the Ctrl group. The mean concentration of MBL was 5.11 ng/ml in the CM group, but 0.38 ng/ml in the Ctrl group. The mean concentration of FB was 5.73 ng/ml in the CM group, but 1.88 ng/ml in the Ctrl group. Moreover, CSF concentrations of C1q, MBL and FB were found to be correlated to CSF protein levels (r = 0.5804 for C1q, *p*-value =0.0479, r = 0.7061 for MBL, *p*-value = 0.0003, and r = 0.6716, *p*-value =0.009). However, There were no

Table 1 The clinical characteristics of participants

	Ctrl	CM	*p* value
Gender, M/F	9/4	28/14	0.5740
Age (means ± SEM, years old)	46.38 ± 11.15	44.86 ± 14.14	0.7233
Blood WBC (means ± SEM, $10^6/mm^3$)	6.98 ± 2.67	8.20 ± 3.75	0.2981
CSF WBC (median, $10^3/mm^3$)	2	9	0.0022
CSF Protein (median, mg/l)	387.5	883	0.0006
Blood Sugar (median, mmol/l)	5.4	6.9	0.5631
CSF Glucose (median, mmol/l)	2.65	2.70	0.4762
CSF Chloride (median, mmol/l)	121	120	0.3703

CM: cryptococcal meningitis group
Ctrl: control group

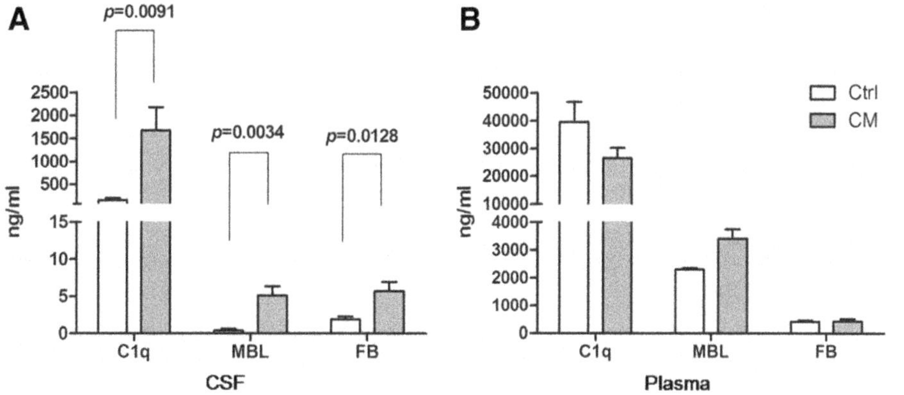

Fig. 1 The concentrations of C1q, MBL and FB in plasma and CSF samples. The white bar represented Ctrl group and the gray bar represented CM group. **a** CSF concentrations of C1q, MBL and FB were significantly higher in the CM group than those in the Ctrl group. **b** There were no significant differences in plasma concentrations of three complement components among the Ctrl and CM groups

statistical significances of the plasma concentrations of C1q, MBL and FB between the CM and Ctrl groups (Fig. 1b), suggesting that increased concentrations of C1q, FB and MBL in CSF is a localized phenomenon.

The concentrations of complement components C2, C3, C4 and C5 in plasma and CSF samples

We further examined the concentrations of C2, C3, C4 and C5 in the plasma and CSF samples. There were no statistical significances of the concentrations of these complement factors in both plasma and CSF samples between the two groups (Fig. 2a and b).

C3 activation in CSF and plasma in CM

The complement system activation is mediated through the CP, AP and LP pathways. Each pathway converges at the C3 convertase level resulting in C3 cleavage. To further assess whether the C3 activation is involved in CM, levels of C3 breakdown products in CSF and those in simultaneously collected blood plasma samples were evaluated by Western blot. C3 cleavage fragments iC3b was detected in CM group from both plasma and CSF samples (Fig. 3).

The concentrations of sC5b-9 in plasma and CSF samples

To determine the complement terminal pathway activation, we examined the concentrations of sC5b-9 in plasma and CSF samples in Ctrl and CM groups. There was no significant difference in plasma concentrations of sC5b-9 between the two groups. However, the CSF concentrations of sC5b-9 in CM group was significantly higher than that in the Ctrl group ($p = 0.0064$) (Fig. 4).

The concentrations of C4BP, FI and FH in plasma and CSF

The complement system is regulated by some key fluid regulators, such as C4BP, FI and FH. We next measured the concentrations of these factors in plasma and CSF samples. There were no significant differences in the plasma concentrations of C4BP, FI and FH expressed between Ctrl and CM groups (Fig. 5a). The concentrations of C4BP and FI in CSF were also similar in both Ctrl and CM groups (Fig. 5b). However, the CSF concentrations of FH increased significantly in CM group compared to the Ctrl group ($p = 0.0303$) (Fig. 5b).

The levels of IL-12 in the plasma and in CSF samples

We next investigated the levels of IL-12 because it may plays an important role in host defense in CM [23]. As

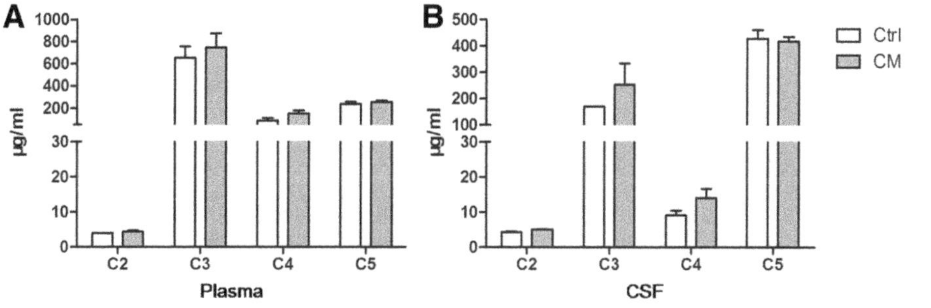

Fig. 2 The concentrations of C2, C3, C4 and C5 were detected in both plasma (**a**) and CSF (**b**) samples. There were no significant differences between the CM and Ctrl groups

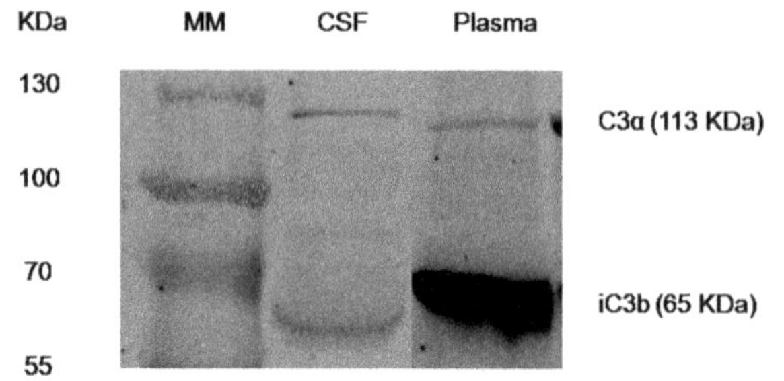

Fig. 3 C3 cleavage fragments were analyzed by western blot. Approximately 20 μl of CSF and 2 μl of plasma samples were subjected to SDS-PAG. The immunoreactive bands corresponding to C3α and iC3b are denoted. Prominent iC3b band was found in the CSF and plasma samples in CM patients. A representative is shown

shown in Fig. 6, though the plasma levels of IL-12 were similar between the Ctrl and CM groups, the CSF levels of IL-12 were significantly higher in CM group than that in Ctrl group ($p = 0.0121$) (Fig. 6).

Discussion

In this study, we showed elevated CSF concentrations of C1q, MBL, FB, sC5b-9 and FH in CM patients compared to that in the control group and the common complement pathway factors iC3b in both CSF and plasma samples of CM patients. Our data suggest that the increased CSF complement system activity might indicate its important roles in host defense and pathogenesis in CM.

Though the importance of the complement system to *C. neoformans* infection is well established, it is not clear how the complement system responds to pathogens in CM clinically. The brain may represent its own characteristics not like other organ when infected with *Cryptococcus*. There are few publications in this field. Our data demonstrated that complement components including the initiators of three complement pathways (C1q, FB and MBL), other complement factors (C2, C3, C4, C5) and regulators (FH, FI, C4BP) were present in CSF in CM. Moreover, CSF levels of C1q, MBL, and FB were significantly higher compared with that in control group. In this study, we showed C3 and the complement terminal pathways were activated in CSF during CM. Cleavage of C3 generates the key opsonins, C3b and iC3b for phagocytosis [24]. Activation of the complement terminal pathway results in releasing anaphylatoxins C5a, and formation of a membrane attack complex to lyse the target cells. Meanwhile, sC5b-9 as the final product of complement activation was significantly higher in CSF in CM group than that in the control group. Our results were similar with the report from Mook-Kanamori et.al [6], which demonstrated that CSF levels of C1q, MBL, FH and sC5b-9 were significantly elevated during pneumococcal and meningococcal meningitis. Thus our data suggest an important role of the complement system in host protection against CM as well. C1q, MBL and FB each separately initiates the classical, lectin and alternative pathway, and plays a key role in the innate immune system. C1q also take part in the clearance of apoptotic cells during inflammation resolution [25, 26]. Significantly elevated CSF levels of C1q, MBL and FB in CM patients may reflect all of the three pathway activations are involved in CM.

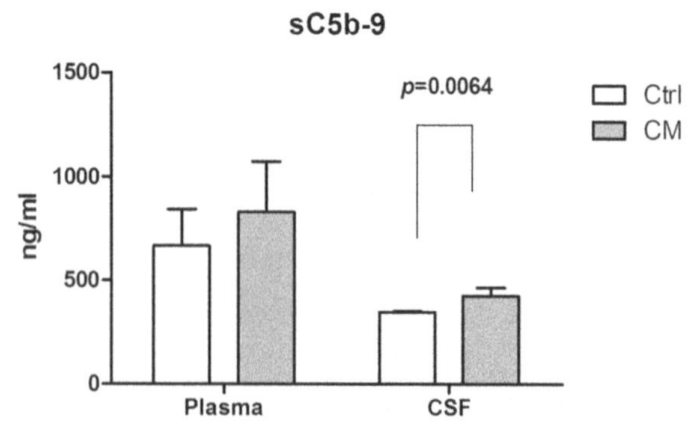

Fig. 4 The concentrations of sC5b-9 in plasma and CSF. The concentration of sC5b-9 in CSF increased significantly in CM group compared to the Ctrl group and the *p* value was 0.0064

The differences of complement components between the CM and Ctrl groups were only detected in CSF samples, not in the plasma samples. This indicates that local inflammatory responses impact significantly on activity of the complement system in CSF. The brain as a well-developed organ of CNS is shielded by the blood–brain-barrier (BBB) with tight junction formations. BBB is a structural and functional barrier formed by the microvascular endothelium, astrocytes and pericytes. The complement system has taken part in various developmental and regenerative processes, and is integrated with multiple biological systems and pathways in many researches [27]. We think that the elevated CSF complement factors of patients with CM have leaked from the plasma because the CSF complement levels of C1q, MBL and FB were significantly correlated with the total concentrations of CSF protein. It is well known that a non-specific increase in permeability of the blood-CSF barrier during meningitis results in a rise in CSF protein concentrations including all the plasma proteins [28]. However, complement factors can be synthesized locally in the CNS [29]. Astrocyte and glial cell are the main sources of complement in CNS [30, 31]. Previous study using Reibergram method demonstrates that C3 and C4 were synthesized locally during bacterial meningitis. Further studies using Reibergram are needed to determine whether intrathecal synthesis of complement factors is, at least in part, responsible for the increased levels of CSF complement factors in CM.

However, complement has been described as a double-edged sword since activation of the complement system

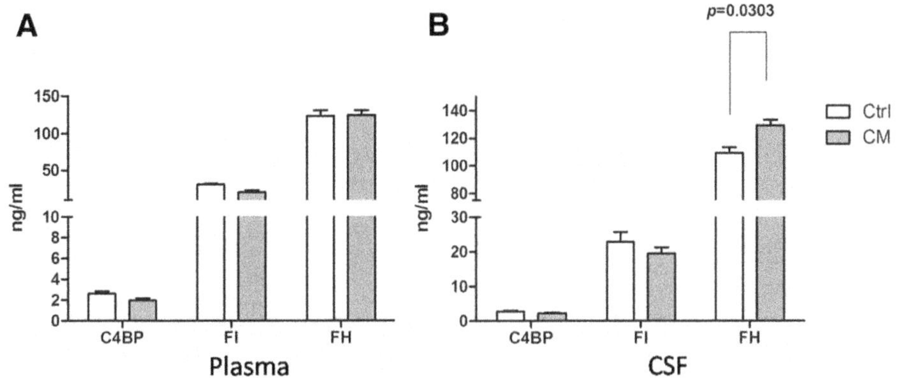

Fig. 5 The concentrations of C4BP, FI and FH in CSF and plasma. **a** There were no significant differences in plasma concentrations of C4BP, FI and FH between the two groups. **b** There were no significant differences in CSF concentrations of C4BP and FI between the two groups. However, CSF levels of FH in CSF was significantly higher in CM group than that in Ctrl group

significantly contributes to the pathogenesis of various acute and chronic inflammatory diseases [32]. Adequate regulation of the complement system is a central component of the system's ability to control unintended complement activation on host cells. The expression of regulator also can be detected in CSF, such as C4BP, FI, and FH. Their amounts are nearly the same in CSF and plasma. However, CSF FH concentrations were obviously higher in CM than that in the control group. FH regulates the AP both in the fluid phase and on cell surfaces. Expression of FH regulators indicates the balance also exits to control the degree of activation of complement. The role of the complement system activation in host defense and neuro-inflammation in CM is not fully understood. Elucidating which components of the complement system are important in both protective and inflammatory roles in CM to drive development of CM-specific immunotherapies.

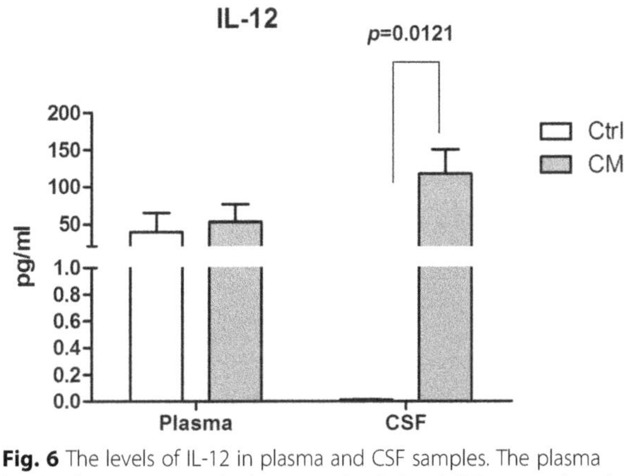

Fig. 6 The levels of IL-12 in plasma and CSF samples. The plasma levels of IL-12 were similar between the Ctrl and CM groups, but the CSF levels of IL-12 significantly increased compared to in CM group that in the Ctrl group

It is well known that a Th1-driven cell-mediated response is necessary for the control of *C. neoformans* infections. Beenhouwer and his colleagues found that the relative inherent susceptibilities of the mouse strains to *C. neoformans* were as follows: $IL\text{-}12^{-/-} > IL\text{-}6^{-/-} >$ C57BL/6 $>> IL\text{-}10^{-/-}$ [33]. In the present study, the CSF concentrations of IL-12 were significantly higher in CM group than that in Ctrl group. In mirror with other reports, our data indicated a protective role of IL-12 in CM. Exploring underlying mechanisms in regulation of IL-12 production and the cross talk with the complement system in CM would provide a new perspective for treatment of CM.

Conclusion

In conclusion, our data revealed the presence of the complement components and the complement activation in CSF in non-HIV patients with CM, and suggested an important role of complement factors C1q, MBL, FB, FH and sC5b-9 in the pathogenesis of CM. Further studies are warranted to confirm the pathophysiological role of these complement factors in CM and to stimulate the development of new therapeutic strategies for CM by directing treatment to specific pathways within the complement cascade.

Abbreviations

AP: Alternative pathway; BBB: Blood–brain-barrier; C1INH: C1 inhibitor; C4BP: C4 binding protein; CM: Cryptococcal meningitis; CNS: Central nervous system; CP: Classical pathway; CSF: Cerebrospinal fluid; Ctrl: Control patients; ELISA: Enzyme-linked immunosorbent assay; FB: Factor B; FH: Factor H; FI: Factor I; IL: Interleukin; LP: Lectin pathway; MBL: Mannose binding lectin; PVDF: Polyvinylidene difluoride; SDS-PAGE: Sodium dodecyl sulfate polyacrylamide gel electrophoresis; TBST: Tris-buffered saline

Acknowledgements

We thank Dr. Hua Hua Tong from the Ohio State University for helpful suggestions and criticism.

Funding
The study was supported by Shanghai Health and Family Planning Commission (award number 201440578).

Authors' contributions
LS, JZ performed the experiments. YW, MZ aided in the data analysis as well as drafted the manuscript. HZ, QC contributed reagents/material. QL conceived, designed, executed, evaluated the experiments and wrote the paper. All authors read and approved the final manuscript.

Competing interests
The authors declare that they have no competing interests.

Consent for publication
Not applicable.

Author details
[1]Department of Thoracic Intensive Care Units, Shanghai Pulmonary Hospital, Shanghai, China. [2]Department of Infectious Diseases, Huashan Hospital, Fudan University, Shanghai, China. [3]Central Laboratory, Huashan Hospital, Fudan University, Shanghai, China.

References
1. Sloan DJ, Parris V. Cryptococcal meningitis: epidemiology and therapeutic options. Clin Epidemiol. 2014;6:169–82.
2. Park BJ, Wannemuehler KA, Marston BJ, Govender N, Pappas PG, Chiller TM. Estimation of the current global burden of cryptococcal meningitis among persons living with HIV/AIDS. AIDS. 2009;23(4):525–30.
3. Fang W, Fa Z, Liao W. Epidemiology of Cryptococcus and cryptococcosis in China. Fungal Genet Biol. 2015;78:7–15.
4. Merle NS, Noe R, Halbwachs-Mecarelli L, Fremeaux-Bacchi V, Roumenina LT. Complement system part II: role in immunity. Front Immunol. 2015;6:257.
5. Rupprecht TA, Angele B, Klein M, Heesemann J, Pfister HW, Botto M, et al. Complement C1q and C3 are critical for the innate immune response to Streptococcus pneumoniae in the central nervous system. J Immunol. 2007;178(3):1861–9.
6. Mook-Kanamori BB, Brouwer MC, Geldhoff M, Ende A, van de Beek D. Cerebrospinal fluid complement activation in patients with pneumococcal and meningococcal meningitis. J Infect. 2014;68(6):542–7.
7. Woehrl B, Brouwer MC, Murr C, Heckenberg SG, Baas F, Pfister HW, et al. Complement component 5 contributes to poor disease outcome in humans and mice with pneumococcal meningitis. J Clin Invest. 2011;121(10):3943–53.
8. Goonetilleke UR, Scarborough M, Ward SA, Hussain S, Kadioglu A, Gordon SB. Death is associated with complement C3 depletion in cerebrospinal fluid of patients with pneumococcal meningitis. MBio. 2012;3(2):e00272–11.
9. Munshi MA, Rella A, Poeta MD. Fungal Infection of the CNS. In: García-Moncó JC, editor. London: CNS Infections; 2014. p.119–37.
10. Voelz K, May RC. Cryptococcal interactions with the host immune system. Eukaryot Cell. 2010;9(6):835–46.
11. Rhodes JC, Wicker LS, Urba WJ. Genetic control of susceptibility to Cryptococcus neoformans in mice. Infect Immun. 1980;29(2):494–9.
12. Diamond RD, May JE, Kane M, Frank MM, Bennett JE. The role of late complement components and the alternate complement pathway in experimental cryptococcosis. Proc Soc Exp Biol Med. 1973;144(1):312–5.
13. Rhodes JC. Contribution of complement component C5 to the pathogenesis of experimental murine cryptococcosis. Sabouraudia. 1985;23(3):225–34.
14. Macher AM, Bennett JE, Gadek JE, Frank MM. Complement depletion in cryptococcal sepsis. J Immunol. 1978;120(5):1686–90.
15. Truelsen K, Young T, Kozel TR. In vivo complement activation and binding of C3 to encapsulated Cryptococcus neoformans. Infect Immun. 1992;60(9):3937–9.
16. Diamond RD, May JE, Kane MA, Frank MM, Bennett JE. The role of the classical and alternate complement pathways in host defenses against Cryptococcus neoformans infection. J Immunol. 1974;112(6):2260 70.
17. Sun D, Zhang M, Liu G, Wu H, Zhu X, Zhou H, et al. Real-time imaging of interactions of neutrophils with Cryptococcus neoformans demonstrates a crucial role of complement C5a-C5aR signaling. Infect Immun. 2015;84(1): 216–29.
18. Kozel TR, Highlson B, Stratton CJ. Localization on encapsulated Cryptococcus neoformans of serum components opsonic for phagocytosis by macrophages and neutrophils. Infect Immun. 1984;43(2):574–9.
19. Kelly RM, Chen J, Yauch LE, Levitz SM. Opsonic requirements for dendritic cell-mediated responses to Cryptococcus neoformans. Infect Immun. 2005;73(1):592–8.
20. Ou XT, Wu JQ, Zhu LP, Guan M, Xu B, Hu XP, et al. Genotypes coding for mannose-binding lectin deficiency correlated with cryptococcal meningitis in HIV-uninfected Chinese patients. J Infect Dis. 2011;203(11):1686–91.
21. Perfect JR, Dismukes WE, Dromer F, Goldman DL, Graybill JR, Hamill RJ, et al. Clinical practice guidelines for the management of cryptococcal disease: 2010 update by the infectious diseases society of America. Clin Infect Dis. 2010;50(3):291–322.
22. De Pauw B, Walsh TJ, Donnelly JP, Stevens DA, Edwards JE, Calandra T, et al. Revised definitions of invasive fungal disease from the European Organization for Research and Treatment of Cancer/Invasive Fungal Infections Cooperative Group and the National Institute of Allergy and Infectious Diseases Mycoses Study Group (EORTC/MSG) Consensus Group. Clin Infect Dis. 2008;46(12):1813–21.
23. Decken K, Köhler G, Palmer-Lehmann K, Wunderlin A, Mattner F, Magram J, et al. Interleukin-12 is essential for a protective Th1 response in mice infected with Cryptococcus neoformans. Infect Immun. 1998;66(10):4994–5000.
24. Li Q, Li YX, Douthitt K, Stahl GL, Thurman JM, Tong HH. Role of the alternative and classical complement activation pathway in complement mediated killing against Streptococcus pneumoniae colony opacity variants during acute pneumococcal otitis media in mice. Microbes Infect. 2012; 14(14):1308–18.
25. Kouser L, Madhukaran SP, Shastri A, Saraon A, Ferluga J, Al-Mozaini M, et al. Emerging and novel functions of complement protein C1q. Front Immunol. 2015;6:317.
26. Fraser DA, Laust AK, Nelson EL, Tenner AJ. C1q differentially modulates phagocytosis and cytokine responses during ingestion of apoptotic cells by human monocytes, macrophages, and dendritic cells. J Immunol. 2009; 183(10):6175–85.
27. Ricklin D, Hajishengallis G, Yang K, Lambris JD. Complement: a key system for immune surveillance and homeostasis. Nat Immunol. 2010;11(9):785–97.
28. Davson H, Oldendorf WH. Symposium on membrane transport. Transport in the central nervous system. Proc R Soc Med. 1967;60(4):326–9.
29. Alawieh A, Elvington A, Tomlinson S. Complement in the homeostatic and ischemic brain. Front Immunol. 2015;6:417.
30. Lévi-Strauss M, Mallat M. Primary cultures of murine astrocytes produce C3 and factor B, two components of the alternative pathway of complement activation. J Immunol. 1987;139(7):2361–6.
31. Gasque P, Fontaine M, Morgan BP. Complement expression in human brain. Biosynthesis of terminal pathway components and regulators in human glial cells and cell lines. J Immunol. 1995;154(9):4726–33.
32. Charchaflieh J, Wei J, Labaze G, Hou YJ, Babarsh B, Stutz H, et al. The role of complement system in septic shock. Clin Dev Immunol. 2012;2012:407324.
33. Beenhouwer DO, Shapiro S, Feldmesser M, Casadevall A, Scharff MD. Both Th1 and Th2 cytokines affect the ability of monoclonal antibodies to protect mice against Cryptococcus neoformans. Infect Immun. 2001;69(10):6445–55.

7

Acute vision loss in post-partum period as presenting symptom of HIV-associated cryptococcal meningitis

Aniruddha More, Ravindra Kumar Garg*, Hardeep Singh Malhotra, Neeraj Kumar and Ravi Uniyal

Abstract

Background: Acute vision loss in the post-partum period can occur due to many reasons. Eclampsia, posterior reversible encephalopathy syndrome (PRES), pituitary apoplexy, and central serous retinopathy are some of the important causes. Cryptococcal meningitis as a cause of acute vision loss in the post-partum period has not been mentioned in literature.

Case presentation: A 25-year-old female presented to us with acute bilateral complete vision loss in the post-partum period. Her serum was tested positive for HIV antibodies. Cerebrospinal fluid (CSF) examination revealed cryptococcal meningitis. She was started on amphotericin B, antiretroviral drugs, and steroids. Though symptoms of meningitis resolved after treatment no significant improvement in vision was observed at 3 months.

Conclusions: Cryptococcal meningitis may be considered as one of the causes of acute vision loss in pregnant/post-partum females with human immunodeficiency virus (HIV) positivity.

Keywords: Acquired immune deficiency syndrome, Human immunodeficiency virus, Meningitis, Optic nerve

Background

Approximately, 36.7 million people globally were suffering from HIV infection at end of 2015 [1]. About 17.4 million women were suffering from HIV infection worldwide in 2014 [2]. HIV infection in pregnancy has become the most common complication of pregnancy in some developing countries. In pregnancy immune function is suppressed in HIV infected as well as non-infected subjects [3]. There is a reduction in immunoglobulin, reduced complement levels and a significant decrease in cell-mediated immunity during pregnancy [3]. This leads to increased susceptibility of pregnant females to opportunistic infections like tuberculosis and cryptococcal meningitis. Cryptococcal disease is very uncommonly seen in HIV infected pregnant females and to date only three cases of HIV infection with cryptococcal meningitis have been reported during the peripartum period [4]. Symptoms of cryptococcal meningitis include fever, headache, nausea/vomiting, altered sensorium, and multiple cranial nerve palsies. Vision loss is seen in 33–47 % of patients [5]. Seven percent of HIV infected individuals suffer from cryptococcal meningitis in the course of their illness out of which only 1.9 % have cryptococcal meningitis as the presenting symptom [5, 6]. Complete bilateral vision loss as presenting symptom of HIV related cryptococcal meningitis is extremely rare [7]. Similar presentations in post-partum female, as it was in our case, are unique and high index of suspicion is necessary for accurate diagnosis.

* Correspondence: garg50@yahoo.com
Department of Neurology, King George Medical University, Lucknow PIN-226003, Uttar Pradesh, India

Case presentation

A 25- year-old previously healthy pregnant female in 36th week of her gestation presented in labour to the department of Obstetrics & Gynecology of our hospital. Before admission she was having mild to moderate headache of 10 days duration which was associated with mild fever with intermittent high grade spikes which used to subside on administration of antipyretic medications.

Her serum tested positive, by ELISA, for antibodies towards HIV. She delivered a still-born baby vaginally. She was apparently asymptomatic for 2 days, besides fever and headache which were relieved by antipyretics and analgesics. On the 3rd day post-partum day, she woke up in the morning realizing that she was not able to see from both eyes; the loss of vision was painless and symmetrical. She was transferred to the department of Neurology unit of our hospital for further evaluation. On clinical examination, her vitals and level of consciousness were normal. Her visual acuity was significantly reduced and she could only perceive light in both eyes. Her pupils were completely dilated and not reacting to light. Fundus examination revealed bilateral edematous optic discs suggestive of papillitis. Other cranial nerves were normal on examination. Motor and sensory system examination were normal. Plantar reflex was bilaterally flexor. She had neck stiffness and Kerning's sign was positive. Urgently a CT scan of her head was done which showed no significant abnormality and then her CSF examination was done based on her clinical signs. Her CSF opening pressure was mildly elevated (200cms of H_2O). CSF examination showed mild pleocytosis (35 cells/mm^3) with lymphocytic predominance, mildly elevated proteins (76.5 mg%) and low sugars (32.7 mg% with corresponding blood glucose of 117 mg%). Her CSF was tested positive for Cryptococcus by India ink staining (Fig. 1). The CSF showed a titre of 1:100 for cryptococcal antigen by latex agglutination method. Since she was diagnosed with cryptococcal meningitis she was categorized as having stage 4 disease according to WHO clinical staging for HIV/AIDS. All other hematological and biochemical parameters were within normal limits. Her CD4 counts were done which turned out to be 166 cells/mm^3. The plasma HIV-RNA levels were not performed in this case. As per National AIDS Control Guidelines of India prior HIV-RNA levels assessment, before starting antiretroviral drugs, is not mandatory. Her MRI was planned to evaluate the cause of her blindness which showed signal intensity changes in bilateral optic nerve and (cryptococcoma/cryptococcal) infiltration in bilateral ganglio-capsular region (soap-bubble appearance) (Fig. 2). She was initiated on amphotericin-B 0.7 mg/kg/day IV once daily (slow infusion) and intravenous methylprednisolone 1 gm IV once daily (for 5 days), and an antiretroviral regimen consisting of zidovudine (300 mg once daily), lamivudine (150 mg once daily), and nevirapine (200 mg once daily) was planned. She received amphotericin B for 21 days after which she was started on tablet fluconazole 400 mg per day which was continued for 8 weeks. Antiretroviral medications were started after completion of intravenous antifungal medications. Her headache improved with treatment and she became afebrile. Repeat CSF examination was negative for Cryptococci by India ink staining. Though she showed significant improvement in meningitic symptoms, her vision did not show any significant improvement even at end of 3 months of her illness.

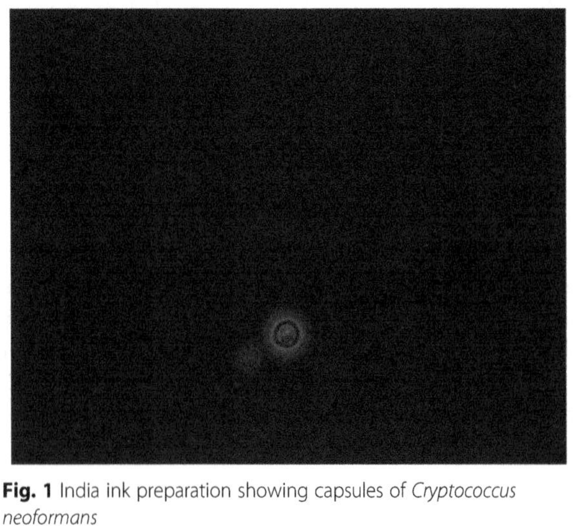

Fig. 1 India ink preparation showing capsules of *Cryptococcus neoformans*

Discussion

Acute vision loss in the post-partum period is reported due to severe preeclampsia/eclampsia (in which vision loss could be due to exudative retinal detachment, hypertensive retinopathy and cortical blindness) [8], PRES which can cause reversible acute vision loss [9], pituitary apoplexy [10], posterior ischemic optic neuropathy [11], anterior ischemic optic neuropathy [12], cortical venous sinus thrombosis [13], and central serous retinopathy [14]. Cryptococcal meningitis as a cause of acute vision loss in the post-partum period has not yet been reported in literature.

Vision loss in HIV infected individuals can be due to infectious and non-infectious causes [15–17]. HIV retinopathy is the most common non-infectious ocular complication. Amongst infectious causes cytomegalovirus retinitis is considered as the most common ocular infection. Neuro-ophthalmic lesions affected 6 % of individuals of acquired immunodeficiency states of which most common cause was cryptococcal meningitis. Approximately 25 to 50 % patients with cryptococcal meningitis demonstrate a neuro-ophthalmic complication. In a cross-sectional analysis looking at the ophthalmic complications in the pre-HAART (Highly Active Anti-Retroviral Therapy) and HAART period, it has been suggested that despite of an advancement in terms of treatment the difference between the two treatment protocols has not been significant (pre-HAART (41.67 %) versus HAART (38 %). Of significance was the fact that the odds of development of ophthalmic

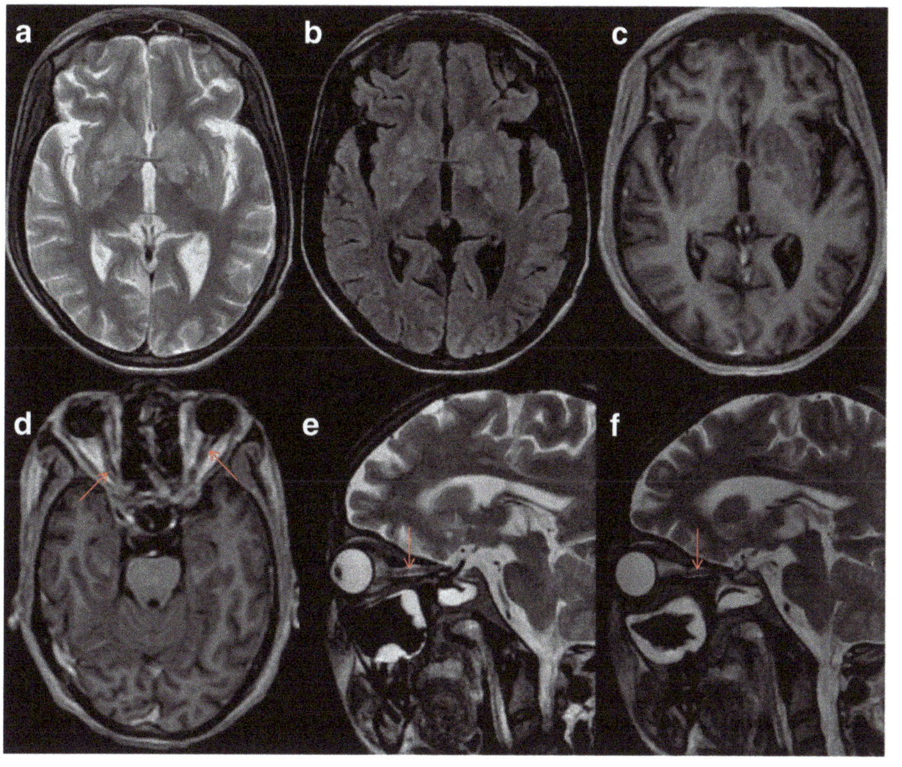

Fig. 2 MRI of the brain depicts hyperintense signal intensity changes in the basal ganglia on axial T2-weighted (**a**) and FLAIR (**b**) sequences. There is no suggestion of contrast uptake in the basal ganglia (**c**) while both optic nerves demonstrate enhancement (**d**) on SPGR-GAD sequence. T2-weighted para-sagittal orbital sections show hyperintensity in the right (**e**) and the left (**f**) optic nerves (arrows)

complications with a CD4 count of >200 cells/μL were significantly higher (4.87) during the HAART period [17]. Since most patients with ophthalmic complications have been noted to present in WHO stage 3 and 4, it has been recommended that regular ophthalmic assessments are done in patients with HIV positivity.

Cryptococcal meningitis is one of potentially fatal opportunistic infection seen in HIV infected individuals. The causative agent is *Cryptococcus neoformans*, an encapsulated fungus commonly isolated from pigeon droppings. Humans are infected by inhalation of organism [18]. Human to human transmission is yet to be documented [19]. Signs and symptoms of cryptococcal meningitis include headache (80–92 %), meningeal signs (50–80 %), nausea/vomiting (40–80 %), fever (36–67 %), cranial nerve palsies (28–60 %), vision disturbances (33–47 %), confusion/somnolence (33–40 %), ataxia/gait disturbance (26–40 %), papilledema (28–33 %), seizures (13–15 %) [5].

Vision loss in cryptococcal meningitis can be rapid (<3 days) occurring as rapidly as 12 h or can occur slowly (>3 days) over weeks to months [20]. Possible mechanisms of rapid visual loss include direct invasion of optic nerve by Cryptococcus, optic neuritis, and opto-chiasmatic arachnoiditis while a possible mechanism for slow vision loss has been attributed to raised intracranial pressure [20]. Factors predicting vision loss are presence of papilledema, high CSF opening pressure, and a positive India ink preparation. In cases with acute vision loss despite of giving antifungals and steroids no substantial improvement in vision is expected and these cases tend to have a poor prognosis for visual recovery. In cases with slow visual loss therapeutic measures to reduce intracranial pressure like shunting or optic nerve sheath fenestration have been shown to halt vision loss and shown improvement in some cases [20].

Vision loss in our patient was most probably due to infiltration of optic nerve by Cryptococcus causing optic neuritis and acute vision loss. This was supported by fact that her MRI showed enhancement of both optic nerves and presence of papillitis on ophthalmoscopy with cryptococcal infiltration in both ganglio-capsular regions. This also explains her poor recovery of vision despite of receiving steroids as noted in previous studies (Table 1). The general belief that pregnancy is a state of immune suppression may not hold true in all patients. Pregnancy, indeed, is a state of an altered immune status which may respond to different stimuli variably. Thus, in the background of pregnancy and a HIV positive state, this rare manifestation of Cryptococcus appears to have evolved [21].

Table 1 A review of published cases of vision loss in Cryptococcal meningitis (Cases, reported after year 2000 and those who had a MRI done, were included)

Reference	HIV status	Summary of case	MRI	Suggested cause of vision loss	Outcome
Ng et al. [22]	Positive	A 39-year-old Chinese man presented with bitemporal headache, giddiness and vomiting over a period of 2 days. There was no Cryptococcus detected by Indian ink examination of the CSF but CSF culture grew Cryptococcus neoformans. The patient was treated with amphotericin, and then to fluconazole.	Normal	increased intracranial pressure	irreversible blindness in both eyes
	Positive	A 36-year-old Chinese man presented with subacute onset of severe headache and confusional state. CSF microscopy with Indian ink examination showed Cryptococcus. Eight days after starting IV amphotericin, he complained of bilateral blurring of vision and had a seizure. A repeat lumbar puncture showed raised opening CSF pressure of more than 40 cm and 20 mL of CSF was withdrawn. During follow up, concentric diminution of visual field in both eyes was recorded. A lumbo-peritoneal shunt was done.	CT was normal	Increased intracranial pressure	Normal vision
Mohan et al. [23]	Positive	A 41-year-old male with a history of cryptococcal meningitis admitted with severe headache. On the 6th day, He had complete loss of hearing, vision loss as well as bilateral facial palsy and bilateral sixth nerve palsy. Bilateral papilledema was seen. CSF opening pressure was 460 mm H2O. Amphotericin and Flucytosine were given. Repeated lumbar punctures were done but pressure remained over 500 mm H2O. Ommaya reservoir placed. There was dramatic clinical improvement of the patient.	Hydrocephalus	Increased intracranial pressure	Regained his vision partially
Hong et al. [7]	Positive	A 58-year-old man presented with acute vision loss. Patient had normal CSF opening pressure and fundus. He received antiretroviral and antifungal agents.	Normal	Possibly, direct fungal infiltration of the optic nerve, optic chiasm, or optic tracts	Vision improved
Milman et al. [24]	Positive	25-year-old patient developed headaches, seizures, altered mental status, and visual loss. Lumbar puncture showed markedly increased opening CSF pressure; cryptococcal organisms were identified by India ink preparation and in culture. Despite treatment with amphotericin and fluconazole, visual loss progressed.	leptomeningeal and optic nerve enhancement without hydrocephalus	increased intracranial pressure	Improved with bilateral optic nerve sheath fenestration.

Table 1 A review of published cases of vision loss in Cryptococcal meningitis (Cases, reported after year 2000 and those who had a MRI done, were included) *(Continued)*

Muslikhan et al. [25]	Negative	A 17-year-old boy presented with blurring of vision in both eyes and diplopia for 3 weeks. Extraocular muscles movement showed bilateral sixth nerve palsies. Discs were hyperaemic and slightly elevated. Lumbar puncture revealed high opening pressure >300 mmH(2)O. CSF showed *Cryptococcus neoformans*. IV amphotericin and fluconazole were given.	CT scan of the brain was normal	high intracranial pressure	His vision was improved to 6/6 in both eyes with recovery of peripheral visual field.
De Socio et al. [26]	Positive	A 32-year-old man with disseminated Cryptococcosis was being treated with antiretroviral therapy. On day 7 he had a unilateral vision loss.	retrobulbar neuritis	IRIS leading to optic nerve neuritis following anti-retroviral therapy	At 3 months, vision was normal After starting ART and IV methyl-prednisolone
Duggan and Walls [27]	Positive	A 39-year-old man with AIDS presented with recent onset of headache, dizziness, and syncope. CSF showed *C neoformans*. Amphotericin and flucytosine were started. On day 2, the patient had several episodes of complete loss of vision bilaterally. Drainage of CSF to decrease ICP resulted in the immediate return of vision. External ventricular drain was placed and later optic nerve sheath fenestration.	optic nerve edema or neuritis	high intracranial pressure	permanent vision loss
	Positive	A 39-year-old African female with AIDS presented with headache, neck pain, and altered mental status of 3 days. CSF showed *C neoformans*. On hospital day 2, the patient complained of sudden complete loss of vision bilaterally. Retinal microvasculopathy was noted.	Normal	Retinal microvasculopathy	Patient died
Espino Barros Palau et al. [28]	Out of three cases one was HIV positive	A 46-year-old male had bilateral optic atrophy. He had been well until 3 months prior when he experienced vision loss, headache, nausea, and fever.	Normal	Intracranial hypertension	serial lumbar drain
		A 43-year-old female presented with 3 weeks of headache, horizontal diplopia, and bilateral vision loss. Patient had renal transplantation requiring immunosuppression in 2005. CSF opening pressure was markedly elevated. Amphotericin B and flucytosine were initiated.	Diffuse leptomeningeal enhancement and punctate areas of enhancement in the pons and basal ganglia.		
		A 35-year-old male presented with 1 month of bilateral progressive vision loss. Ophthalmoscopy showed peripapillary subretinal fluid extending into the macula bilaterally. Both optic discs had edema. CSF opening pressure was elevated. Amphotericin B and flucytosine were started.	Multiple T2-hyperintense lesions throughout the cerebral hemispheres, brainstem, and cerebellum as well as with leptomeningeal enhancement.		

Table 1 A review of published cases of vision loss in Cryptococcal meningitis (Cases, reported after year 2000 and those who had a MRI done, were included) *(Continued)*

Portelinha et al. [29]	Negative	A 52-year-old woman with headaches, vomiting and fatigue for 3 weeks. She was diagnosed with cryptococcal meningitis and treated with antifungal therapy. She also had decreased vision in the left eye, bilateral sixth nerve palsy and papilloedema. A ventriculo-peritoneal shunt was placed and methylprednisolone was started.	Signs of intracranial hypertension as well as multiple parenchymal lesions and optic nerve sheath enhancement.	high intracranial pressure and optic nerve fungal infiltration	In spite of the control of intracranial pressure there was a decrease in vision in the right eye and deterioration of visual fields.
Ghatalia et al. [30]	Positive	A 34 year old man of vision loss in a patient with Cryptococcal meningitis and normal ICP.	Abnormal circumferential enhancement within the bilateral optic nerve sheaths.	IRIS leading to optic nerve neuritis	Vision improved with corticosteroids
Merkler et al. [31]	Negative	A 38-year-old woman presented with bilateral vision loss. Empiric steroids resulted in improvement in visual acuity, while tapering steroids, she had visual loss again.	Multiple areas of ill-defined enhancement in the optic chiasm and tracts.	Invasion of the optic apparatus by *Cryptococcus neoformans*	One year later, symptom free.

Conclusions

Cryptococcal meningitis may be considered as one of causes of acute vision loss in HIV-infected pregnant females with suggestive symptoms; needless to say that a high index of suspicion should be kept to diagnose the condition. Though prognosis of visual recovery is poor in cases of acute vision loss, early therapeutic measures to relieve intracranial pressure may potentially halt the progression while some recovery may be observed in cases with slowly progressive vision loss.

Abbreviations

AIDS: Acquired immune deficiency syndrome; ART: Antiretroviral therapy; CSF: Cerebrospinal fluid; CT: Computed tomography; HAART: Highly Active Anti-Retroviral Therapy; HIV: Human immunodeficiency virus; ICP: Intracranial pressure; IRIS: Immune Reconstitution Inflammatory Syndrome; IV: Intravenous; MRI: Magnetic Resonance Imaging; PRES: Posterior reversible encephalopathy syndrome

Acknowledgement

None.

Funding

Not applicable.

Authors' contributions

AM Case evaluation, contributing in work up of the patient and writing the manuscript. RKG Case evaluation, contributing in work up of the patient and writing the manuscript. HSM Review of literature and writing the manuscript. NK Review of literature and writing the manuscript. RU Case evaluation, contributing in work up of the patient and writing the manuscript. All authors read and approved the final manuscript.

Competing interests

On behalf of all authors, the corresponding author states that there is no conflict of interest.

Consent for publication

Written informed consent was obtained from the patient/legal guardian.

References

1. Unaids.org. Fact sheet 2016 | UNAIDS [Internet]; 2016. Available from: http://www.unaids.org/en/resources/fact-sheet. Cited 19 Jun 2016.
2. World Health Organization. Number of women living with HIV [Internet]; 2016. Available from: http://www.who.int/gho/hiv/epidemic_status/cases_adults_women_children/en/. Cited 19 Jun 2016.
3. Minkoff H. Pregnancy and HIV infection. In: Minkoff H, DeHovitz JA, Duerr A, editors. HIV infection in women. New York: Raven; 1995. p. 173–88.
4. Nayak S, Talwani R, Gilliam B, Taylor G, Ghosh M. Cryptococcal Meningitis in an HIV-Positive Pregnant Woman. J Int Assoc Physicians AIDS Care (Chic). 2011;10:79–82.
5. Giberson TP, Kalyan-Raman K. Cryptococcal meningitis: initial presentation of acquired immunodeficiency syndrome. Ann Emerg Med. 1987;16:802–4.
6. Johnston SR, Corbett EL, Foster O, Ash S, Cohen J. Raised intracranial pressure and visual complications in AIDS patients with cryptococcal meningitis. J Infect. 1992;24:185–9.
7. Hong YJ, Jung S, Kim JY, Kwon SB, Song KB, Hwang SH, Min YK, Kwon KH, Lee BC. Complete Binocular Blindness as the First Manifestation of HIV-Related Cryptococcal Meningitis. J Clin Neurol. 2007;3:212–4.
8. Waziri-Erameh MJ, Omoti AE, Edema OT. Bilateral total loss of vision following eclampsia—a case report. Afr J Reprod Health. 2003;7:106–8.
9. Lee VH, Wijdicks EF, Manno EM, Rabinstein AA. Clinical spectrum of reversible posterior leukoencephalopathy syndrome. Arch Neurol. 2008;65:205–10.
10. Boellis A, di Napoli A, Romano A, Bozzao A. Pituitary apoplexy: an update on clinical and imaging features. Insights Imaging. 2014;5:753–62.
11. Rishi K, Puri M. Posterior Ischaemic Optic Neuropathy Following Vaginal Delivery. Webmed Central Ophthalmol. 2012;3:WMC003307. doi:10.9754/journal.wmc.2012.003307.
12. Giridhar P, Freedman K. Nonarteritic Anterior Ischemic Optic Neuropathy in a 35-Year-Old Postpartum Woman With Recent Preeclampsia. JAMA Ophthalmol. 2013;131:542–4.
13. Femi OL, Mohammed H, Musa BM, Ibrahim DA, Gwaram BA, Dutse AI. Puerperal superior sagittal sinus thrombosis and pulmonary embolism: A case report and review of literature. J Basic Clin Reprod Sci. 2014;3:64–7. Downloaded from: http://www.jbcrs.org/article.asp?issn=2278-960X;year=2014;volume=3;issue=1;spage=64;epage=67;aulast=Femi. Assessed on 29 Jun 2016.
14. Gass JD. Central serous chorioretinopathy and white subretinal exudation during pregnancy. Arch Ophthalmol. 1991;109:677–81.
15. Jabs DA. Ocular manifestations of HIV infection. Trans Am Ophthalmol Soc. 1995;93:623–83.
16. Martin-Odoom A, Bonney EY, Opoku DK. Ocular complications in HIV positive patients on antiretroviral therapy in Ghana. BMC Ophthalmol. 2016;16:134.
17. Agarwal A, Singh R, Sharma A, Gupta V, Dogra MR. Ocular Manifestations in Patients with Human Immunodeficiency Virus Infection in the Pre-HAART Versus the HAART Era in the North Indian Population. Ocul Immunol Inflamm. 2016;24:1–9. [Epub ahead of print] http://dx.doi.org/10.3109/09273948.2015.1133837.
18. Sabetta JR, Andriole VT. Cryptococcal infections of the central nervous system. Med Clin North Am. 1985;69:333–44.
19. Braude AI, Davis CE, Fierer J, editors. Infectious Diseases and Medical Microbiology. Philadelphia: WB Saunders Company; 1986. p. 564–70.
20. Rex JH, Larsen RA, Dismukes WE, Cloud GA, Bennett JE. Catastrophic visual loss due to Cryptococcus neoformans meningitis. Medicine (Baltimore). 1993;72:207–24.
21. Mor G, Cardenas I. The immune system in pregnancy: a unique complexity. Am J Reprod Immunol. 2010;63:425–33.
22. Ng CW, Lam MS, Paton NI. Cryptococcal meningitis resulting in irreversible visual impairment in AIDS patients—a report of two cases. Singap Med J. 2000;41:80–2.
23. Mohan S, Ahmed SI, Alao OA, Schliep TC. A case of AIDS associated cryptococcal meningitis with multiple cranial nerve neuropathies. Clin Neurol Neurosurg. 2006;108:610–3.
24. Milman T, Mirani N, Turbin RE. Optic nerve sheath fenestration in cryptococcal meningitis. Clin Ophthalmol. 2008;2:637–9.
25. Muslikhan Y, Hitam WH, Ishak SR, Mohtar I, Takaran J. Cryptococcus meningitis in an immunocompetent teenage boy presented early with diplopia. Int J Ophthalmol. 2010;3:92–4.
26. De Socio GV, Bernini L, Menduno P, Pitzurra L, Leone F, Baldelli F. Monolateral visual loss due to cryptococcal meningitis. J Int Assoc Physicians AIDS Care (Chic). 2011;10:76–8.
27. Duggan J, Walls HM. Ocular complications of cryptococcal meningitis in patients with HIV: report of two cases and review of the literature. J Int Assoc Physicians AIDS Care (Chic). 2012;11:283–8.
28. Espino Barros Palau A, Morgan ML, Foroozan R, Lee AG. Neuro-ophthalmic presentations and treatment of Cryptococcal meningitis-related increased intracranial pressure. Can J Ophthalmol. 2014;49(5):473–7. doi:10.1016/j.jcjo.2014.06.012
29. Portelinha J, Passarinho MP, Almeida AC, Costa JM. Bilateral optic neuropathy associated with cryptococcal meningitis in an immunocompetent patient. BMJ Case Rep. 2014;2014. doi:10.1136/bcr-2013-203451
30. Ghatalia PA, Vick A, Vattoth S, Roberson GH, Pappas PG. Reversible blindness in cryptococcal meningitis with normal intracranial pressure: case report and review of the literature. Clin Infect Dis. 2014;59:310–3.
31. Merkler AE, Gaines N, Baradaran H, Schuetz AN, Lavi E, Simpson SA, Dinkin MJ. Direct Invasion of the Optic Nerves, Chiasm, and Tracts by Cryptococcus neoformans in an Immunocompetent Host. Neurohospitalist. 2015;5:217–22.

8

Comparison of clinical features and prognostic factors in HIV-negative adults with cryptococcal meningitis and tuberculous meningitis

Junyan Qu, Taoyou Zhou, Cejun Zhong, Rong Deng and Xiaoju Lü*

Abstract

Background: The incidence of cryptococcal meningitis (CM) and tuberculous meningitis (TBM) have gradually increased in recent years. These two types of meningitis are easily misdiagnosed which leads to a poor prognosis. In this study we compared differences of clinical features and prognostic factors in non-HIV adults with CM and TBM.

Methods: We retrospectively reviewed the medical records of CM and TBM patients from January 2008 to December 2015 in our university hospital in China. The data included demographic characteristics, laboratory results, imaging findings, clinical outcomes.

Results: A total of 126 CM and 105 TBM patients were included. CM patients were more likely to present with headache, abnormal vision and hearing, and they might be less prone to fever and cough than TBM patients ($P < 0.05$). Higher percentage of CM patients presented with cerebral ischemia/infarction and demyelination in brain MRI than TBM patients ($P < 0.05$). CM patients had lower counts of WBC in CSF, lower total protein in CSF and serum CD4/CD8 ratio than TBM patients ($P < 0.05$). After three months of treatment, CM group have worse outcome than TBM group ($P < 0.05$). Multivariate analysis showed that age more than 60y (OR = 4.981, 95% CI: 1.955–12.692, $P = 0.001$), altered mentation (OR = 5.054, 95% CI: 1.592–16.046, $P = 0.006$), CD4/CD8 ratios < 1 (OR = 8.782, 95% CI: 2.436–31.661, $P = 0.001$) and CSF CrAg ≥ 1:1024 (OR = 4.853, 95% CI: 1.377–17.098, $P = 0.014$) were independent risk factors for poor prognosis for CM patients. For TBM patients, hydrocephalus (OR = 7.290, 95% CI: 1.630–32.606, $P = 0.009$) and no less than three underlying diseases (OR = 6.899, 95% CI: 1.766–26.949, $P = 0.005$) were independent risk factors, headache was a protective factor of prognosis.

Conclusions: Our study provided some helpful clues in the differential diagnosis of non-HIV patients with CM or TBM and identified some risk factors for the poor prognosis of these two meningitis which could help to improve the treatment outcome. Further studies are worth to be done.

Keywords: Cryptococcal meningitis, Tuberculous meningitis, Clinical features, Prognostic factors, HIV negative

* Correspondence: lvxj33966@126.com
Center of Infectious Disease, West China Hospital, Sichuan University, 37 Guoxue Lane, Chengdu 610041, China

Background

Many organisms such as *meningococcus*, *Mycobacterium tuberculosis* and *Cryptococcus neoformans* can result in meningitis. With increasing use of immune suppressive medication use in rheumatologic conditions, oncology, and organ transplantation, the incidence of Cryptococcal meningitis (CM) and tuberculous meningitis (TBM) are rising [1, 2].

CM and TBM are the two most common types of chronic infectious meningitis, especially in developing countries, and may have similar clinical manifestations and cerebrospinal fluid (CSF) findings [3, 4]. Although mortality has decreased significantly in recent years, with the advent of new antimicrobial drugs, diagnostic techniques and treatment strategies, it remains high [3, 5–7]. CM and TBM are easily misdiagnosed due to vague clinical syndromes associated with these conditions [3, 6]. Delay of diagnosis and treatment are directly related to a poor prognosis [3, 8]. Early diagnosis CM and TBM, especially TBM, remain challenges for clinicians.

CM and TBM are common in human immunodeficiency virus (HIV) infected patients, but they are also seen in patients with other forms of immunosuppression and apparently immunocompetent individuals [9]. Some studies have sought to identify clinical features in order to distinguish TBM from CM in human HIV infected patients [10, 11]. Data on how to identify CM and TBM according to clinical profiles in HIV negative patients are scarce. In this retrospective study, we aimed to compare the demographic features, clinical presentations, laboratory data, radiographic findings, therapeutic outcomes and prognostic factors of HIV negative TBM and CM patients who were admitted to a university hospital from 2008 to 2015 in China.

Methods

Study population

The retrospective study was conducted between January 2008 and December 2015, in West China Hospital, Sichuan University, China (a 4,300-bed academic tertiary care hospital). Patients aged 14 years or older with confirmed diagnosis of CM or clinical or confirmed diagnosis of TBM were included. Exclusion criteria were age under 14 years, HIV positive with infected, pregnant mothers, CM combined with TBM, and cases lacking follow-up for anti-tuberculosis or anti-fungal treatment.

The diagnosis of CM and TBM were made by clinical and laboratory findings. Symptoms and signs of meningitis including one or more of the following: headache, vomiting, fever, neck stiffness, convulsions, focal neurological deficits, altered mentation. Laboratory assessments for CM included CSF culture, CSF India ink testing, and CSF cryptococcal antigen testing (CrAg). Patients with TBM included definite TBM and clinical diagnosis of TBM. The diagnostic criteria of definite TBM was clinical findings plus one or more of the following: acid-fast bacilli seen in the CSF, *M. tuberculosis* cultured from the CSF, or a CSF positive commercial nucleic acid amplification test. The clinical diagnosis of TBM based on the clinical algorithm [12], which modified according to Marais' definitions [13]. All enrolled patients were divided into CM and TBM groups.

Altered mentation in CM and TBM refers to general changes in brain function, such as confusion, amnesia, loss of alertness, loss of orientation, defects in judgment and unusual behavior. Which were confirmed by psychiatrists.

Laboratory studies

Laboratory tests such as complete blood counts, blood biochemistry, interferon gamma release assays (IGRAs), peripheral blood T lymphocyte subset measurements and HIV test were done at the department of laboratory medicine of our hospital. Lumbar puncture (LP) and tuberculin skin test (TST) of suspected CM or TBM cases were performed before initial treatment. CSF was sent for WBC, glucose, protein, chloride, India ink stain, CSF cryptococcal antigen titers, TB smear, TB PCR, fungal and *M. tuberculosis* cultures. These tests were done at the discretion of the treating physicians. Fluorescence quantitative PCR was used to detect TB DNA in CSF. The rapid liquid culture mediums were used to detect *M. Tuberculosis*. Fungal culture of CSF was performed on Sabouraud dextrose agar (SDA) and incubated at 30°C to obtain cryptococcus isolates. The CSF cryptococcal antigen titers were determined by Latex Cryptococcal Antigen Detection System (Immuno-Mycologics, Inc., Norman, USA). The test utilizes latex particles coated with anti-cryptococcal antibody, which will reacts with the cryptococcal capsular polysaccharide antigen causing a visible agglutination. Brain magnetic resonance imaging (MRI) or computed tomography (CT) examinations and chest CT were performed at the discretion of the physicians.

Treatment strategies

All the patients received treatments after they got the diagnoses. Time of diagnosis was the time from onset of symptoms to treatment. HIV negative CM patients were treated with amphotericin B (0.7–1 mg/kg/d), 5-flucytosine (100 mg/kg/d) with or without fluconazole (800 mg/day)/voriconazole (loading dose, 6mg/kg/12h, maintenance dose, 4mg/kg/12h) for 6–12 weeks of induction therapy, and then fluconazole (400 mg/day) for 8 weeks of consolidation therapy, fluconazole (200 mg/day) for more than 6 months of maintenance therapy according to the guidelines for the management of cryptococcal disease and our experiences [5, 14]. Only three patients with CM received voriconazole. Because amphotericin B was contraindicated in some patients with kidney disease or renal inadequacy emerged after use of amphotericin B in another patient. Continuous lumbar drainage subarachnoid were applied to the CM patients with persistent high intracranial pressure. The treatment regimen for TBM patients who had not been treated with chemotherapy consisted of three months of isoniazide (INH), rifampin (RIF), pyrazinamide (PZA), and streptomycin (SM)/ethambutol (EMB), followed by INH and RIF [15, 16]. The total treatment course was at least 12 month. Second-line treatment regimens were given after failure to first-line TB chemotherapy according to the guideline and patients' situation [15, 16].

Data collection

We retrospectively reviewed the medical records of patients involved in this study. We obtained demographic characteristics, underlying diseases, use of steroids, symptoms and signs on admission, duration of initial symptoms to diagnosis or treatment, laboratory data, brain MRI /CT findings and clinical outcomes. The clinical outcomes were evaluated after three-month of treatment. Risk factors for the prediction of poor of HIV negative CM and TBM patients were also evaluated. All data were verified by two authors independently.

Ethical considerations

The study was approved by the Ethics Committee of West China Hospital, Sichuan University, which waived the need for informed consent because all the data used in this study were routinely obtained and no additional procedures were carried out.

Statistical analysis

Statistical analyses were performed using SPSS version 17.0 software package (SPSS Inc., Chicago, USA). The Shapiro-Wilk normality test was used for testing normality for all quantitative variables. Continuous variables were presented as mean ± standard deviation or median with interquartile ranges (IQR). Signifcance testing was carried out using Student's *t* test for normally distributed data and Mann-Whitney *U* test for non-normal data. Chi-square test or Fisher exact test was used for categorical variables. Risk factors for three-month treatment outcomes of CM or TBM were identified using a logistic regression model. All variables were initially tested by univariate analysis and those with a $P < 0.05$ were entered stepwise into multivariate analysis by using the forward conditional method. Then the regression equations for predicting the probability of poor prognosis of CM or TBM were established. Receiver operating characteristic (ROC) curves were plotted for these two predicted models with the Medcalc software version 11.5.1.0 (Medcalc software bvba, Belgium). Predictive accuracy was assessed by calculating the areas under the ROC curves (AUC). An AUC of > 0.8 was considered very good. A two-tailed $P < 0.05$ was considered statistically significant.

Results

Patient characteristics

From January 2008 to December 2015, a total of 126 CM patients and 105 TBM patients without HIV infection were included in this retrospective study. The clinical characteristics of these patients were shown in Table 1. There was no significant difference between CM and TBM patients in gender.

Most patients with CM were from 30 to 60 years (65/126, 51.6%), but most of TBM patients were aged under 30 years (54/105, 51.4%). Among CM patients, the most common initial symptoms were headache (118/126, 96.7%), followed by fever (71/126, 56.3%), vomiting (71/126, 56.3%) and altered mentation (51/126, 40.5%). The most common presenting symptoms of TBM patients were also headache (87/105, 82.9%), fever (72/105, 68.6%) and vomiting (47/105, 44.8%). CM patients were more likely to present with headache, abnormal vision and hearing, and less likely to present with fever and cough than TBM patients ($P < 0.05$).

The most frequently underlying diseases, factors or complications of CM patients were corticosteroid use (22/126, 17.5%), pulmonary infection (22/126, 17.5%), hepatobiliary diseases (15/126, 11.9%) and diabetes mellitus (13/126, 10.3%). However, tuberculosis outside CNS was the most common in TBM patients, especially disseminated tuberculosis (27/62, 43.5%, data not shown). Twenty percent of patients had no underlying condition.

Laboratory data and radiological findings

Laboratory data and radiographic findings are prior to shown in Table 2. The CSF WBC and total protein in CM patients were lower than those of TBM group ($P < 0.05$). There was no statistical difference in CSF glucose, chloride level and opening pressure in LP between the two groups. In HIV negative CM group, CD4/CD8 ratio in serum was significantly decreased compared to the TBM group.

Brain MRI was performed in 84.9% (107/126) patients with CM and 76.2% (80/105) patients with TBM. Other patients were examined by head CT. The most common manifestations were cerebral ischemia, demyelination, meningeal enhancement and encephalitis in these two groups. A total of 15.9% (20/126) patients in CM group and 11.4% (12/105) in TBM group had normal image findings. A higher percentage of CM patients presented with cerebral ischemia/infarction and demyelination than TBM patients ($P < 0.05$), but encephalitis and cerebral edema were more common in TBM patients ($P < 0.05$).

Table 1 Demographic and clinical features in HIV negative patients with cryptococcal meningitis (CM) and tuberculous meningitis (TBM)

Variables	CM (*N*=126)	TBM (*N*=105)	*P*-value
Sex			
Male	79(62.7%)	57(54.3%)	0.227
Female	47(37.3%)	48(45.7%)	
Age (years)			
≤30	29(23.0%)	54(51.4%)	**<0.001**
31–60	65(51.6%)	35(33.3%)	
>60	32(25.4%)	16(15.2%)	
Presenting symptoms and signs			
Headache	118(96.7%)	87(82.9%)	**0.012**
Fever	71(56.3%)	72(68.6%)	**0.038**
Vomiting	71(56.3%)	47(44.8%)	0.263
Altered mentation	51(40.5%)	43(41.0%)	0.524
Abnormal vision	35(27.8%)	12(11.4%)	**0.002**
Cough	7(5.6%)	24(22.9%)	**<0.001**
Seizure	14(11.1%)	6(5.7%)	0.111
Abnormal hearing	14(11.1%)	3(2.9%)	**0.014**
Apopsychia	6(4.8%)	2(1.9%)	0.208
Dyspnea	5(4.0%)	1(1.0%)	0.155
Meningeal signs	89(70.6%)	68(64.8%)	0.209
Pathological signs	22(17.5%)	23(21.9%)	0.247
Underlying diseases, factors or complications			
Corticosteroid medication	22(17.5%)	6(5.7%)	**0.005**
Pnumonary infection	22(17.5%)	13(12.4%)	0.188
Hepatobiliary diseases	15(11.9%)	12(11.4%)	0.539
Tuberculosis outside CNS	12(9.5%)	62(59.0%)	**<0.001**
Immune system disease	11(8.7%)	6(5.7%)	0.269
Hypertension	11(8.7%)	3(2.9%)	0.054
Diabetes mellitus	13(10.3%)	10(9.5%)	0.510
Chronic lung disease	6(4.8%)	3(2.9%)	0.348
Multiple organ dysfunction syndrome	6(4.8%)	1(1.0%)	0.095
Renal transplantation	4(3.2%)	2(1.9%)	0.431
Hematology disease	3(2.4%)	1(1.0%)	0.382
Others	13(10.2%)	12(11.4%)	0.571
None	29(23.0%)	20(19.0%)	0.284
Time from onset of symptoms to treatment (d)			
0–30	48(38.1%)	56(53.3%)	**<0.001**
31–60	47(37.3%)	33(31.4%)	
61–90	19(15.1%)	13(12.4%)	
>90	12(9.5%)	3(2.9%)	
Outcome Improved	80(63.5%)	81(77.1%)	0.031
Worse/Died	46(36.5%)	24(22.9%)	

CM and TBM specific test results are shown in Table 3. For CM patients, latex agglutination CrAg titer were positive in 99.2% (125/126) of them. The positive rates of CSF India ink stain and CSF culture for *C. neoformans* in CM patients were 77.8% (98/126) and 79.3% (100/126), respectively. IGRA had higher positive rate than other detection methods in TBM patients ($P < 0.05$).

Treatment outcome

A total of 38.1 and 53.3% of patients with CM and TBM received treatment within 30 days after the onset of clinical symptoms, respectively. And the proportion of patients with a duration of more than 2 month was higher in the CM group than TBM group (26.6% vs. 15.2%, $P = 0.100$), but there was no significant difference. After three months of treatment, 63.5% (80/126) of CM patients and 77.1% (81/105) of TBM patients had improved ($P = 0.031$).

Risk factors for poor treatment outcome of HIV negative CM and TBM patients

Univariate analysis revealed that the factors impacting the prognosis of CM patients were age, altered mentation, demyelination, CD4/CD8 ratios < 1 and CSF CrAg ≥ 1:1024. Multivariate analysis showed that age, altered mentation, CD4/CD8 ratios < 1 and CSF CrAg ≥ 1:1024 were independent risk factors for poor prognosis. For TBM patiens, multiple regression analysis showed that hydrocephalus (OR = 7.290, 95% CI: 1.630–32.606, P =0.009) and no less than three underlying diseases (OR = 6.899, 95% CI: 1.766–26.949, $P = 0.005$) were the risk factors, and headache was a protective factor of prognosis, as shown in Table 4.

ROC curve for the prognostic index derived from the logistic regression models

Prediction models for the probability of poor prognosis in patients with CM and TBM are shown in Appendix 1. The ROC curves of the models of CM and TBM are shown in Additional file 1: Figure S1.

Discussion

Many patients with CM and TBM were misdiagnosed or had a delay in diagnosis. Fever, headache, vomiting, altered mentation and meningeal irritation were the most common initial symptoms of both CM and TBM patients. However, CM patients were more likely to suffer headache, vision and hearing damage, TBM patients were more prone to have fever and cough. These results were fairly consistent with previous reports [9, 17, 18]. One review showed headache (87%), fever (74%), meningeal irritation (67%), vomiting (61%) and altered mentation (26%) as the most common clinical manifestations of CM [9]. One study showed that among

Table 2 Laboratory data and radiographic findings in HIV negative patients with cryptococcal meningitis (CM) and tuberculous meningitis (TBM)

Variables	CM (*N*=126)	TBM (*N*=105)	*P*-value
CSF			
WBC (cells/mm^3), Median (IQR)	80.00 (20.00–200.00)	120.00 (59.00–295.00)	**0.005**
Total protein (mg/dL), Median (IQR)	0.83 (0.58–1.32)	1.53(0.99–2.66)	**<0.001**
Glucose (mmol/L), Median (IQR)	1.57 (0.80–2.56)	1.78(1.10–2.35)	0.694
Chloride (mmol/L), (mean±SD)	118.11±6.67	111.40±7.59	0.169
Open pressure > 220mm H_2O	98 (77.78%)	75 (71.4%)	0.289
Serum			
Albumin(g/L), (mean±SD)	37.77±5.29	36.61±5.20	0.688
WBC (×10^9/L), (mean±SD)	8.89±3.51	7.46±3.45	0.701
Neutrophile (%)	78.44±10.85	75.92±11.33	0.690
Hemoglobin (g/L), (mean±SD)	122.83±23.05	118.50±22.71	0.548
CD3$^+$ T lymphocyte (%)	65.11±14.25	70.96±13.20	0.533
CD4$^+$ T lymphocyte (%)	28.71±10.46	34.77±11.27	0.542
CD8$^+$ T lymphocyte (%)	25.40±8.57	25.19±10.26	0.139
CD4/CD8 ratio	1.22±0.59	1.71±1.12	**0.003**
Brain images (CT/MRI)			
Cerebral ischemia/infarction	55 (43.7%)	30 (28.6%)	**0.028**
Demyelination	30 (23.8%)	14 (9.5%)	**0.046**
Meningeal enhancement	23 (18.3%)	20 (16.0%)	0.877
Hydrocephalus	16 (12.7%)	17(16.2%)	0.709
Encephalitis	14 (11.1%)	40 (38.1%)	**<0.001**
Cerebral edema	4 (3.17%)	13 (12.4%)	**0.010**
Others	4 (3.17%)	8 (7.6%)	0.147
Normal	20 (15.9%)	12 (11.4%)	0.347

CSF cerebrospinal fluid, *WBC* white blood count, *MRI* magnetic resonance imaging

patients without HIV, those with CM were more likely to present headache, altered mentation, vision and hearing damage as compared to those with TBM [18].

Although CM and TBM are often considered as an opportunistic infection in patients with HIV, they are also seen in individuals with apparently normal immune function. In this study, corticosteroid medication, hepatobiliary diseases (abnormal liver function for various reasons, such as chronic hepatitis, cirrhosis) and diabetes mellitus occupied the top three underlying diseases and factors for CM patients. A study reviewed 3698 cryptococcosis cases that found the most common underlying diseases were HIV infection, tuberculosis, liver disease, systemic lupus erythematosus and diabetes mellitus, while 17% had no underlying diseases [9]. Another study showed the commom underlying disease of HIV negative CM patients were hepatobiliary diseases, hypertension, cancer and diabetes mellitus [7]. Sixty-two TBM patients, 27 of them were disseminated tuberculosis, in this study were known to have pulmonary

Table 3 The positive rate of pathogens and other serological tests for diagnosis of cryptococcal meningitis (CM) and tuberculous meningitis (TBM) in HIV negative patients

Variables	CM (*N*=126)	Variables	TBM (*N*=105)
India ink stain	98 (77.8%)	TB smearing	5 (4.8%)
CSF fungal culture	100 (79.3%)	TB DNA	59 (56.2%)
India ink stain & fungal culture	72 (57.1%)	Mycobacterium tuberculosis culture	9 (8.6%)
CrAg	125 (99.2%)	IGRA	94 (89.5%)
CrAg titer ≥1:1024	73 (57.9%)	TST	62 (60.0%)

CSF cerebrospinal fluid, *CrAg* cryptococcal antigen, *TST* tuberculin skin test, *IGRA* interferon gamma release assay

Table 4 Risk factors associated with poor prognosis of HIV negative cryptococcal meningitis (CM) and tuberculous meningitis (TBM) patients

Cryptococcal meningitis (CM)						
Variables	Univariate analysis			Multivariate analysis		
	Odds ratio	95% CI	*P*-value	Odds ratio	95% CI	*P*-value
Ages>60y	5.946	2.493–14.183	<0.001	4.981	1.955–12.692	0.001
Altered mentation	4.533	1.763–11.656	0.002	5.054	1.592–16.046	0.006
Demyelination	7.270	2.560–20.646	<0.001			
CD4/CD8 ratio<1	8.475	2.831–25.378	<0.001	8.782	2.436–31.661	0.001
CrAg titer ≥1:1024	5.338	1.769–16.103	0.003	4.853	1.377–17.098	0.014
Tuberculous meningitis (TBM)						
Fever	9.659	1.208–77.252	0.033			
Headache	0.139	0.042–0. 459	0.001	0.125	0.032–0.497	0.003
Hydrocephalus	3.692	1.062–12.839	0.040	7.290	1.630–32.606	0.009
Underlying diseases or factors≥3	6.817	1.927–19.869	0.002	6.899	1.766–26.949	0.005

HIV human immunodeficiency virus, *CrAg* cryptococcal antigen, *CI* confidential intervals

tuberculosis. Gu et al. also found 30.1% of TBM patients derived their TBM from disseminated tuberculosis [17]. TBM is the most severe form of extrapulmonary tuberculosis, it can occur in isolation or along with a pulmonary focus. TBM and disseminated tuberculosis are usually due to hematogenous dissemination of the tubercle bacillus [19].

In CM and TBM patients, the most common manifestations on brain imagines were cerebral ischemia/infarction, meningeal enhancement, hydrocephalus, which consistent with previous reports [3, 5, 20]. Demyelination were seen on some patients' head MRI or CT. Of course, MR imaging is more sensitive in depicting demyelination than head CT. In this study, demyelination was more commom for CM patients than in prior reports [5, 20]. Another study showed that gadolinium-enhancing white matter lesions found on brain MRI of CM patients. Biopsy revealed the lesions of resembled demyelinating were cryptococci, non-specific inflammatory changes or small perivascular lymphocyte collections. Which possibly be leukoencephalopathy or immune response to the pathogen [21]. In addition, our patients showed evidence of cerebral ischemia or encephalitis more often than previous studies [9, 18], this was likely related to the increased sensitivity of MRI with diffusion-weighted imaging.

Patients with TBM presented with higher CSF WBC and total protein than CM patients, similar to prior studies [18]. A low ratio of CD4/CD8 was also found in the apparently healthy CM patients, it's possible those patients may have some undetectable underlying disease.

In our study, multivariate analysis showed that age >60 years, altered mentation, CD4/CD8 ratios < 1 and CSF CrAg ≥ 1:1024 were closely correlated with poor outcome of CM patients. Previous studies showed there were many poor prognostic factors for CM, including Cryptococcus growth from sites other than CSF, altered mentation, intracranial pressure (ICP) >400 mmH_2O, CSF glucose < 40 mg/dl, high CSF CrAg titer, decreased CSF/blood glucose ratio, papilledema, chronic use of corticosteroids or other immunosuppressants, absence of headache and low GCS score [7, 20, 22–24]. Our study showed that CrAg test was highly specific to the diagnosis of cryptococcal meningitis, and it also had prognostic value, similar to previous studies [25]. Though middle-aged people made up a greater percentage of our CM patients, mortality was increased with patients aged greater than than 60 years, possibly related to a decreased immune response to pathogens declines with age [26].

For TBM patients, poor outcome was related to hydrocephalus and more than three underlying diseases in the present study. Hydrocephalus, optochiasmatic arachnoiditis, microbiologically confirmed TBM have been associated with poor outcome of TBM in previous studies [27, 28]. Early diagnosis and treatment improve prognosis. We found no literature showing that more than three underlying diseases was correlated with poor outcome of TBM. It might be because these studies did not include this factor. On admission, there were 17.1% TBM patients had no headache. Headache was a protective factor for TBM in this study. The inflammation that occurs in the subarachnoid space during meningitis can largely be attributed to the response of the immune system to bacteria, which leads to headache [29]. Patients without headache probably means they have weak immune response. So they had poor outcome.

There were some limitations concerning this study. Because our study was a retrospective research, the medical records about epidemiological contact history were incomplete, so we did not analyse relevant contents. In addition, there were three patients with CM using voriconazole because they could not tolerate the adverse effect of amphotericin B or they complicated renal disease. But just three patients used non standard treatments, which might not affect the statistic results.

Conclusions

We found that compared to patients with TBM, CM patients were more likely to present with headache, vision and hearing damage, cerebral ischemia and de-myelination. TBM patients were more likely to have fever, cough, encephalitis and cerebral edema. CM patients had lower CSF WBC, total protein, and CD4/CD8 ratio than those of TBM patients. Prognosis was poorer for CM patients than TBM patients. Age, altered mentation, CD4/CD8 ratios < 1 and CSF CrAg ≥ 1:1024 were independent risk factors for poor prognosis of HIV negative CM patients. Hydrocephalus and no less than three underlying diseases were the risk factors, and headache was a protective factor for HIV negative patients with TBM. Our prediction models may be helpful for making treatment plan and prognosis assessment. Of course, specific identification of the offending microorganism is considered to be the gold standard in diagnosing infectious diseases. More work needs to be done to develop more rapid, sensitive and specific diagnosis methods and more effective treatments for patients CM and TBM, and the prognosis can be improved accordingly.

Appendix 1

Prediction models for the probability of poor prognosis in patients with cryptococcal meningitis (CM) and tuberculous meningitis (TBM)

Prediction model for the probability of poor prognosis in CM: $P_{CM}=e^x/(1 + e^x)$, x = −6.360 + (1.606 × age) + (1.620 × altered mentation) + (2.173 × CD4/CD8 ratios) + (1.579 × CSF CrAg titer). Prediction model for the probability of poor prognosis in TBM: $P_{TBM}=e^x/(1 + e^x)$, x = −0.658 + (1.931 × underlying diseases) + (1.987 × hydrocephalus) + (−2.079 × headache). Where the following are used: *e* is the natural logarithm; age>60y, altered mentation, CD4/CD8 ratios<1, CSF CrAg titer ≥1:1024, underlying diseases≥3 and headache are scored as 1 or otherwise as 0; hydrocephalus was derived from the imaging report (1: yes, 0: no). The ROC curves of the risk index models for predicting poor prognosis of CM or TBM are shown in Additional file 1: Figure S1. The AUC of CM was 0.872 (95% CI: 0.786–0.932). The appropriate cut off point was selected at P_{CM}=0.5127, and the model achieved a sensitivity of 69.44%, a specificity of 91.23%. The AUC of TBM was 0.802 (95% CI: 0.700–0.882), the appropriate cut off point was 0.3209 for P_{TBM} with a sensitivity of 57.89% and a specificity of 88.89%.

Abbreviations

5-FC: 5-flucytosine; AIDS: Acquired immune deficiency syndrome; AMB: Amphotericin B; CM: Cryptococcal meningitis; CNS: Central nervous system; CrAg: Cryptococcal antigen; CSF: Cerebrospinal fluid; CT: Computed tomography; EMB: Ethambutol; HIV: Human immunodeficiency virus; IGRA: Interferon gamma release assay; INH: Isoniazide; LP: Lumbar puncture; MRI: Magnetic resonance imaging; PCR: Polymerase chain reaction; PZA: Pyrazinamide; RIF: Rifampin; TBM: Tuberculous meningitis; TST: Tuberculin skin test; WBC: White blood cell count

Acknowledgments
The authors thank the staff in Information Center of West China Hospital, Sichuan University for data retrieval. The authors would like to thank Dr Hui Ye for helpful in study design and discussion.

Funding
This research received no specific grant from any funding agency in the public, commercial, or not-for-profit sectors.

Authors' contributions
XJL had full access to all the data in the study and takes responsibility for the integrity of the data and the accuracy of the analysis and will act as the guarantor. All authors participated in study conception, design and interpretation. JYQ wrote the initial draft. TYZ revised the manuscript critically for important intellectual content. CJZ and RD participated in acquisition and analysis of data, and critical review. All authors have seen and approved the final version.

Competing interests
The authors declare that they have no competing interests.

Consent for publication
Not applicable.

References

1. Christensen AS, Andersen AB, Thomsen VO, Andersen PH, Johansen IS. Tuberculous meningitis in Denmark: a review of 50 cases. BMC Infect Dis. 2011;11:47.
2. Pyrgos V, Seitz AE, Steiner CA, Prevots DR, Williamson PR. Epidemiology of cryptococcal meningitis in the US: 1997–2009. Plos One. 2013;8(2):390–6.
3. Thwaites GE, van Toorn R, Schoeman J. Tuberculous meningitis: more questions, still too few answers. Lancet Neurol. 2013;12(10):999–1010.
4. Lee HG, William T, Menon J, Ralph AP, Ooi EE, Hou Y, et al. Tuberculous meningitis is a major cause of mortality and morbidity in adults with central nervous system infections in Kota Kinabalu, Sabah, Malaysia: an observational study. BMC Infect Dis. 2016;16:296.
5. Perfect JR, Dismukes WE, Dromer F, Goldman DL, Graybill JR, Hamill RJ, et al. Clinical practice guidelines for the management of cryptococcal disease: 2010 update by the infectious diseases society of America. Clin Infect Dis. 2010;50(3):291–322.
6. Yao Y, Zhang JT, Yan B, Gao T, Xing XW, Tian CL, et al. Voriconazole: a novel treatment option for cryptococcal meningitis. Infect Dis (Lond). 2015;47(10):694–700.
7. Lee YC, Wang JT, Sun HY, Chen YC. Comparisons of clinical features and mortality of cryptococcal meningitis between patients with and without human immunodeficiency virus infection. J Microbiol Immunol Infect. 2011;44(5):338–45.
8. Guo J, Zhou J, Zhang S, Zhang X, Li J, Sun Y, et al. A case-control study of risk factors for HIV-negative children with cryptococcal meningitis in Shi Jiazhuang. China BMC Infect Dis. 2012;12:376.

9. Yuchong C, Fubin C, Jianghan C, Fenglian W, Nan X, Minghui Y, et al. Cryptococcosis in China (1985–2010): review of cases from Chinese database. Mycopathologia. 2012;173(5–6):329–35.
10. Cohen DB, Zijlstra EE, Mukaka M, Reiss M, Kamphambale S, Scholing M, et al. Diagnosis of cryptococcal and tuberculous meningitis in a resource-limited African setting. Trop Med Int Health. 2010;15(8):910–7.
11. Patel VB, Singh R, Connolly C, Kasprowicz V, Zumla A, Ndungu T, et al. Comparison of a clinical prediction rule and a LAM antigen-detection assay for the rapid diagnosis of TBM in a high HIV prevalence setting. PLoS One. 2010;5:e15664.
12. Nhu NT, Heemskerk D, DA T d, Chau TT, Mai NT, Nghia HD. Evaluation of GeneXpert MTB/RIF for diagnosis of tuberculous meningitis. J Clin Microbiol. 2014;52(1):226–33.
13. MarMarais S, Pepper DJ, Marais BJ, Török ME. HIV-associated tuberculous meningitis–diagnostic and therapeutic challenges. Tuberculosis (Edinb). 2010;90(6):367–74.
14. Saag MS, Graybill RJ, Larsen RA, Pappas PG, Perfect JR, Powderly WG, et al. Practice guidelines for the management of cryptococcal disease. Infectious Diseases Society of America. Clin Infect Dis. 2000;30(4):710–8.
15. American Thoracic Society. Treatment of tuberculosis. Morb Mortal Wkly Rep. 2003;52(RR-11):1–77.
16. World Health Organization. Treatment of tuberculosis: guidelines. 4th ed. 2010.
17. Gu J, Xiao H, Wu F, Ge Y, Ma J, Sun W. Prognostic factors of tuberculous meningitis: a single-center study. Int J Clin Exp Med. 2015;8(3):4487–93.
18. Zhang B, Lv K, Bao J, Lu C, Lu Z. Clinical and laboratory factors in the differential diagnosis of tuberculous and cryptococcal meningitis in adult HIV-negative patients. Intern Med. 2013;52(14):1573–8.
19. Galimi R. Extrapulmonary tuberculosis: tuberculous meningitis new developments. Eur Rev Med Pharmacol Sci. 2011;15(4):365–86.
20. Xu XG, Pan WH, Bi XL, Fang W, Chen M, Zhu Y, et al. Comparison of clinical features in patients with persistent and nonpersistent cryptococcal meningitis: twelve years of clinical experience in four centers in China. CNS Neurosci Ther. 2013;19(8):625–31.
21. Wilcox RA, Thyagarajan D, Kempster P. Two cases of Cryptococcus meningitis presenting as leukoencephalopathy prior to amphotericin therapy. Eur J Neurol. 2007;14(3):350–2.
22. Zheng H, Li M, Luo Y, Wang D, Yang J, Chen Q, et al. A retrospective study of contributing factors for prognosis and survival length of cryptococcal meningoencephalitis in Southern part of China (1998–2013). BMC Infect Dis. 2015;15:77.
23. Lessells RJ, Mutevedzi PC, Heller T, Newell ML. Poor long-term outcomes for cryptococcal meningitis in rural South Africa. S Afr Med J. 2011;101(4):251–2.
24. Majumder S, Mandal SK, Bandyopadhyay D. Prognostic markers in AIDS-related cryptococcal meningitis. J Assoc Physicians India. 2011;59:152–4.
25. Lin TY, Yeh KM, Lin JC, Wang NC, Peng MY, Chang FY. Cryptococcal disease in patients with or without human immunodeficiency virus: clinical presentation and monitoring of serum cryptococcal antigen titers. J Microbiol Immunol Infect. 2009;42(3):220–6.
26. Pourgheysari B, Khan N, Best D, Bruton R, Nayak L, Moss PA. The cytomegalovirus-specific CD4+ T-cell response expands with age and markedly alters the CD4+ T-cellrepertoire. J Virol. 2007;81(14):7759–65.
27. Sharma P, Garg RK, Verma R, Singh MK, Shukla R. Incidence, predictors and prognostic value of cranial nerve involvement in patients with tuberculous meningitis: a retrospective evaluation. Eur J Intern Med. 2011;22(3):289–95.
28. Jha SK, Garg RK, Jain A, Malhotra HS, Verma R, Sharma PK. Definite (microbiologically confirmed) tuberculous meningitis: predictors and prognostic impact. Infection. 2015;43(6):639–45.

9

Meningitis in a Chinese adult patient caused by *Mycoplasma hominis*

Menglan Zhou[1,2†], Peng Wang[1†], Sharon Chen[3], Bin Du[4], Jinlong Du[5], Fengdan Wang[6], Meng Xiao[1], Fanrong Kong[3] and Yingchun Xu[1*]

Abstract

Background: *Mycoplasma hominis*, a well known cause of neonatal infection, has been reported as a pathogen in urogenital infections in adults; however, central nervous system (CNS) infections are rare. We report here the first case of *M. hominis* meningitis in China, post neurosurgical treatment for an intracerebral haemorrhage in a 71-year-old male.

Case presentation: We describe a 71-year-old man who developed *M. hominis* meningitis after neurosurgical treatment and was successfully treated with combined azithromycin and minocycline therapy of 2 weeks duration, despite delayed treatment because the Gram stain of cerebrospinal fluid (CSF) yielded no visible organisms. The diagnosis required 16S rDNA sequencing analysis of the cultured isolate from CSF. Literature review of *M. hominis* CNS infections yielded 19 cases (13 instances of brain abscess, 3 of meningitis, 1 spinal cord abscess and 1 subdural empyema each). Delay in diagnosis and initial treatment failure was evident in all cases. With appropriate microbiological testing, antibiotic therapy (ranging from 5 days to 12 weeks) and often, multiple surgical interventions, almost all the patients improved immediately.

Conclusions: Both our patient findings and the literature review, highlighted the pathogenic potential of *M. hominis* together with the challenges prompted by rare infectious diseases in particular for developing countries laboratories with limited diagnostic resources.

Keywords: *Mycoplasma hominis*, Post-operative infection, Meningitis, Hospital acquired pneumonia, Case report

Background

Mycoplasma hominis, initially described as pleuropne umonia-like organism, is a commensal of the human oral cavity, respiratory tract, and genitourinary tract [1–3]. However, its role in the pathogenesis of infections in adult patients, especially extragenital infections such as central nervous system (CNS) infection, post-operative wound infections, mediastinitis, and septic arthritis [2, 4–7], has been difficult to determine. *M. hominis*, which does not possess a cell wall and hence is not identifiable by Gram staining of clinical specimens, is difficult to detect [3, 8, 9]. Culturing *M. hominis* which is fastidious in nature, is both resource- and time-consuming because specialized media and incubation conditions are required. Direct 16S rDNA PCR amplification/sequencing on clinical specimens may be performed but sensitivity is moderate at best, and not all laboratories perform this test [2, 3, 8]. The true incidence of *M. hominis* infections is thus probably underestimated and delayed diagnosis leads to delayed treatment with suboptimal outcomes [10].

CNS infections due to *M. hominis* are rare in patients other than neonates. To the best of our knowledge, only 19 cases of such infections have been reported in the English literature (Table 1). We herein report a case of *M. hominis* meningitis in which the organism was detected in the cerebrospinal fluid (CSF) following

* Correspondence: xycpumch@139.com
†Equal contributors
[1]Department of Clinical Laboratory, Peking Union Medical College Hospital, Chinese Academy of Medical Sciences, Beijing 100730, People's Republic of China
Full list of author information is available at the end of the article

Table 1 Literature reports of CNS infections caused by *Mycoplasma hominis* in non-neonatal patients (1950-2016.7)

No.	Author & year	Pt age(years), sex	Pt Country	HU	Tr	SI	Clinical manifestation	Days to Dx after Ad	Dx basis	Antibiotics used prior to diagnosis	Final antibiotic regimen	Otc	Ref
1	Paine et al. [14]	20, M	USA	N	Y	Y	fever, headache, a stiff neck	18	C	S + P + St	Sm	CR	[14]
2	Payan et al. [15]	29, M	USA	Y	Y	Y	fever, loss of consciousness	23	C	O + Cp + N + C	T + E	CR	[15]
3	Madoff S et al. [16]	11, F	USA	N	N	Y	fever	26	GIT + IRT	V + E	Mc	De	[16]
4	McMahon et al. [24]	76, M	USA	N	N	Y	fever, unresponsive	18	C	P + G	none	De	[24]
5	Kersten RC et al. [17]	20, M	USA	Y	Y	Y	fever, comatose	19	C	A + M + Su + V + Cf	M + Cf + Az + Am + Cl	Re	[17]
							NM	35	C	Az + Am + Cl	M + Cf + D + Cd	CR	[17]
6	Cohen & Kubak. [25]	18, F	USA	N	Y	Y	fever, altered mental status	20	C	E	D + Ci + C	CR	[25]
7	Zheng et al. [18]	22, F	USA	N	N	Y	fever, left-sided weakness and numbness	18	IRT + IBA	Ct + N + Ca + M	none	CR	[19]
8	Douglas et al. [19]	17, F	Australia	N	Y	Y	fever, headache, photophobia, nausea, vomiting	13	C + 16S	A + Ca + E	D + Cd	CR	[19]
9	House P et al. [20]	40, F	Spain	N	N	Y	headache, left facial weakness, nausea, afebrile	12 + "several"	C + 16S	V + Cf + M	Ci + M	CR	[20]
10	Kupila L et al. [21]	40, M	Finland	N	Y	Y	haematuria and urine retention, confused	14	16S	none	T	CR	[21]
11	McCarthy & Looke. [3]	48, M	Australia	N	N	Y	fever	36	C + 16S	Cz + V	Ga + Cd	CR	[3]
12	McCarthy & Looke. [3]	17, F	Australia	N	Y	Y	fever	17	C	V + Me	Ga + Mo	CR	[3]
13	Al Masalma et al. [22]	41, F	Russia	N	N	Y	vertigo, coma headache, hemiparesis	10	16S	V + Me	D	CR	[22]
14	Lee et al. [8]	48, F	Netherlands	Y	Y	Y	fever	15	16S	F + V	Mo	CR	[8]
15	Henao-Martínez et al. [10]	40, M	Somalia	N	Y	Y	fever	17	C + 16S	V + PT + Ct + M	D	CR	[10]
16	Pailhorie 's et al. [23]	43, M	France	N	Y	Y	fever, delirium tremens	13	Vitek MS + 16S	Me + V + Fo	L + D	CR	[23]
17	Whitson WJ [2]	17, M	USA	Y	Y	Y	fever, bicep and deltoid weakness	32	C	PT + V + Ct + M	D + Mo	CR	[2]
18	Hos NJ [27]	21, F	Germany	N	N	Y	fever, neck pain, nausea, vomiting,	31	C + 16S	A + Ct	Mo	CR	[27]
19	Reissier S [26]	39, M	France	N	Y	Y	afbrile, loss of consciousness	33	C + 16S + RT-PCR	PT + Li + Ct + Me + V	Mo	De	[26]
20	Present study	79, M	China	N	N	Y	fever, anepia and right-sided weakness	17	16S	Me + V + CF	Az + D + Mi	CR	

Ad admitted, *C* culture, *CR* clinical recovery, *De* death, *Dx* diagnosis, *GIT* growth inhibition test, *HU* hormone use, *IBA* immunoblot assay, *IRT* immunofluo-rescence test, *Otc* outcome, *Re* recurrence, *Ref* reference, *SI* surgical intervention, *16S* 16S rDNA sequencing, *RT-PCR* real-time PCR, *Tr* trauma, yrs: years

Ampicillin, (*A*) amoxicillin, (*Am*) azithromycin, (*Az*) chloramphenicol, (*C*) cefazolin, (*Ca*) clindamycin, (*Cd*) cefotaxime, (*Cf*) ciprofloxacin, (*Ci*) clavulanate potassium, (*Cl*) cephalothin (*Cp*), ceftriaxone (*Ct*), ceftazidime (*Cz*), cefoperazone/ sulbactam (*CF*), doxycycline (*D*), erythromycin (*E*),flucloxacillin (*F*), fosfomycin (*Fo*),gentamicin (*G*), gatifloxacin (*Ga*),levofloxacin (*L*), linezolid (*Li*), metronidazole (*M*), methacycline (*Mc*), meropenem (*Me*), minocyline (*Mi*), moxifloxacin (*Mo*),nafcillin (*N*), oxacillin (*O*),penicillin (*P*), piperacillin/tazobactam (*PT*), sulfadiazine (*S*), streptomycin (*Sm*), sulfathiazole (*St*), sulbactam (*Su*), tetracycline (*T*), vancomycin (*V*)

neurosurgical intervention for cerebral haemorrhage. This is the first reported case of meningitis in an adult caused by *M. hominis* from China.

Case presentation

History and first admission

The patient was a 71-year-old man with a history of hypertension for 2 years who suddenly developed aphasia, and right-sided weakness and numbness while lifting water and was sent to the local hospital immediately on 21 September 2014. A cerebral computed tomography (CT) scan identified a cerebral hemorrhage rupturing into the ventricular system. He underwent craniotomy and evacuation of the hematoma. One week after the surgery, the patient developed hospital-acquired pneumonia, which was complicated by respiratory failure despite treatment with broad-spectrum antibiotics of imipenem.

MICU admission

The patient was soon transferred to the medical intensive care unit (MICU) of Peking Union Medical College Hospital (PUMCH) on October 14. On admission, he was febrile, comatose (Glasgow Coma Score of 9), dyspneic, and hypotensive. Mechanical ventilation was started after endotracheal intubation.

Examination on MICU & anti-infectious therapy

Empiric antibiotic treatment consisting of meropenem (2.0 g intravenously q8h) and vancomycin (1.0 g intravenously q12h) was initiated for hospital-acquired pneumonia. A lumbar puncture showed an opening pressure > 33 cmH_2O, 1201 x 10^6/L red cells, 201 x 10^6/L white cells (79 % polymorphonuclear forms), an undetectable glucose concentration, protein 2.32 g/L, and chloride 128 mmol/L. No organisms were seen on Gram stain of the CSF. A cerebral CT showed an extensive left temporal hematoma and moderate lateral ventricle enlargement (Fig. 1a).

During his stay in ICU, repeated cultures of tracheal aspirates grew multidrug resistant (MDR) *Acinetobacter baumannii*, which was only susceptible to cefoperazone/sulbactam, and intermediately susceptible to tigecycline and minocycline. A follow-up chest CT scan revealed a thick-walled cavity in the right lower lobe (Fig. 1b). As a result, meropenem was changed to cefoperazone/sulbactam (3.0 g q8h), while the dose of vancomycin was increased to 1.5 g q12h to optimize the serum trough level (Fig. 2).

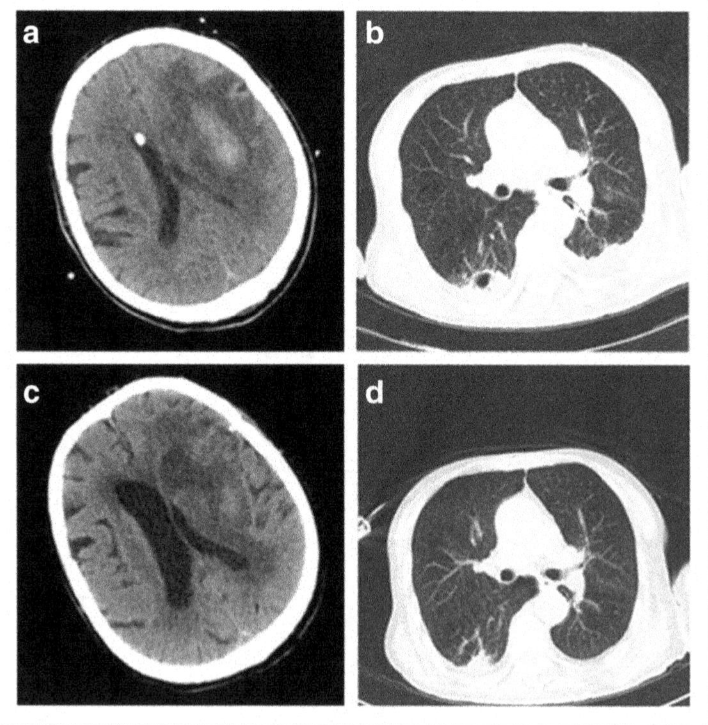

Fig. 1 Computed tomography (CT) scans of the patient's brain and lung during hospitalization. **a**. Cerebral CT scan revealed an extensive left hematoma in the temporal region of the hemispheres and moderate lateral ventricle enlargement with a drainage tube in it. The hematoma was surrounded by brain edema, narrowed gyri and the right-shifted cranial midline. **b**. Thoracic CT scan (lung windows) revealed a cavity with a wall of 7-mm thick surrounded by patchy shadowing in the right lower lobe. **c**. After 30 days of therapy, resolving brain swelling was seen in the CT scan with decreased edema. **d**. After 30 days of therapy, thoracic CT scan (lung window) revealed that the area of cavitation had decreased substantially

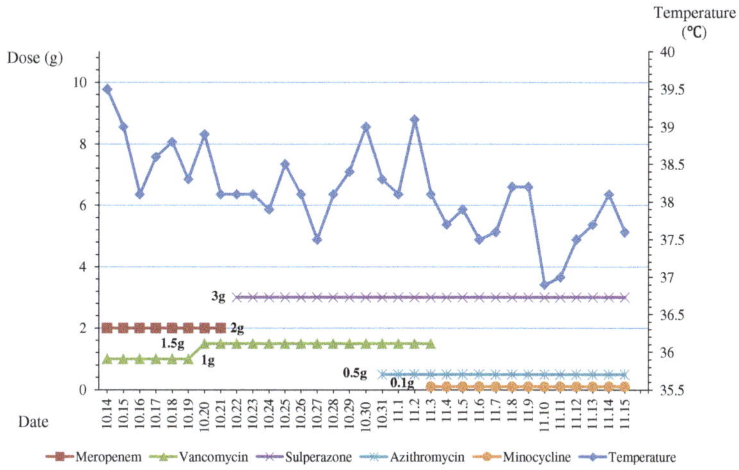

Fig. 2 The correlation between the change of body temperature and the use of antibiotics during hospitalization

Etiological examination

Microbiology laboratory examination

CSF specimens were plated onto 5 % sheep blood agar and chocolate agar and were incubated at 37 °C under aerobic and anaerobic conditions, and in air with 5 % CO_2. On October 30, cultures revealed non-hemolytic, semi-translucent pinpoint colonies on sheep blood agar plate after 4 days of incubation under anaerobic conditions (Fig. 3). Gram-stain smears of the CSF sample showed no evidence of bacteria.

MALDI-TOF analysis of the cultured isolate

Two systems of the matrix-assisted laser desorption/ionization–time of flight mass spectrometry (MALDI-TOF MS) were used, i.e. the MALDI Biotyper (Bruker) and VITEK MS IVD (bioMérieux) as instructed by the manufacturer. The spectra were analyzed by using the MALDI Biotyper database library V.3.3.1.2 and the VITEK® MS IVD v2.0 database respectively. Both MALDI Biotyper and VITEK MS IVD consistently yielded no identifying profile and assigned "no identification" to this isolate.

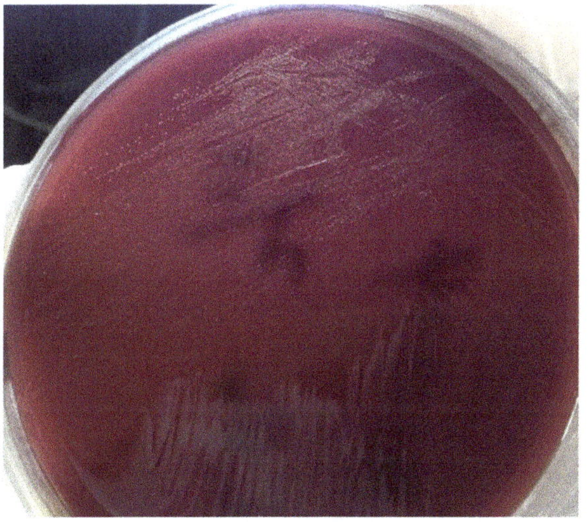

Fig. 3 Non-hemolytic, semi-translucent pinpoint colonies of *M. hominis* were shown on 5 % blood sheep agar after 4 days of incubation

16S rDNA gene identification

Bacterial DNA was obtained from isolates by using QIAamp DNA minikit (Qiagen, Hilden, Germany) following the manufacturer's instructions starting from 200 μL of bacterial pellet suspension about 2-3 McFarland followed by a series of extracting steps with different reagents. Amplification of the 16S rDNA gene was performed by broad-range bacterial polymerase chain reaction (PCR) assay using the universal primers: 27 F (5'-AGAGTTTGATCCTGGCTCAG-3') and 1522R (5'-AAGGAGGTGATCCAGCCGCA-3') as described before [11, 12]. Purified PCR products and sequencing primers (the same as for amplification) were mixed and sent to Ruibiotech (Beijing, China) for sequencing. Species identification was performed by comparing the obtained sequences against those in the GenBank database using the BLASTn software (http://www.ncbi.nlm.nih.gov/blast). By querying 16S rDNA sequences against those in the GenBank database, the isolate best matched with 3 *M. hominis* reference strains (GenBank accession numbers: CP011538.1, NR_041881.1 and CP009652.1) with an identity of 100 % (1385/1385), followed by *Mycoplasma equirhinis*, with an identity of 97 % (1314/1353). All *M. hominis* 16S rDNA nucleotide sequences available in GenBank till 2015 ($n = 10$) are summarized in Additional file 1.

Post-treatment course

On November 2, the microbiology laboratory reported isolation from the CSF sample of *M. hominis*, which was susceptible to doxycycline, and intermediately suscepible to azithromycin by the bioMérieux® SA *Mycoplasma* IST2 kit (Biomerieux, France). Combination therapy with azithromycin (0.5 g qd) and minocycline (100 mg q12h) was then started (Fig. 2). On November 16, 14 days after appropriate antimicrobial therapy was started, the patient was transferred back to the local hospital. Repeated brain and chest CT scans before discharge showed marked improvement of the cerebral edema and size of the brain swelling (Fig. 1c), and almost complete resolution of the pulmonary cavity and pleural effusion (Fig. 1d).

Discussion

A PubMed search was performed using the following key words: "*Mycoplasma hominis*" AND "encephalitis" OR "cerebritis" OR "cephalitis" OR "neuraxitis" OR "phrenitis" OR "meningitis" OR "brain abscess" OR "cranial infection" OR "myelitis" OR " polyradiculoneuritis " OR "spinal cord infection". A total of 58 manuscripts were found, most reporting *M. hominis* infection in neonates, which most likely arising from contact with maternal genital flora [13]. By carefully reading all the papers, we found that there were only 19 reported non-neonatal-associated cases of CNS infection caused by *M. hominis*; none was reported from China (Table 1). Of these 20 cases, brain abscess was the most common CNS infections ($n = 13$) [3, 10, 14–23], followed by meningitis ($n = 4$) [8, 24–26], spinal cord abscess ($n = 1$) [2], subdural empyema ($n = 1$) [27], (Table 1).

Current microbiological analysis, mostly based on direct examination and culture of pus specimens, underestimate the role of fastidious microorganisms, such as *M. hominis* [22], in CNS infections. Predisposing host factors such as immunosuppression, malignancy, trauma, and manipulation or surgery of the genitourinary tract are considered to be risk factors for extra-genital infections caused by this microorganism [8, 15, 17, 18, 28]. In most *M. hominis* brain infections thus far described, patients usually presented with prior head trauma or had undergone neurosurgical procedures [8, 10, 14, 15, 17, 19, 21, 23–27]. This was also the case in our patient who had an intracererbal haematoma evacuated 7 days prior to developing meningitis.

Three routes of intracranial infection are typically considered: direct contamination during trauma, direct contamination during surgery, or seeding of the cerebral site secondary to bacteraemia due to genitourinary manipulation [21, 23]. In traumatized brain tissue where CNS capillaries are damaged, *M. hominis* can easily reach the ischemic brain tissue through blood circulation. In our case, the patient was exposed to the aforementioned last 2 hypothetical sources. Cerebral hemorrhage was cured by a neurosurgical intervention, but he also underwent urinary catheterization after the coma during hospitalization. Therefore, we were unable to definitively identify the source of infection.

Identification of *M. hominis* infections by culture is challenging due to the slow growth of the colonies and the absence of cell wall, which contributes to a negative result on Gram staining [10], as in our patient. Moreover, even when culture is successful, it is difficult to rule out the possibility of contamination. Although *M. hominis*, being less fastidious than other mycoplasmas, is able to grow on conventional blood agar medium, specific laboratory methods are required for its identification. In most reports of cerebral infections, 16S rDNA sequencing is required for definitive identification as was the case here [8]. It has been recently highlighted that MALDI-TOF MS could be useful for the rapid identification of *M. hominis* [23, 29]. However, we were unable to identify *M. hominis* by MALDI TOF MS even though the spectra of this species is represented in the VITEK® MS IVD v2.0 database. In this regard, similar results were also found for the MALDI Biotyper by Nulens E and his colleges [30]. Thus, further improvement of *M. hominis* spectra database seems necessary. Nevertheless, neither the Bruker nor Vitek database misidentified the strain as another species.

Since cases of intracranial infections caused by *M. hominis* are rare, clinicians usually fail to consider the diagnosis in the absence of microbiological evidence. In addition, it is difficult to distinguish brain abscesses or meningitis caused by mycoplasmas from those caused by bacteria or viruses, due to the lack of specific clinical manifestations. This may lead to delayed initiation of antimicrobial therapy with serious clinical consequence [31], as *M. hominis* is not susceptible to most first-line antibiotics used to treat brain abscesses [21]. The possibility of a *M. hominis* infection should be suspected when Gram stain reveals abundant neutrophils but no bacteria, and empirical treatment shows poor efficacy during this period.

In all previously published case studies of *M. hominis* brain abscesses, treatment involved abscess drainage, debridement, and specific antimicrobial therapy. The importance of surgical treatment is evident from a case report of a patient who responded to surgical therapy alone [32]. Infections caused by *Mycoplasma* spp. (i.e. a microorganism lacking both cell wall and folic acid synthesis) require ad-hoc antibiotic treatment [33, 34]. There are no CLSI (Clinical and Laboratory Standards Institute) and EUCAST (European Committee on Antimicrobial Susceptibility Testing) breakpoints for *M. hominis* at present. Nevertheless, the organism is generally considered to be susceptible to tetracyclines, lincosamides, streptogramins and quinolones, but not to the macrolides although tetracyclines-resistant *M. hominis* has been reported [10, 35–37]. However, poor passage through the blood brain barrier could lead to low antibiotic concentrations in the brain, with the possible major exception of fourth generation quinolones that, besides exhibiting low MICs for *M. hominis*, do possess reasonable CSF penetration [35–43]. Because of the tendency for chronic and often latent infection, long-term antimicrobial treatment against *M. hominis* is warranted. However, surgical drainage and debridement remain the key to recovery, since patients may respond to surgical treatment alone [29].

In our case, initial treatment with meropenem and vancomycin showed little efficiency since a low-grade fever still persisted (as shown in Fig. 2). MDR *A. baumannii* was also isolated from the lower respiratory tract possibly due to nosocomial infection. Persistent fever despite various antibiotic treatment with meropenem, vancomycin, and cefoperazone/sulbactam, as well as the satisfactory response to azithromycin and minocycline, strongly suggested that *M. hominis*, rather than *A. baumannii* was the primary pathogen in our patient.

Conclusions

The prevalence of brain infections caused by *M. hominis* may be increasing, presenting a diagnostic and therapeutic challenge to clinicians. We reported here the first case of meningitis caused by *M. hominis* in an adult in China, who was successfully treated with azithromycin and minocycline. The pathogenic potential of *M. hominis*, the need for early diagnosis, and the importance of initial appropriate chemotherapy must be highlighted also in developing countries, where the challenges in diagnostic capacity for clinical laboratories are greater.

Abbreviations

BBB: Blood brain barrier; CLSI: Clinical and laboratory standards institute; CNS: Central nervous system; CSF: Cerebrospinal fluid; CT: Computed tomography; EUCAST: European committee on antimicrobial susceptibility testing; MALDI-TOF MS: Matrix-assisted laser desorption/ionization-time of flight mass spectrometry; MDR: Multidrug resistant; MICU: Medical intensive care unit; PCR: Polymerase chain reaction; PUMCH: Peking union medical college hospital

Acknowledgements

We thank Dr. Zhihong Guan from the Department of neurology, Peking Union Medical College Hospital, Chinese Academy of Medical Sciences, Beijing, China where the patient is in care.

Authors' contributions

MZ, PW, FK and YCX conceived and designed the experiments. MZ, PW, JD, MX and FW collected the information about the case, contributed to the acquisition, analysis and interpretation of data. MZ, SC, BD and FK wrote and revised the manuscript. All authors read and approved the final manuscript.

Competing interests

The authors report no conflict of interest concerning the materials or methods used in this study or the findings specified in this paper.

Consent for publication

Written informed consent was obtained from the patient for publication of this Case report. A copy of the written consent is available for review by the Editor of this journal.

Author details

[1]Department of Clinical Laboratory, Peking Union Medical College Hospital, Chinese Academy of Medical Sciences, Beijing 100730, People's Republic of China. [2]Graduate School, Peking Union Medical College, Chinese Academy of Medical Sciences, Beijing, China. [3]Centre for Infectious Diseases and Microbiology Laboratory Services, Pathology West, Westmead Hospital, University of Sydney Darcy Road, Westmead, New South Wales 2145, Australia. [4]Department of Medical Intensive Care Unit, Peking Union Medical College Hospital, Chinese Academy of Medical Sciences, Beijing, China. [5]Department of Clinical Laboratory, Fu Xing Hospital, Capital Medical University, Beijing, China. [6]Department of Radiology, Peking Union Medical College Hospital, Chinese Academy of Medical Sciences, Beijing, China.

References

1. Dienes L, Edsall G. Observations on the L-organism of Klieneberger. Proc Soc Exp Biol Med. 1937;36:740–4.
2. Whitson WJ, Ball PA, Lollis SS, Balkman JD, Bauer DF. Post-operative *Mycoplasma hominis* infections after neurosurgical intervention. J Neurosurg Pediatr. 2014;14:212–8.
3. McCarthy KL, Looke DF. Successful treatment of post-neurosurgical intracranial *Mycoplasma hominis* infection using gatifloxacin. J Infect. 2008;57:344–6.
4. Pastural M, Audard V, Bralet MP, Rémy P, Salomon L, Tankovic J, et al. *Mycoplasma hominis* infection in renal transplantation. Nephrol Dial Transplant. 2002;17:495–6.
5. Mattila PS, Carlson P, Sivonen A, Savola J, Luosto R, Salo J, et al. Life-threatening *Mycoplasma hominis* mediastinitis. Clin Infect Dis. 1999;29:1529–37.
6. Flouzat-Lachaniette CH, Guidon J, Allain J, Poignard A. An uncommon case of *Mycoplasma hominis* infection after total disc replacement. Eur Spine J. 2013;22 Suppl 3:S394–8.
7. Taylor-Robinson D. Infections due to species of *Mycoplasma* and *Ureaplasma*: an update. Clin Infect Dis. 1996;23:671–82.
8. Lee EH, Winter HL, van Dijl JM, Metzemaekers JD, Arends JP. Diagnosis and antimicrobial therapy of *Mycoplasma hominis* meningitis in adults. Int J Med Microbiol. 2012;302:289–92.
9. Waites KB, Schelonka RL, Xiao L, Grigsby PL, Novy MJ. Congenital and opportunistic infections: *Ureaplasma* species and *Mycoplasma hominis*. Semin Fetal Neonatal Med. 2009;14:190–9.
10. Henao-Martinez AF, Young H, Nardi-Korver JJ, Burman W. *Mycoplasma hominis* brain abscess presenting after a head trauma: a case report. J Med Case Rep. 2012;6:253.
11. Kupila L, Rantakokko-Jalava K, Jalava J, Nikkari S, Peltonen R, Meurman O, et al. Aetiological diagnosis of brain abscesses and spinal infections: application of broad range bacterial polymerase chain reaction analysis. J Neurol Neurosurg Psychiatry. 2003;74:728–33.
12. Drancourt M, Berger P, Raoult D. Systematic 16S rRNA gene sequencing of atypical clinical isolates identified 27 new bacterial species associated with humans. J Clin Microbiol. 2004;42:2197–202.
13. Hata A, Honda Y, Asada K, Sasaki Y, Kenri T, Hata D. *Mycoplasma hominis* meningitis in a neonate: case report and review. J Infect. 2008;57:338–43.
14. Paine TF, Murray R, Perlmutter I, Finland M. Brain abscess and meningitis associated with a pleuropneumonia-like organism: clinical and bacteriological observations in a case with recovery. Ann Intern Med. 1950;32:554–62.
15. Payan DG, Seigal N, Madoff S. Infection of a brain abscess of *Mycoplasma hominis*. J Clin Microbiol. 1981;14:571–3.
16. Madoff S, Hooper DC. Nongenitourinary infections caused by *Mycoplasma hominis* in adults. Rev Infect Dis. 1988;10:602–13.
17. Kersten RC, Haglund L, Kulwin DR, Ma'luf R, DeConciliis C. *Mycoplasma hominis* orbital abscess. Arch Ophthalmol. 1995;113:1096–7.
18. Zheng X, Olson DA, Tully JG, Watson HL, Cassell GH, Gustafson DR, et al. Isolation of *Mycoplasma hominis* from a brain abscess. J Clin Microbiol. 1997;35:992–4.

19. Douglas MW, Fisher DA, Lum GD, Roy J. *Mycoplasma hominis* infection of a subdural haematoma in the peripartum period. Pathology. 2003;35:452–4.
20. House P, Dunn J, Carroll K, MacDonald J. Seeding of a cavernous angioma with *Mycoplasma hominis*: case report. Neurosurgery. 2003;53:749–52.
21. Kupila L, Rantakokko-Jalava K, Jalava J, Peltonen R, Marttila RJ, Kotilainen E, et al. Brain abscess caused by *Mycoplasma hominis*: a clinically recognizable entity? Eur J Neurol. 2006;13:550–1.
22. Al Masalma M, Drancourt M, Dufour H, Raoult D, Fournier PE. *Mycoplasma hominis* brain abscess following uterus curettage: a case report. J Med Case Rep. 2011;5:278.
23. Pailhories H, Rabier V, Eveillard M, Mahaza C, Joly-Guillou ML, Chennebault JM, et al. A case report of *Mycoplasma hominis* brain abscess identified by MALDI-TOF mass spectrometry. Int J Infect Dis. 2014;29:166–8.
24. McMahon DK, Dummer JS, Pasculle AW, Cassell G. Extragenital *Mycoplasma hominis* infections in adults. Am J Med. 1990;89:275–81.
25. Cohen M, Kubak B. *Mycoplasma hominis* meningitis complicating head trauma: case report and review. Clin Infect Dis. 1997;24:272–3.
26. Reissier S, Masson R, Guérin F, Viquesnel G, Petitjean-Lecherbonnier J, Pereyre SInt J, et al. Fatal nosocomial meningitis caused by *Mycoplasma hominis* in an adult patient: case reportand review of the literature. Infect Dis. 2016;48:81–3.
27. Hos NJ, Bauer C, Liebig T, Plum G, Seifert H, Hampl J. Autoinfection as a cause of postpartum subdural empyema due to *Mycoplasma hominis*. Infection. 2015;43(2):241–4. doi:10.1007/s15010-014-0713-2. Epub 2014 Dec 10.
28. Simberkoff MS, Toharsky B. Mycoplasmemia in adult male patients. JAMA. 1976;236:2522–4.
29. Pereyre S, Tardy F, Renaudin H, Cauvin E, Del Prá Netto Machado L, Tricot A, et al. Identification and subtyping of clinically relevant human and ruminant mycoplasmas by use of matrix-assisted laser desorption ionization-time of flight mass spectrometry. J ClinMicrobiol. 2013;51:3314–23.
30. Nulens E, Van Praet J, Selleslag D, Van Landschoot T, Dekeyzer D, Descheemaecker P, et al. A disseminated *Mycoplasma hominis* infection in a patient with an underlying defect in humoral immunity. Infection. 2016;44(3):379–81.
31. Brouwer MC, Tunkel AR, McKhann GM, van de Beek D. Brain abscess. N Engl J Med. 2014;371:447–56.
32. Mossad SB, Rehm SJ, Tomford JW, Isada CM, Taylor PC, Rutherford I, et al. Sternotomy infection with *Mycoplasma hominis*: a cause of "culture negative" wound infection. J Cardiovasc Surg. 1996;37:505–9.
33. McCormack WM. Susceptibility of mycoplasmas to antimicrobial agents: clinical implications. Clin Infect Dis. 1993;17 Suppl 1:S200–1.
34. Krausse R, Schubert S. In-vitro activities of tetracyclines, macrolides, fluoroquinolones and clindamycin against *Mycoplasma hominis* and *Ureaplasma* spp. isolated in Germany over 20 years. Clin Microbiol Infect. 2010;16:1649–55.
35. Kenny GE, Cartwright FD. Susceptibilities of *Mycoplasma hominis, M. pneumoniae*, and *Ureaplasma urealyticum* to GAR-936, dalfopristin, dirithromycin, evernimicin, gatifloxacin, linezolid, moxifloxacin, quinupristin-dalfopristin, and telithromycin compared to their susceptibilities to reference macrolides, tetracyclines, and quinolones. Antimicrob Agents Chemother. 2001;45:2604–8.
36. Redelinghuys MJ, Ehlers MM, Dreyer AW, Lombaard HA, Kock MM. Antimicrobial susceptibility patterns of *Ureaplasma* species and *Mycoplasma hominis* in pregnant women. BMC Infect Dis. 2014;14:171.
37. Mardassi BB, Aissani N, Moalla I, Dhahri D, Dridi A, Mlik B. Evidence for the predominance of a single tet(M) gene sequence type in tetracycline-resistant *Ureaplasma parvum* and *Mycoplasma hominis* isolates from Tunisian patients. J Med Microbiol. 2012;61(Pt9):1254–61.
38. Cottagnoud P, Tauber MG. Fluoroquinolones in the treatment of meningitis. CurrInfect Dis Rep. 2003;5:329–36.
39. Lutsar I, Friedland IR, Wubbel L, McCoig CC, Jafri HS, Ng W, et al. Pharmacodynamics of gatifloxacin in cerebrospinal fluid in experimental cephalosporin-resistant pneumococcal meningitis. Antimicrob Agents Chemother. 1998;42:2650–5.
40. Scotton PG, Pea F, Giobbia M, Baraldo M, Vaglia A, Furlanut M. Cerebrospinal fluid penetration of levofloxacin in patients with spontaneous acute bacterial meningitis. Clin Infect Dis. 2001;33:e109–11.
41. Shimada J, Nogita T, Ishibashi Y. Clinical pharmacokinetics of sparfloxacin. Clin Pharmacokinet. 1993;25:358 69.
42. Lutsar I, McCracken Jr GH, Friedland IR. Antibiotic pharmacodynamics in cerebrospinal fluid. Clin Infect Dis. 1998;27:1117–27.
43. Kanellakopoulou K, Pagoulatou A, Stroumpoulis K, Vafiadou M, Kranidioti H, Giamarellou H, et al. Pharmacokinetics of moxifloxacin in non-inflamed cerebrospinal fluid of humans: implication for a bactericidal effect. J Antimicrob Chemother. 2008;61:1328–31.

10

Cerebrospinal fluid in tuberculous meningitis exhibits only the L-enantiomer of lactic acid

Shayne Mason[1*], Carolus J. Reinecke[1], Willem Kulik[2], Arno van Cruchten[2], Regan Solomons[3] and A. Marceline Tutu van Furth[4]

Abstract

Background: The defining feature of the cerebrospinal fluid (CSF) collected from infants and children with tuberculous meningitis (TBM), derived from an earlier untargeted nuclear magnetic resonance (NMR) metabolomics study, was highly elevated lactic acid. Undetermined was the contribution from host response (L-lactic acid) or of microbial origin (D-lactic acid), which was set out to be determined in this study.

Methods: In this follow-up study, we used targeted ultra-performance liquid chromatography–electrospray ionization–tandem mass spectrometry (UPLC–ESI–MS/MS) to determine the ratio of the L and D enantiomers of lactic acid in these CSF samples.

Results: Here we report for the first time that the lactic acid observed in the CSF of confirmed TBM cases was in the L-form and solely a response from the host to the infection, with no contribution from any bacteria. The significance of elevated lactic acid in TBM appears to be that it is a crucial energy substrate, used preferentially over glucose by microglia, and exhibits neuroprotective capabilities.

Conclusion: These results provide experimental evidence to support our conceptual astrocyte–microglia lactate shuttle model formulated from our previous NMR-based metabolomics study — highlighting the fact that lactic acid plays an important role in neuroinflammatory diseases such as TBM. Furthermore, this study reinforces our belief that the determination of enantiomers of metabolites corresponding to infectious diseases is of critical importance in substantiating the clinical significance of disease markers.

Keywords: Cerebrospinal fluid (CSF), Enantiomers, L- and D-lactic acid, Tuberculous meningitis (TBM), Ultra-performance liquid chromatography–electrospray ionization–tandem mass spectrometry (UPLC–ESI–MS/MS)

Background

Lactic acid is a common metabolite and occurs as two, optically active stereoisomers (enantiomers) — L-lactic acid and D-lactic acid.

In humans, the L enantiomer is considered the normal, physiological form of lactic acid. The endogenous D form is also found in humans, but in nanomolar amounts due to methylglyoxal metabolism [1], which converts acetone derivatives to glutathione. The D enantiomer typically originates from gut microbiota, such that it can be detected in the blood and urine up to the millimolar range. Elevation of D-lactic acid typically occurs as a result of gut trauma or gastrointestinal disorder, for example, in jejuno-ileal bypass for obesity [2], appendicitis [3, 4], inflammatory bowel syndrome [5], and even in patients with chronic fatigue syndrome [6] and type 2 diabetes [5]. The main source of elevated D-lactic acid in urine, however, is in patients with short bowel syndrome [7].

It is known that the gut possesses its own unique microbiotic environment; it is also generally believed that the brain is a fairly sterile environment without its own microbiota, with the microglia in the circulating cerebrospinal fluid (CSF) actively eliminating any

* Correspondence: nmr.nwu@gmail.com
[1]Centre for Human Metabolomics, Faculty of Natural Sciences, North-West University (Potchefstroom Campus), Private Bag X6001, Potchefstroom 2531, South Africa
Full list of author information is available at the end of the article

microbial incursions beyond the blood–brain barrier (BBB). However, in pathological conditions where an invading pathogen successfully transgresses the BBB and an infection occurs in the central nervous system (CNS), any subsequent metabolic perturbations may be difficult to trace and interpret. In the case of bacterial meningitis, in which bacteria infect the meninges, with disastrous consequences due to neuroinflammation, there have been numerous reports of highly acidotic CSF owing to the presence of lactic acid [8–10]. A unique form of bacterial meningitis, caused by *Mycobacterium tuberculosis* (Mtb), is tuberculous meningitis (TBM). What makes this form of meningitis unique, and dangerous, is that it has a slow, insidious onset which often leads to accumulated damage due to neuroinflammation, resulting in irreparable neural damage, or even death. It is a disease that is difficult to diagnose in its early stages and fatal if recognized at a late stage. Of the various CSF diagnostic markers for TBM, lactic acid is one that has been reported in a limited number of studies [11–13]. In a previous study we examined a cohort of infants and children with TBM by means of an untargeted ^{1}H nuclear magnetic resonance (NMR)-based metabolomics approach [14]. The most noticeable feature that we detected was highly elevated lactic acid (7.36 ± 2.36 mM) in the CSF of these cases compared to the normal, age-related reference range (1.65 ± 0.63 mM) [15]. The presence of highly elevated lactic acid in CSF is not unique to meningitis cases: in patients with cerebral malaria there was significantly higher CSF lactic acid recorded (9.0 ± 5.3 mM [16]; 6.0 ± 1.0 mM [17]) in those who died compared to survivors. Yao et al. [18] reported that CSF lactic acid levels reflect the severity of metabolic impairment of the brain in patients with hepatic encephalopathy. Thus, knowledge of increased CSF lactic acid levels in response to neuropathology is not new; however, distinguishing the respective roles of the L and D forms has not been attempted hitherto.

In our NMR-based metabolomics study [14] the high levels of lactic acid, together with several other statistically significant metabolites, led to the formulation of the hypothesis: 'The host's response to neural infection results in an "astrocyte–microglia lactic acid shuttle" (AMLS) that operates in neuroinflammatory diseases, such as TBM'; thereafter, a conceptual model describing the AMLS was constructed. We are therefore seeing that lactic acid, previously considered an unimportant by-product of CNS metabolism, is now receiving more attention as it appears to play an essential role in normal neural homeostasis — in the astrocyte–neuron lactic acid shuttle (ANLS) [19] — and possibly has an important role in neuropathological states. For example, lactic acid is neuroprotective in cerebral ischemia [20], a condition often associated with TBM.

In the present investigation, we used the CSF samples collected in our previous study and employed a derivatization method adapted from Scheijen et al. [5] to differentiate the enantiomers of lactic acid present. We analysed the samples using the highly sensitive, targeted method of ultra-performance liquid chromatography–electrospray ionization–tandem mass spectrometry (UPLC–ESI–MS/MS). We report here for the first time that highly lactic acidotic CSF from infants and children with confirmed TBM exhibits only the L-enantiomer — hence it is a response solely by the host to the infection — and then discuss the relevance of the phenomenon of elevated lactic acid in this example of a neuroinflammatory disease.

Methods

Sampling

The experimental group consisted of infants and children (<13 years of age) ($n = 20$) from the Western Cape region of South Africa, who were directed from local clinics to the paediatric unit of Tygerberg Hospital, Cape Town, on suspicion of meningitis, based on clinical symptoms. Upon admission to hospital, a lumbar CSF sample was taken for differential diagnosis, a portion of which was stored at −80 °C for this study, which was used to confirm a diagnosis of TBM. A diagnosis of TBM was based on the procedure of the uniform research case definition of Marais et al. [21], practiced in our clinical setting. Only children with 'definite' and 'probable' TBM were included in the present patient group. TBM was classified as 'definite' when CSF demonstrated acid-fast bacilli on microscopy, a positive Mtb culture and/or passed a positive CSF Mtb commercial nucleic acid amplification test in a child with symptoms or signs suggestive of the disease. TBM was classified as 'probable' according to a scoring system based on clinical, CSF and neuroimaging criteria, as well as evidence of extraneural TB. Clinical details of the patients are described in the Supplementary Information of Mason et al. [14]. For the purpose of the present study the stage of TBM, as well as the glucose concentration in 16 out of the 20 CSF samples, were made available, as shown in Fig. 2. We also collected a urine sample from our subjects upon admission to hospital. Urine is often the biofluid of choice for investigating the various potential sources of lactic acid, as well as providing for a non-invasive mode of sample collection. A limitation in using urine remains the unpredictable fluctuation in the concentration of targeted metabolites linked to the disease state of the patients. Written consent was obtained from the caregiver and assent if the child was older than 7 years and competent to do so. This study was approved by the Human Research Ethics Committee of Stellenbosch University, South Africa (study no. N11/01/006) — informed consent and assent forms are given as additional information in Additional file 1.

Chemicals

The chemicals used as standards were: sodium L-lactic acid ≥99.0 % (Sigma-Aldrich 71718, CAS: 867-56-1); sodium D-lactic acid ≥99.0 % (Sigma-Aldrich 71716, CAS: 920-49-0); sodium L-lactic acid-3,3,3-d3 (CDN isotopes D-2646, CAS: 79-33-4).

The following chemicals were used in sample preparation and analyses: (+)-O,O'-Diacetyl-L-tartaric anhydride (DATAN) (Sigma-Aldrich 358924, CAS: 6283-74-5); acetonitrile HPLC supragrade (Biosolve 01203502, CAS: 75-05-8); MilliQ water (Millipore, CAS: 7732-18-5); acetic acid 100 % (Merck 1.00063.1000, CAS: 64-19-7); ammonium formate (Sigma-Aldrich 25204, CAS: 540-69-2); dichloromethane (Lab-Scan AR1040A, CAS: 75-09-2); perchloric acid (Sigma-Aldrich 244252, CAS: 7601-90-3); formic acid 98–100 % (Merck 1.00264.1000, CAS: 64-18-6).

Sample preparation and UPLC-ESI-MS/MS analysis

A dilution series of L- and D-lactic acid and a 2.5 mM L-lactic acid-d_3 internal standard (IS) solution were prepared in advance for the calibration curve. A fresh diacetyl-L-tartaric anhydride (DATAN) derivatization solution was prepared by dissolving 250 mg of DATAN in 4 mL dichloromethane and 1 mL acetic acid. Samples were prepared by combining 50 μL CSF / 100 μL urine with 20 μL internal standard solution and 300 μL acetonitrile (ACN) in an Eppendorf tube. Samples were vortexed and centrifuged for 10 min at 3000 RPM in order to remove proteins and other macromolecules. The supernatant was transferred to a clean glass vial and dried under nitrogen gas at 40 °C. To this, 100 μL DATAN solution was added, vortexed and incubated at 75 °C for 30 min. Once again the solution was dried under nitrogen gas at 40 °C and then reconstituted in 200 μL ACN / H_2O (1/2 v / v) for UPLC-ESI-MS/MS analysis. For the UPLC: eluent A (2.5 mM ammonium formate, pH = 3.6) and eluent B (100 % acetonitrile) were used. Samples were analysed on a Waters Acquity UPLC hyphenated to a Quattro premier XE triple quadrupole mass spectrometer using negative ion electrospray ionization — details given in Additional file 1.

After derivatization with DATAN, L- and D-lactic acid were separated from each other on the UPLC column and measured by MS/MS in MRM mode. Use of solvent delay time avoided the introduction of salts in the MS. Results were quantified in terms of the stable isotope-labelled analogue of L-lactic acid. The peak areas corresponding to component-specific transitions were converted via calibration lines to concentrations.

Results

Using a spiked sample containing both the L and D forms of lactic acid, and comparing the chromatogram qualitatively with the stable isotope (L-lactic acid-d_3), it was evident that the UPLC–ESI–MS/MS method used in this study was able to differentiate between the two enantiomers (Fig. 1a and b). We were therefore able to identify and quantify the lactic acid content of the CSF samples from the 20 TBM cases, as described in the 'Methods' section. These results revealed that the lactic acid was exclusively in the L-form — no D-isomer was detected (Fig. 1c) — with a mean concentration of 5.2 mM (SD = 2.6; range: 1.5–10.5 mM).

We also compared the total lactic acid concentrations in the corresponding samples with those derived from the UPLC–ESI–MS/MS method used in the current study and with those from the NMR method of Mason et al. [14], and found a strong linear relationship between the two sets of results ($r = 0.93$), with a statistically significant positive correlation (0.86) and a statistically strong validation of the fit with an R^2 value of 0.73. These data therefore confirm that both methods are highly comparable, demonstrating high reproducibility.

Of the 20 CSF samples examined, a clinician reported glucose values for 16 samples. Figure 2 is a scatterplot, showing both the lactic acid and glucose concentrations of the CSF, with the corresponding stage of the TBM disease. This figure illustrates the inverse relationship between lactic acid and glucose, together with the patient severity outcome after treatment. Additional statistics (shown in Additional file 1) support existing knowledge that glucose is significantly correlated with TBM stage and outcome severity. While L-lactic acid reached high concentrations in CSF samples in some patients from the present group (well above the reference ranges), the L-lactic acid did not correlate with statistical significance with the TBM stage or outcome severity — an observation that may, however, relate to the small sample size of the present group.

In addition to the CSF, the urine was examined of 7 patients upon admission to hospital. Both the L and D forms of lactic acid were detectable (illustrated in Fig. 1d), but in small amounts. The mean urine lactic acid was determined to be 98.4 μM for the L form (SD = 37.4; range: <50–155 μM) and 47.4 μM for the D form (SD = 56.7; range: nd–148 μM). The contribution of D-lactic acid from the gut microbiota cannot be distinguished from any possible influence of the Mtb, and the small amount of urinary lactic acid was well within the normal range. We conclude that urine is not a suitable biofluid for monitoring and assessing lactic acid for diagnostic purposes in TBM.

Discussion

In the present investigation we identified and quantified the L and D enantiomers of lactic acid in the CSF of 20

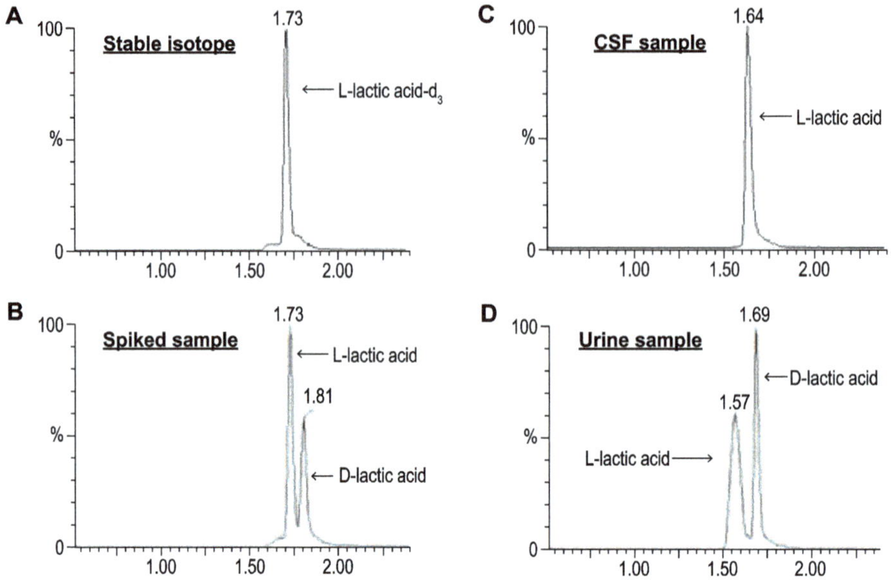

Fig. 1 Representative chromatograms depicting **a** definitive identification of L-lactic acid using the stable isotope (L-lactic acid-d_3); **b** clear differentiation of L and D forms of lactic acid in the spiked sample; **c** in CSF, complete lack of D form of lactic acid with only the L form present; and **d** presence of both L and D forms of lactic acid in urine

cases of infants and children with confirmed TBM, using UPLC–ESI–MS/MS. This study was motivated by our NMR-based metabolomics study [14], in which the most prominent feature of the CSF of these TBM cases was highly elevated lactic acid. We therefore sought to determine the source and form of the lactic acid — was it a response from the host (which would generate the L-isomer), of microbial origin (which produces the D-isomer), or both? Because NMR is incapable of distinguishing the enantiomers of lactic acid, we conducted this follow-up study with the means to identify the separate isomers.

We have shown that both enantiomers were detectable in urine samples, but the elevated lactic acid in the CSF samples of the TBM patients consisted of only L-lactic acid, and hence was produced exclusively by the host with no contribution from the Mtb. Moreover, Fig. 2 shows that as the TBM disease progressed into later stages there was a drop in patient prognosis (i.e., increased outcome severity). Generally, in more advanced TBM stages, fewer energy substrates are available for microglia activity and decreased protection of neurons from the lactic acid. During this period, irreversible

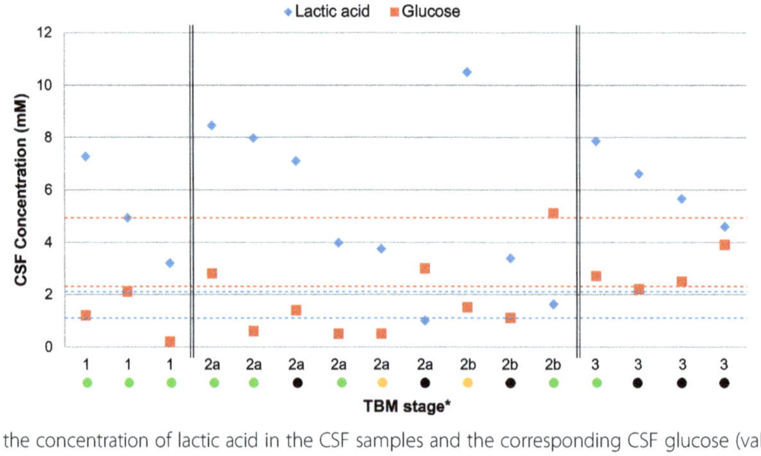

Fig. 2 Scatterplot showing the concentration of lactic acid in the CSF samples and the corresponding CSF glucose (values not reported in text) over different stages of TBM disease (*dashed lines indicate respective reference ranges*). Outcome severity: *green circle* = normal; *yellow circle* = mild neurological problems (e.g., learning difficulties, visual impairment); *black circle* = severe neurological problems (e.g., partial paralysis, severe motor impairment, cranial nerve palsy). *TBM stage: 1 = Glasgow coma score (GCS) 15 and no focal neurology; 2a = GCS 15 plus focal neurology; 2b = GCS 11–14 with focal neurology; 3 = GCS <11

neurological damage can begin to occur. Lactic acid boosts energy production in the brain and increases neuroprotection, thus potentially improving the prognosis of patients, especially those at high risk. TBM patients in late stages of the disease who exhibit CSF with low lactic acid and glucose may be beyond help as the accumulated neural damage and lack of energy substrate can be fatal.

The origin and rationale of high levels of lactic acid produced by the host in response to a neuroinflammatory disease such as TBM is unclear. Interconversion of lactic acid and pyruvate occurs via lactate dehydrogenase, with increased lactic acid typically being associated with anaerobic respiration. Thus, elevated levels of lactic acid in the CSF due to neuroinflammation could be due to hypoxia caused by ischemia, or by increased glucose levels and hence increased flow through the glycolysis pathway. However, in TBM cases there are typically low levels of glucose in the CSF [22], corresponding to a CSF to serum glucose ratio less than 0.5 or an absolute CSF glucose concentration of less than 2.2 mM. Furthermore, several studies have shown no correlation between CSF lactic acid levels and cerebral blood flow (i.e., they are unrelated to ischemia) [23–25]. Thus, elevated lactic acid in CSF of TBM cases is unlikely to be due to anaerobic respiration but instead is possibly a product of temporarily increased flux in the glycolysis pathway.

The results reported here also provide experimental evidence which supports our proposed AMLS hypothesis [14]. The hypothesis postulates that, when the brain is in crisis due to neuroinflammatory-inducing infection, energy flow in brain metabolism is shifted away from the neurons and shunted towards the microglia. Hence, in neuroinflammatory infectious diseases, such as TBM, lactic acid produced by glycolysis in astrocytes participates in the activated immune response and, in association with ketones and gluconeogenic amino acids, is collectively directed from the neurons preferentially into microglia where it enters the mitochondrial citric acid cycle. This process contributes to oxidative phosphorylation and hence produces high levels of adenosine triphosphate (ATP) and forms of reactive oxygen species, such as hydrogen peroxide, required for degradation of the invading pathogen.

Further studies are needed to advance our understanding of the dynamics involved in this lactic acid phenomenon — for example: determining the rate at which microglia produce lactic acid under neuroinflammatory conditions such as TBM; an in vitro scenario testing whether a high level of lactic acid within the microglia reduces the uptake of interstitial lactic acid due to concentration gradients, accounting for the high concentrations of lactic acid in the CSF; more in-depth studies into transporters that shuttle lactate, namely, monocarboxylate transporters; and, in a clinical setting, determining the impact of adjunctive treatments involving direct infusion of sodium lactate into the CSF of advanced stage TBM patients.

While simple in design and execution, this study provides important information not reported before. The implications of these results are compelling in that the levels of lactic acid in the CSF, produced by the host, should be carefully considered by the clinician, especially regarding neuroinflammatory diseases. The reason for this is that lactic acid is used preferentially over glucose in such cases [26–30], provides a boost in neuroprotection [31, 32], and aids microglia energy demands in their bactericidal actions. Thus lactic acid has a potential beneficial role in the clinical management of neurological disorders [33].

Conclusions

In summary, we have shown that the contribution from Mtb in the form of D-lactic acid in all our TBM-infected CSF cases was not demonstrable. The lactic acid consisted solely of the L-form, with the host being responsible for its high concentrations in the CSF. Beyond this study, the ramifications of determining the enantiomers — and by doing so the origin — of particular metabolites holds importance for future research. Knowledge of what is produced by the host and what is of microbial origin could revolutionize treatment regimes and allow us to understand disease pathogenesis and progress better. Therefore adaptation of the method presented should be made routine for common, optically active markers of disease to determine their respective enantiomers, particularly in the field of metabolomics.

Abbreviations

ACN, acetonitrile; AMLS, astrocyte–microglia lactic acid shuttle; ANLS, astrocyte–neuron lactic acid shuttle; ATP, adenosine triphosphate; BBB, blood–brain barrier; CNS, central nervous system; CSF, cerebrospinal fluid; D-, dextrorotary; DATAN, diacetyl-L-tartaric anhydride; IS, internal standard; L-, levorotary; MRM, multiple reaction monitoring; Mtb, *Mycobacterium tuberculosis*; NMR, ^{1}H nuclear magnetic resonance; SD, standard deviation; SI, supplementary information; TB, tuberculosis; TBM, tuberculous meningitis; UPLC–ESI–MS/MS, ultra-performance liquid chromatography–electrospray ionization–tandem mass spectrometry

Acknowledgements

S.M. and R.S. are recipients of a Desmond Tutu-NRF-VU doctoral fellowship for a joint PhD study between the Vrije Universiteit in Amsterdam, the Netherlands and North-West University (Potchefstroom), and the University of Stellenbosch, South Africa, respectively. Research funding for this project is provided by the Technological Innovation Agency (TIA) of the Department of Science and Technology of South Africa. Opinions expressed and conclusions arrived at, are those of the authors and are not necessarily to be attributed to the funding body TIA.

Authors' contributions

RS is the paediatrician who collected the samples and clinical information, and treated the patients. WK and AvC supervised and conducted the experimental work. CJR and AMTvF are the supervisors of SM and directed and contributed to the paper. SM analysed the results and wrote the manuscript. All authors contributed in the revision of the manuscript and approved the final version.

Competing interests

The authors declare that they have no competing interests.

Consent for publication

N/A – all data are anonymous and consent to publish abides according to the informed consent.

Author details

[1]Centre for Human Metabolomics, Faculty of Natural Sciences, North-West University (Potchefstroom Campus), Private Bag X6001, Potchefstroom 2531, South Africa. [2]Laboratory Genetic Metabolic Diseases, Department of Clinical Chemistry, Academic Medical Center, University of Amsterdam, Amsterdam, The Netherlands. [3]Department of Paediatrics and Child Health, Faculty of Medicine and Health Sciences, Stellenbosch University, PO Box 19063, Tygerberg 7505, South Africa. [4]Department of Paediatric Infectious Diseases–Immunology and Rheumatology, Vrije Universiteit Medical Centre, De Boelelaan 1117, 1081HV Amsterdam, The Netherlands.

References

1. Ewaschuk JB, Naylor JM, Zello GA. D-lactate in human and ruminant metabolism. J Nutr. 2005;135(7):1619–25.
2. Stolberg L, Rolfe R, Gitlin N, Merritt J, Mann Jr L, Linder J, et al. D-Lactic acidosis due to abnormal gut flora: diagnosis and treatment of two cases. N Engl J Med. 1982;306:1344–8.
3. Duzgun AP, Bugdayci G, Sayin B, Ozmen MM, Ozer MV, Coskun F. Serum D-lactate: a useful diagnostic marker for acute appendicitis. Hepatogastroenterology. 2006;54(77):1483–6.
4. Çaglayan F, Çakmak M, Çaglayan O, Çavusoglu T. Plasma D-lactate levels in diagnosis of appendicitis. J Invest Surg. 2003;16:233–7.
5. Scheijen JL, Hanssen NM, van de Waarenburg MP, Jonkers DM, Stehouwer CD, Schalkwijk CG. L (+) and D (−) lactate are increased in plasma and urine samples of type 2 diabetes as measured by a simultaneous quantification of L (+) and D (−) lactate by reversed-phase liquid chromatography tandem mass spectrometry. Exp Diabetes Res. 2012;2012:234812.
6. Sheedy JR, Wettenhall RE, Scanlon D, Gooley PR, Lewis DP, McGregor N, et al. Increased D-lactic acid intestinal bacteria in patients with chronic fatigue syndrome. In Vivo. 2009;23(4):621–8.
7. Kowlgi NG, Chhabra L. D-Lactic acidosis: an underrecognized complication of short bowel syndrome. Gastroenterol Res Pract. 2015;2015:476215. doi:10.1155/2015/476215.
8. Genton B, Berger JP. Cerebrospinal fluid lactate in 78 cases of adult meningitis. J Intensive Care Med. 1990;16:196–200.
9. Huy NT, Thao NT, Diep DT, Kikuchi M, Zamora J, Hirayama K. Cerebrospinal fluid lactate concentration to distinguish bacterial from aseptic meningitis: a systemic review and meta-analysis. Crit Care. 2010;14:R240.
10. Abro AH, Abdou AS, Ustadi AM, Saleh AA, Younis J, Doleh WF. CSF lactate level: a useful diagnostic tool to differentiate acute bacterial and viral meningitis. JPMA J Pak Med Assoc. 2009;59(8):508–11.
11. Thwaites GE, Chau TTH, Stepniewska K, Phu NH, Chuong LV, Sinh DX, et al. Diagnosis of adult tuberculous meningitis by use of clinical and laboratory features. Lancet. 2002;360:1287–92.
12. Thwaites GE, Caws M, Chau TTH, Dung NT, Campbell JI, Phu NH, et al. Comparison of conventional bacteriology with nucleic acid amplification (amplified mycobacterium direct test) for diagnosis of tuberculous meningitis before and after inception of antituberculosis chemotherapy. J Clin Microbiol. 2004;42:996–1002.
13. Torok ME, Chau TTH, Mai PP, Phong ND, Dung NT, Chuong LV, et al. Clinical and microbiological features of HIV-associated tuberculous meningitis in Vietnamese adults. PLoS One. 2008;3:e1772.
14. Mason S, van Furth AM, Mienie LJ, Engelke UF, Wevers RA, Solomons R, et al. A hypothetical astrocyte–microglia lactate shuttle derived from a 1H NMR metabolomics analysis of cerebrospinal fluid from a cohort of South African children with tuberculous meningitis. Metabolomics. 2015;11:822–37.
15. Leen WG, Willemsen MA, Wevers RA, Verbeek MM. Cerebrospinal fluid glucose and lactate: age-specific reference values and implications for clinical practice. PLoS One. 2012;7:e42745.
16. White N, Looareesuwan S, Phillips R, Warrell D, Chanthavanich P, Pongpaew P. Pathophysiological and prognostic significance of cerebrospinal-fluid lactate in cerebral malaria. Lancet. 1985;325:776–8.
17. Medana IM, Hien TT, Day NP, Nguyen HP, Nguyen THM, Van Chu'ong L, et al. The clinical significance of cerebrospinal fluid levels of kynurenine pathway metabolites and lactate in severe malaria. J Infect Dis. 2002;185:650–6.
18. Yao H, Sadoshima S, Fujii K, Kusuda K, Ishitsuka T, Tamaki K, et al. Cerebrospinal fluid lactate in patients with hepatic encephalopathy. Eur Neurol. 1987;27:182–7.
19. Pellerin L, Magistretti PJ. Sweet sixteen for ANLS. J Cereb Blood Flow Metab. 2011;32:1152–66.
20. Castillo X, Rosafio K, Wyss MT, Drandarov K, Buck A, Pellerin L, et al. A probable dual mode of action for both L-and D-lactate neuroprotection in cerebral ischemia. J Cereb Blood Flow Metab. 2015;35(10):1561–9.
21. Marais S, Thwaites G, Schoeman JF, Török ME, Misra UK, Prasad K, et al. Tuberculous meningitis: a uniform case definition for use in clinical research. Lancet Infect Dis. 2010;10(11):803–12.
22. Thwaites G, Fisher M, Hemingway C, Scott G, Solomon T, Innes J. British Infection Society guidelines for the diagnosis of tuberculosis of the central nervous system in adults and children. J Infect. 2009;59:167–87.
23. Brodersen P, Jørgensen EO. Cerebral blood flow and oxygen uptake, and cerebrospinal fluid biochemistry in severe coma. J Neurol Neurosurg Psychiatry. 1974;37:384–91.
24. DeSalles AA, Kontos HA, Becker DP, Yang MS, Ward JD, Moulton R, et al. Prognostic significance of ventricular CSF lactic acidosis in severe head injury. J Neurosurg. 1986;65:615–24.
25. De Salles AA, Muizelaar PJ, Young HF. Hyperglycemia, cerebrospinal fluid lactic acidosis, and cerebral blood flow in severely head-injured patients. Neurosurgery. 1987;21:45–50.
26. Schurr A, West CA, Rigor BM. Lactate-supported synaptic function in the rat hippocampal slice preparation. Science. 1988;240:1326–8.
27. Schurr A, Payne RS, Miller JJ, Rigor BM. Glia are the main source of lactate utilized by neurons for recovery of function posthypoxia. Brain Res. 1997;774:221–4.
28. Schurr A, Payne RS, Miller JJ, Rigor BM. Brain lactate is an obligatory aerobic energy substrate for functional recovery after hypoxia: further in vitro validation. J Neurochem. 1997;69:423–6.
29. Schurr A, Payne RS, Miller JJ, Rigor BM. Brain lactate, not glucose, fuels the recovery of synaptic function from hypoxia upon reoxygenation: an in vitro study. Brain Res. 1997;744:105–11.
30. Schurr A, Payne RS, Tseng MT, Miller JJ, Rigor BM. The glucose paradox in cerebral ischemia: new insights. Ann N Y Acad Sci. 1999;893:386–90.
31. Cater HL, Benham CD, Sundstrom LE. Neuroprotective role of monocarboxylate transport during glucose deprivation in slice cultures of rat hippocampus. J Physiol. 2001;531:459–66.
32. Cater HL, Chandratheva A, Benham CD, Morrison B, Sundstrom LE. Lactate and glucose as energy substrates during, and after, oxygen deprivation in rat hippocampal acute and cultured slices. J Neurochem. 2003;87:1381–90.
33. Taher M, Leen WG, Wevers RA, Willemsen MA. Lactate and its many faces. Eur J Paediatr Neurol. 2016;20(1):3–10.

11

The dubious value of cerebrospinal fluid adenosine deaminase measurement for the diagnosis of tuberculous meningitis

Pieter Ekermans[1,3*], Adriano Dusé[2] and Jaya George[1]

Abstract

Background: The diagnosis of tuberculous meningitis (TBM) can be extremely difficult in the absence of culture confirmation. Cerebrospinal fluid (CSF) adenosine deaminase (ADA) can potentially assist in this regard, although its current value remains unclear. The literature on the usefulness of CSF ADA in TBM diagnosis is inconsistent, especially from an analytical point of view.

Methods: A retrospective analysis of clinical and laboratory data relating to all CSF ADA requests during 2009 and 2010 in a South African quaternary healthcare setting was performed. A CSF ADA cut-off for TBM diagnosis was calculated using receiver operating characteristic curve analysis. The performance of CSF ADA in different infective and non-infective categories was assessed.

Results: In total, 3548 CSF ADA requests were considered over the 2-year period. Of these, 1490 were for patients for whom both a CSF ADA and a mycobacterial culture were requested. The optimal cut-off was calculated at 2.0 U/L (AUC = 0.86; 95% CI = 0.82 – 0.89; p-value < 0.01; sensitivity of 85.9% (95% CI of 77.0 – 92.3) and specificity of 77.7% (95% CI of 75.4 – 79.8%); positive likelihood ratio = 3.85 and negative likelihood ratio = 0.18). At this cut-off 13 TBM cases were missed.

Conclusion: An optimal cut-off for routine use could not be established as too many TBM cases were missed. Specimen integrity, lack of ADA assay standardisation and overlap in performance of the assay in different diagnostic categories affect interpretation.

Keywords: Tuberculosis, Meningitis, Adenosine deaminase, Giusti, Pre-analytical, Youden

Background

The diagnosis of tuberculous meningitis (TBM) in general can be extremely difficult in the absence of culture confirmation. A non-definitive test such as cerebrospinal fluid (CSF) adenosine deaminase (ADA) could potentially assist in the regard, although its current value for the diagnosis of TBM remains unclear.

South Africa is a low to middle income country with a heavy burden of infectious diseases, particularly Human Immunodeficiency virus (HIV) and tuberculosis. As the diagnosis of TBM based on culture confirmation can take weeks, clinicians rely heavily on CSF ADA as a rule-in test, because of its fast turn-around time. However, as indicated in Table 1, the sensitivity and specificity of CSF ADA utilised in the diagnostic work-up of suspected TBM patients cited in the literature vary considerably. One of the reasons for this is the different cut-offs used. Mishra and colleagues reported a cut-off of 5 U/L with a sensitivity of 89% and specificity of 92% [1], whilst others have reported a sensitivity of 66.6% and specificity of 90% using a cut-off of 10 U/L [2] and a sensitivity of 100% and specificity of 99% using a cut-off of 20 U/L [3]. Furthermore, additional confounding factors include, among others: differences in the number of participants/specimens [4, 5], ages and HIV-status(where stated) of participants [1, 3, 6–8] and

* Correspondence: ekermansp@ampath.co.za
[1]Department of Chemical Pathology, University of Witwatersrand and National Health Laboratory Service, Johannesburg, South Africa
[3]Department of Chemical Pathology and Department of Clinical Microbiology and Infectious Diseases, School of Pathology, Faculty of Health Sciences, University of Witwatersrand and National Health Laboratory Service, 7 York Road, Johannesburg, South Africa
Full list of author information is available at the end of the article

Table 1 Factors confounding the interpretation of literature on CSF ADA

Factors	Variables			
CSF ADA cut-offs	Study from India [1]	5 U/L	Sensitivity: 89%	Specificity: 92%
	Study from India [2]	10 U/L	Sensitivity: 66.6%	Specificity: 90%
	Study from Finland [3]	20 U/L	Sensitivity: 100%	Specificity: 99%
ADA assay types	Giusti method [8, 10]	Non-Giusti method [6, 11]		In-house method [6, 12]
Total number of participants/specimens	Range: 26 – 417 [4, 5]			
Age of participants	Adults only [3]	Children only [1]		Pooled data for adults and children [6]
Definition of TBM groups	Clinical as well culture evidence was used to group participants [1] Culture-positive cases sometimes was < 10 cases [3, 9]			
Definition of control groups	One infective category: bacterial meningitis only [4]			
	More than one infective category: viral/aseptic meningitis, bacterial meningitis, fungal meningitis [8]			
	Infective and non-infective categories: bacterial meningitis, viral meningitis, hydrocephalus, epilepsy, malignancy, subarachnoid haemorrhage, senile dementia, normal CSF [6]			
HIV status	HIV status is not always specified in the literature [7, 8]			

variable definitions of TBM [1, 3, 9] and selection of control groups [4, 6, 8]. Finally, various methods have been used to measure CSF ADA such as those based on the Giusti method [8, 10] or on non-Giusti methods [6, 11]. Many of the methods used are developed in-house [6, 12] (see Table 1).

In view of the limitations described above, the objective of this study was to determine an appropriate CSF ADA cut-off level in a quaternary healthcare setting in South Africa to assist in the diagnosis of TBM.

Methods

A retrospective study was conducted over a period of two years (2009 and 2010) in which 3495 medical records were reviewed. As some patients had more than one admission the final number of records eligible for analysis was 3548 (see Fig. 1).

All adult and paediatric, male and female, as well as HIV-positive and HIV-negative patients for whom a CSF ADA was requested were included in this study. If a patient had more than one specimen taken during a particular admission period, only the CSF ADA result from the first specimen was considered. If more than one admission occurred during the study period, each admission was considered as a separate event. All data previously captured on the laboratory information system up to and including the admission data from which the CSF ADA test request originates were considered. Any subsequent admissions and associated data where CSF ADA tests were not requested, as well as results emanating from other hospitals were excluded (see Fig. 1).

The cut-off age of 12 years was arbitrarily applied to separate adult and paediatric patients thus including adolescents in the adult patient category.

For the purpose of this study patients were considered HIV-positive based on one of the following criteria: (1) presence of a positive rapid test as well as a positive enzyme-linked immunosorbent assay (ELISA), (2) presence of a positive initial and confirmatory ELISA, and (3) presence of a positive polymerase chain reaction (PCR) for HIV [13]. In addition (1) the presence of an elevated HIV viral load, and (2) positivity for HIV as stated in the patient file (where tests were done at a different laboratory) were used to assign HIV positivity. In patients aged 18 months or younger, only the HIV PCR result was considered to assign positivity to a patient in this age group [13].

A CD4 absolute cell count of 350 x 10^6/L was used to further classify patients according to the 2010 World Health Organisation (WHO) guidelines regarding treatment for HIV [14].

Subjects were categorised as 'Confirmed TBM' and various infective non-tuberculous pathologies (*confirmed infective categories*) according to definitive evidence (including culture, molecular, and/or serological evidence). For a specific breakdown of the cases considered for the 'Confirmed TBM' category, please see Table 2. In addition suspected diagnoses of infective origin were captured separately (*suspected infective categories*) according to the evidence as documented by clinicians in patient files. In cases when CSF ADA was requested as part of a diagnostic work-up, but a non-infectious diagnosis was ultimately made by the clinician, a review of clinical, radiological and histological evidence was performed to exclude the possibility of TBM. The 'Other' category includes pathologies not involving CSF or intracranial anatomy. The 'No diagnosis made' category includes patients where no clinical, radiological or laboratory evidence was found to assign patients to any of the other categories. CSF ADA performance was assessed in all these categories (see Fig. 2).

The Diazyme ADA assay (Diazyme, United States of America) for the measurement of total ADA was used

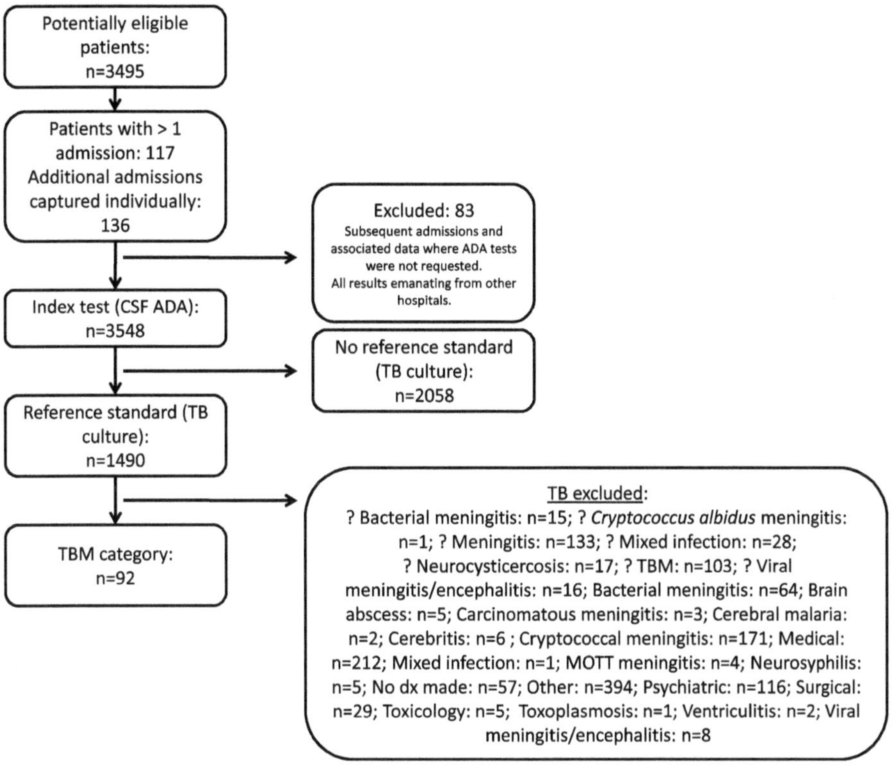

Fig. 1 Flow of participants throughout the study. Key to Fig. 1: ? – Suspected infective categories, dx - diagnosis. *Confirmed infective categories*: refers to all those infective categories where the '?' is omitted. For further breakdown of the 'Confirmed TBM category' please see Table 2

and performed on a Pentra analyser (Horiba Medical Diagnostics, Japan) with colorimetric detection. The clinical decision limit for TBM used at this healthcare facility was 6 U/L as determined in a South African study by Blake and Berman [6].

The median, interquartile range (IQR), the 95% distribution of values and outliers for the CSF ADA results for each of the categories defined for this study were determined.

All CSF ADA test results for the demographic categories were compared using the Mann–Whitney test for non-parametric data [15]. Similarly CSF ADA results for the 'Confirmed TBM' category were compared to all CSF ADA results for patients where culture for *Mycobacterium tuberculosis* complex (TB) on CSF was either not requested or negative, i.e. on the total population for this study ($n = 3548$). Using the Mann–Whitney test, CSF ADA results in the confirmed infective categories were compared between 'Confirmed viral meningitis/encephalitis', 'Confirmed ventriculitis', 'Confirmed bacterial meningitis' and 'Confirmed TBM' groups.

Receiver operating characteristic (ROC) curves and the Youden index were generated to establish the optimal cut-off point for ADA interpretation in patients for whom a CSF specimen was submitted for both mycobacterial culture and ADA determination [16]. Using the optimal cut-off point, sensitivity and specificity, as well as positive and negative likelihood ratios were determined. A p-value of < 0.05 was considered statistically significant.

The dataset ($n = 1490$) was arbitrarily split into a training and validation cohort after random assignment of values to each of the CSF ADA results to assess for overfitting of the model. The ROC curve and Youden index

Table 2 Breakdown of cases considered for the 'Confirmed TBM' category ($n = 92$)

Patients		Reason for assigning patients to the 'Confirmed TBM' category
88 patients	83 patients	Patients admitted to hospital for the first time and were culture positive
	5 patients	Known patients, where culture positivity was determined in a previous admission during the 2009 – 2010 period; the patient still fell within the 9–12 months treatment period; the CSF specimen in the current admission was negative on culture
4 patients		Patients were positive for acid-fast bacilli on microscopy only[a]

[a] These four patients where included due to HIV status (including CD4 count $< 350 \times 10^6$/L) and/or had suspicious radiological findings

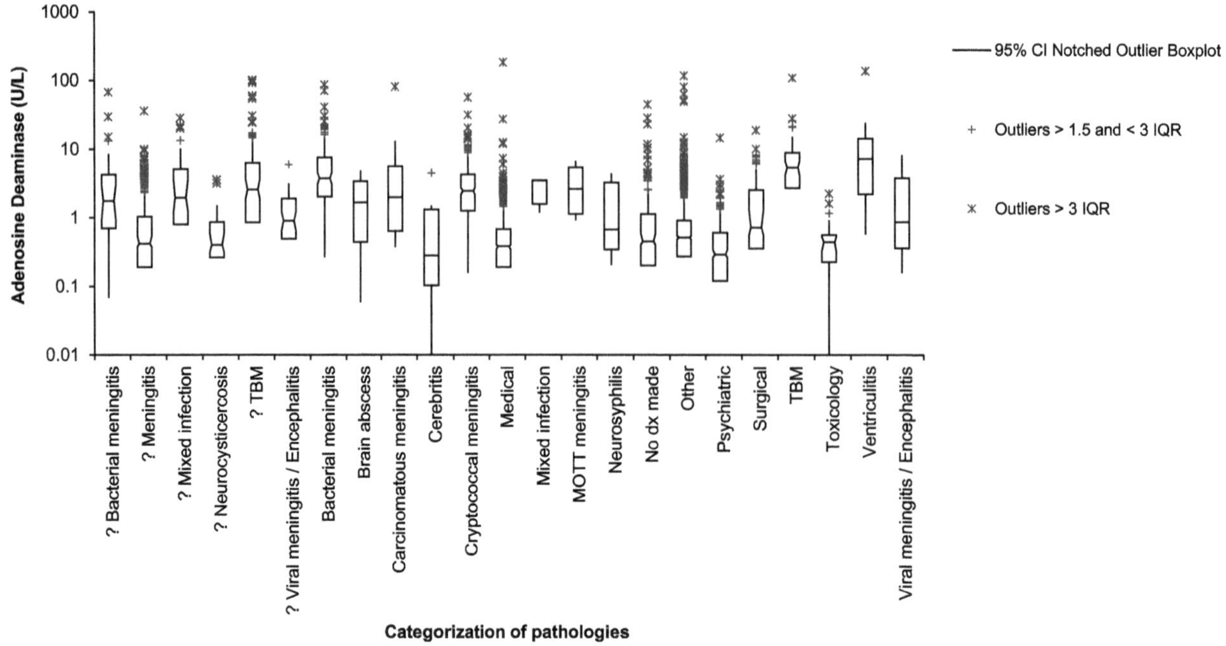

Fig. 2 CSF ADA values for each of the categories. Key to Fig. 2: CI - confidence interval; IQR - interquartile range; ? - Suspected infective categories, dx - diagnosis. *Confirmed infective categories*: refers to all those infective categories where the '?' is omitted

was generated for the training set. The CSF ADA cut-off point determined was applied to the validation set. The same diagnostic accuracy parameters were determined for the validation cohort as above.

For each of the demographic categories from which a CSF sample was submitted for mycobacterial culture and ADA determination, ROC curve analysis was utilised to determine differences in these groups' cut-off point for ADA. The area under the curve (AUC) was used to compare the individual ROC curves [15].

CSF sample integrity as determined by its appearance (clear, turbid, bloodstained and xanthochromic) was used to re-categorise CSF ADA results and these categories were compared by establishing the minimum, median, and maximum values as well as the interquartile ranges (IQRs).

A uniform case definition for diagnosis of TBM as determined by Marais and colleagues was used to re-categorise patients and CSF ADA results were assessed in each of the categories [17]. The CSF ADA result is not included in this definition.

Statistical analyses were performed on Analyse-it (Analyse-it Software, Ltd., United Kingdom).

Results

The majority of the patients in this study were adults ($n = 3170$, 89.3%), of which 2009 individuals (56.6%) were between the ages of 20 and 40 years. Male and female patients were roughly equal in number ($n = 1721$, 48.5% and $n = 1824$, 51.4% respectively). Most patients were HIV-positive (n = 1970, 55.5%). Of the total population, CD4 cell counts for 1456 (41.0%) patients measured ≤ 350 x 10^6/L. Table 3 summarises the demographic characteristics, HIV status and the CD4 cell count as determined by the medical records reviewed ($n = 3548$).

The performance of CSF ADA measurement in each of the infective and non-infective categories is shown in Fig. 2. Figure 2 shows the outlier values in terms of IQR

Table 3 Demographic characteristics, HIV status and the CD4 cell count as determined by the medical records reviewed ($n = 3548$)

Age	Adult patients: $n = 3170$ (89.3%)
	Paediatric patients: $n = 365$ (10.3%)
	No information regarding age available: n = 13 (0.4%)
Sex	Male patients: $n = 1721$ (48.5%)
	Female patients: $n = 1824$ (51.4%)
	No information regarding sex available: n = 3 (0.1%)
HIV status	HIV-positive patients: $n = 1970$ (55.5%)
	HIV-negative patients: $n = 693$ (19.5%)
	No information regarding HIV status available: n = 885 (25%)
CD4 cell count	Patients with CD4 cell count > 350 × 10^6/L: $n = 235$ (6.6%)
	Patients with CD4 cell count ≤ 350 × 10^6/L: $n = 1456$ (41.0%)
	No information regarding CD4 cell count available: n = 1857 (52.3%)

as well as the 95% distribution of the values in each of the categories. Notably the total number of CSF ADA results ($n = 3548$) follow a non-parametric distribution. For the majority of results ($n = 3415$) CSF ADA values were less than 10 U/L. The CSF ADA results in Fig. 2 indicate a considerable overlap, not only in the outliers for each category, but also in each category's 95% distribution of values. Of note the 'Confirmed ventriculitis' category had the widest 95% distribution of values.

In all comparisons of CSF ADA results were higher in adult than paediatric patients ($p < 0.02$), higher in male than female patients ($p < 0.01$), higher in HIV-positive than HIV-negative patients ($p < 0.01$) and higher in patients with CD4 cell counts $\leq 350 \times 10^6$/L as opposed to patients with CD4 cell counts $> 350 \times 10^6$/L ($p < 0.01$).

In Table 4 'Confirmed TBM' CSF ADA results ($n = 92$) are compared to all CSF ADA results for patients where TB culture on CSF was either absent or negative ($n = 3456$). Similar statistically significant results ($p < 0.01$) were obtained from the sub-set analysis of medical records ($n = 1490$) where both culture and ADA was requested on a CSF specimen.

Individually all CSF ADA results in the 'Confirmed cryptococcal meningitis', 'Confirmed bacterial meningitis', 'Confirmed viral meningitis/encephalitis' and 'Confirmed ventriculitis' categories were compared with the 'Confirmed TBM' category (see Table 5). Statistically significant differences were noted in the comparisons between the 'Confirmed TBM' and 'Confirmed cryptococcal meningitis' and 'Confirmed viral meningitis/encephalitis' categories ($p < 0.01$). This however was not the case in the comparison between the 'Confirmed bacterial meningitis' and 'Confirmed TBM' categories ($p = 0.06$) and the 'Confirmed ventriculitis' and 'Confirmed TBM' categories ($p = 0.42$).

ROC curve analysis (see Fig. 3) was performed for all events where both an ADA and culture for TB were requested on a CSF specimen ($n = 1490$) and an AUC of 0.86 (95% CI of 0.82 – 0.89, $p < 0.01$) was obtained. This analysis together with the Youden index indicates that the optimal cut-off of CSF ADA in suspected TBM patients is 2.0 U/L with a sensitivity of 85.9% (95% CI of 77.0 – 92.3) and specificity of 77.7% (95% CI of 75.4 – 79.8%). The positive and negative likelihood ratios were 3.85 and 0.18. It is important to note that, even at this cut-off, 13 of 92 'Confirmed TBM' cases (14.1%) were missed (see Table 6). Target and actual sensitivities and specificities at different CSF ADA levels using this ROC curve are noted in Table 7.

Table 4 Statistical comparison of 'Confirmed TBM' CSF ADA results with all CSF ADA results for patients where TB culture on CSF was absent and or negative (in U/L)

	TBM (n = 92)	Non-TBM (n = 3456)	
Median	5.4000	0.6000	$p < 0.01$
95% CI	4.1000 – 6.6875	0.6000 – 0.6000	
Ranges	0.0000 - 108.0000	0.0000 - 182.5000	

Key to this table: TBM – refers to 'Confirmed TBM' patients; Non-TBM – refers to patients where TB culture on CSF was either not requested or negative

Training and validation cohorts where determined for the dataset $n = 1490$. The AUC of the ROC curve generated for the training cohort was 0.82 (95% CI of 0.76 – 0.88, $p < 0.01$). For this curve the Youden index determined the appropriate CSF ADA cut-off to be 2.20 U/L. When this cut-off was applied to the validation cohort, the sensitivity, specificity, positive and negative likelihood ratios were 87.5% (95% CI of 74.8 – 95.3%), 77.9% (95% CI of 74.6 – 80.9%), 3.96 and 0.16 respectively.

In sub-set ROC analyses performed for each of the 8 categories listed in Table 3, CSF ADA cut-offs were low (<3 U/L). No optimal cut-off could be determined for paediatric patients and HIV-negative patients with suspected TBM (see Table 8).

All CSF ADA requests ($n = 3548$) were re-categorised according to their integrity and are plotted in Fig. 4. The majority of the specimens were clear and colourless ($n = 3003$, 84.6%). Of note is the considerable spread of CSF ADA results for the 'Ungraded xanthochromia' category compared to the 'Clear and colourless' category, both in terms of outliers and 95% distribution of values. When excluding all specimens that were not clear and colourless ($n = 545$, 15.4%), no change was noted in the ROC curve analysis and the same cut-off of 2.0 U/L using the Youden index was determined. Furthermore the overlap in CSF ADA results for the different categories remained.

According to the uniform case definition, 68.5% ($n = 1024$) of cases that had both a CSF ADA and a mycobacterial culture requested, fell in the 'Not TBM' category. Of these cases, 20.2% ($n = 207$) had CSF ADA results ≥ 2 U/L and 6.2% ($n = 63$) had CSF ADA results ≥ 6 U/L (see Table 9).

Discussion

TBM is a challenging diagnosis especially in view of the fact that the diagnostic gold standard, culture, generally performs so poorly. We aimed to assess the performance of ADA in all clinical scenarios where CSF sampling was performed and ADA was requested as part of a patient work-up. To date this study is the largest and most comprehensive analysis of ADA performance in CSF samples.

An unusually low cut-off for CSF ADA of 2.0 U/L was determined. This contrasts with the first South African study on the use of CSF ADA that determined a cut-off of 6.0 U/L to indicate probable TBM [6]. In the current study, a similarly low cut-off value (<3 U/L) was determined for all of the categories according to demography,

Table 5 Individual comparison of CSF ADA between different confirmed infective categories and the 'Confirmed TBM' category

	'Confirmed TBM' ($n = 92$)	'Confirmed cryptococcal meningitis' ($n = 302$)	'Confirmed viral meningitis/ encephalitis' ($n = 14$)	'Confirmed bacterial meningitis' ($n = 134$)	'Confirmed ventriculitis' ($n = 16$)
Median	5.4000	2.4000	0.85000	3.7000	7.1500
95% CI	4.1000 - 6.6875	2.1000 - 2.7000	0.3896 - 3.7147	3.0176 - 4.4648	2.3470 - 13.8145
p-value		$p < 0.01$	$p < 0.01$	$p = 0.06$	$p = 0.42$
Ranges	0.0000 - 108.0000	0.2000 - 56.1000	0.2000 - 8.0000	0.3000 - 86.3000	0.6000 - 135.7000

HIV-status and CD4 count. The non-parametric distribution of the CSF ADA results assessed may have contributed to this unusual finding. Selection bias and ascertainment bias may have been introduced in the way the CSF ADA results were chosen. In addition, CSF ADA performance in the 'Confirmed TBM' category was compared to a significantly larger set of results in patients where TB culture of CSF was negative ($n = 1398$) and may have skewed the ROC curve analysis. Furthermore, pre-analytical and analytical factors may also have contributed. Similar results were obtained when arbitrarily splitting the dataset ($n = 1490$) in a training cohort and a validation cohort. Overfitting of the model is unlikely to have occurred.

It is important to also note than when confirmed TBM ADA results were compared with all ADA results for patients where TB culture on CSF was either not requested or negative, a statistically significant difference was determined (Table 3). However, the maximum CSF ADA value for the 'Non-TBM' category indicated in Table 3 is higher than that for the 'TBM' category. In addition, upon detailed comparison of the individual categories, there is significant overlap regarding each category's 95% distribution of values, as well as their outliers (Fig. 2). This suggests that the CSF ADA result is not reliable for the presumptive diagnosis of TBM. Elevations in non-infectious pathologies have also been noted by other researchers [3, 18].

In clinical practice CSF ADA is used for rule-in purposes. If CSF ADA is used for rule-in/screening purposes the sensitivity should be optimized, but this may result in the cut-off of 2.0 U/L being dropped even further in the current data set. If ADA is used for rule-out purposes the specificity should be optimized, resulting in an elevation of the cut-off with a considerable loss of sensitivity (see Table 7) in the current data set. Given the

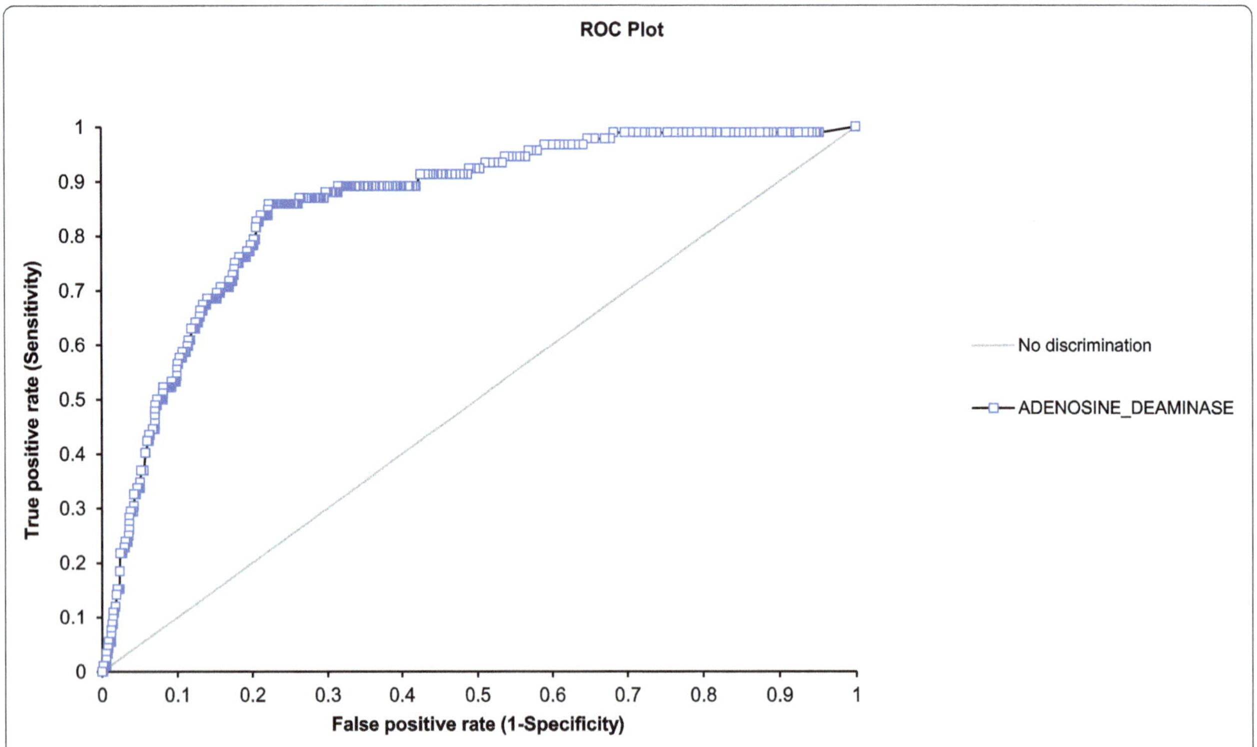

Fig. 3 ROC plot for all patients that had both an ADA and a culture for TB requested on a CSF specimen

Table 6 Sensitivity and Specificity of CSF ADA at a cut-off of 2.0 U/L

ADA	2.0 U/L
Youden index	0.636
True positive (n)	79
True negative (n)	1086
False positive (n)	312
False negative (n)	13
Sensitivity (%)	85.9
95% confidence interval	77.0–92.3
Specificity (%)	77.7
95% confidence interval	75.4–79.8
Positive likelihood ratio	3.85
Negative likelihood ratio	0.18

catastrophic nature of untreated TBM, the consequence of failing to give appropriate therapy in true TBM are considerably worse than the consequences of inadvertently over-treating the disease. The positive likelihood ratio was lower than that published in a recent meta-analysis, whereas the negative likelihood ratio was similar [19]. A positive likelihood ratio of 3.85 does increase the chance of a diagnosis of TBM significantly if there is a high pretest probability of disease. A negative likelihood ratio of 0.18 is of some value if the pretest probability is low as it makes the diagnosis of TBM more than 5-fold less likely. Conversely in all other situations of pretest probabilities, the test is essentially non-contributory. Although these parameters suggest a reasonable performance of CSF ADA, it is of concern that at a cut-off of 2.0 U/L, 13 out of 92 cases of TBM were missed.

When comparing ADA values between prominent infective pathologies (tuberculosis versus other infectious conditions), the absence of a statistically significant difference between the 'Confirmed bacterial meningitis' and 'Confirmed TBM' categories concurred with findings of a number of studies [18, 20, 21]. Similarly there was no statistically significant difference between the 'Confirmed ventriculitis' category and the 'Confirmed TBM' category. CSF ADA results were statistically significantly different between the 'Viral meningitis/encephalitis' and 'Confirmed TBM' categories. This concurred with the research by Donald, et al. [18]. Coovadia, et al. did not find any difference between the 2 categories [21]. A statistically significant difference was found when comparing CSF ADA results between the 'Confirmed cryptococcal meningitis' and 'Confirmed TBM' categories. Rohani, et al. determined a mean CSF ADA result for TBM cases and those with cryptococcal meningitis as 16.33+/−5.66 U/L and 7.26+/−3.80 U/L respectively. Three of the CSF ADA values for cryptococcal meningitis overlapped with the TBM category in this study [22]. In a country like South Africa, where the HIV seroprevalence is high and both TB and cryptococcal infections are important opportunistic co-morbidities, this phenomenon warrants further investigation.

In the 3548 CSF ADA requests reviewed, results for the categories according to demography, HIV status and CD4 cell count yielded a statistically significant difference for all. Statistically significant differences in ADA results in adult and paediatric patients are in keeping with the work by Donald and colleagues [23]. It has been postulated that a difference in immunological reactivity to tubercular antigen between adult and paediatric patients account for this difference [1]. The reason for the difference in CSF ADA performance between male and female patients is not clear from the literature. It was unexpected to find ADA results to be higher in HIV positive patients and patients with CD4 cell counts less than or equal to 350×10^6/L as intuitively it is assumed that cellular responses are impaired in these patients. Co-morbidities may account for this. Information on treatment for HIV was not collected. It is assumed that if cases were on treatment immune reconstitution would be seen, hence elevated values. Although these

Table 7 Target and actual sensitivities and specificities at different CSF ADA levels

Target Sensitivity	First cut-off closest the these targets	Actual Sensitivity	Corresponding Specificity
≥80%	2.3 U/L	81.5%	79.4%
≥85%	2.0 U/L	85.9%	77.7%
≥90%	0.8 U/L	91.3%	57.4%
≥95%	0.5 U/L	95.7%	43%
Target Specificity	First cut-off closest the these targets	Actual Specificity	Corresponding Sensitivity
≥80%	2.4 U/L	80%	78.3%
≥85%	3.3 U/L	85%	68.5%
≥90%	4.5 U/L	90%	55.4%
≥95%	7.3 U/L	95%	33.7%

Table 8 ROC curve results for each of the demographic categories in the population of $n = 1490$

	TBM positive (n)	TBM negative (n)	ROC curve			Sensitivity (%)	Specificity (%)
			AUC	p value	Cut-off (U/L)		
Adult patients	90	1345	0.86	<0.01	2.0/2.2	86.7/85.6	77.8/79.0
Paediatric patients	2	53	0.58	<0.33	0.6	100.0	41.5
Male patients	47	695	0.86	<0.01	2.2 (2.0)	89.4 (89.4)	75.3 (74.1)
Female patients	45	703	0.86	<0.01	2.0	82.2	81.1
HIV positive patients	77	846	0.83	<0.01	2.2 (2.0)	84.4 (85.7)	74.1 (72.8)
HIV negative patients	7	274	0.88	<0.01	0.6	100.0	70.1
Patients with CD4 count ≤ 350 × 10^6/L	58	653	0.83	<0.01	2.0	86.2	74.4
Patients with CD4 count < 350 × 10^6/L	4	114	0.93	<0.01	2.7	100.0	86.0

Cut-offs represented was based on the Youden index. In adult patients the Youden index performed similar for cut-off of 2.0 U/L and 2.2 U/L. In brackets performance at a cut-off of 2.0 U/L is indicated

differences were statistically significant ($p < 0.05$), in all cases the median CSF ADA values were less than 1.0 U/L.

Several pre-analytical and analytical factors limit adequate interpretation of the results from this study. No specific specimen collection and handling procedures are noted in the Diazyme kit package insert (Diazyme, United States of America) regarding CSF samples. There are no guidelines regarding the stability of ADA specifically in CSF samples. It is unclear what the correct specimen volume should be for optimal assay performance. Feres and colleagues mention in their validation of the Diazyme assay for measurement of ADA (Diazyme, United States of America) in CSF that 22 μL was used [24]. This is different from the 5 μL mentioned in the Diazyme kit package insert (Diazyme, United States of America).

It is important to note the effect of sample integrity on ADA. 'Ungraded xanthochromia' accounted for 81 specimens and showed the widest distribution of 95% of their values. Both this category and samples assigned xanthochromia +/− to 2+ (accounting for 52 or 1.5% of

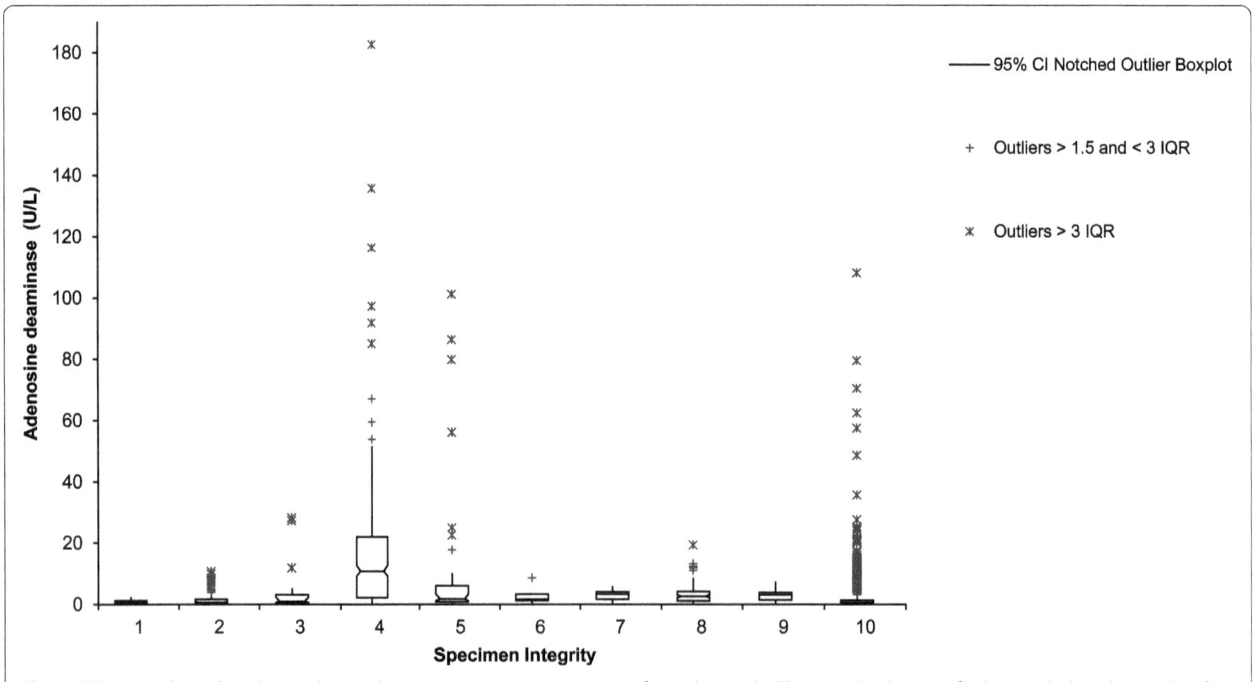

Fig. 4 CSF ADA values plotted according to the specimen integrity comments for each sample. The 95% distribution of values (including the median, first and third IQRs) and the outliers are indicated. Key to this Figure: 1 – ungraded bloodstained ($n = 13$), 2 – bloodstained +/− to 2+ ($n = 196$), 3 – bloodstained 3+ to 4+ ($n = 28$), 4 – ungraded xanthochromia ($n = 81$), 5 – xanthochromia +/− to 2+ ($n = 52$), 6 – xanthochromia 3+ to 4+ ($n = 6$), 7 – ungraded turbid ($n = 11$), 8 – turbid +/− to 2+ ($n = 148$), 9 – turbid 3+ to 4+ ($n = 10$), 10 – clear and colourless ($n = 3003$); CI - confidence interval; IQR – interquartile range

Table 9 CSF ADA results for the clinical research case definition (in U/L) ($n = 1490$)

Categories	Not tuberculous meningitis ($n = 1024$)	Possible tuberculous meningitis ($n = 306$)	Probable tuberculous meningitis ($n = 68$)	Definite tuberculous meningitis ($n = 92$)
Percentage (%)	68.7	20.5	4.6	6.2
ADA Range	0.0 – 135.7	0.0 – 91.8	0.0 – 6.5	0.0 - 108
Median ADA	0.6	0.9	0.7	5.4
Number of cases in each category ADA ≥ 2	$n = 207$, 20.2%	$n = 97$, 31.7%	$n = 15$, 22.1%	
Number of cases in each category ADA ≥ 6	$n = 63$, 6.2%	$n = 32$, 10.5%	$n = 4$, 5.9%	

samples) showed a wide scatter in their outliers, similar to the category for clear and colourless samples (accounting for 3003 or 84.6% of samples). Ungerer and colleagues demonstrated that erythrocytes contribute 100% of ADA-1 (ADA isoform 1) and polymorphonuclear cells contribute 70% ADA-1 and 30% ADA-1 + CP (two ADA isoform 1 molecules connected by a combining protein) to the total ADA activity in cell extracts [25]. This may explain the performance of CSF ADA in the 'Confirmed Ventriculitis' category.

Using a uniform case definition for TBM [17], by weighting the available evidence collected, about two-thirds of cases ($n = 1024$, 68.7%) whom had a CSF ADA and mycobacterial culture requested, fell in the 'Not TBM' category. By applying the CSF ADA cut-off of 2.0 U/L, about a fifth of these cases ($n = 207$, 20.2%) would have been treated if the decision to treat was based on the CSF ADA alone. This is about three times more than the number of patients that would have been treated using a cut-off of 6.0 U/L ($n = 63$, 6.2%). Either way, irrespective of whether a cut-off of 2.0U/L or 6.0 U/L is used, a considerable number of patients would have received unnecessary treatment. The uniform case definition was established after extensive literature review and international expert consensus [17]. Although the current study is subject to limitations, the performance of CSF ADA is such that it simply cannot supersede the uniform case definition (see Table 9).

The measurement of ADA in general is complicated by poor standardisation [26]. Giusti and non-Giusti methods have been documented. Most methods are in-house based. The Diazyme assay (Diazyme, United States of America) is a commercially available assay fit for automated platforms. Bota and colleagues produced and certified enzyme reference material for ADA-1 to be used to compare laboratories and verify performance of calibration material and quality control material. This group utilised ADA purified from human erythrocytes. A commutability study was only performed on pleural fluid samples clear of haemolysis and turbidity [27]. The poor standardisation of ADA measurement makes it difficult to interpret the significance of CSF ADA values in the literature. Both the calibrator and control material supplied by Diazyme (Diazyme, United States of America) are bovine serum albumin based. An important question to resolve is how matrix effects interfere with this assay.

No consensus exists regarding the linear range of this assay. The calibration curve for the Diazyme assay (Diazyme, United States of America) lies between 0 – 50 U/L. However, the package insert for the Diazyme assay (Diazyme, United States of America) states that dilution should occur for samples with results > 200 U/L. Delacour, et al., (2010) performed a linearity study and determined the analytical measurement range to be 0.5 – 120 U/L [28].

Ideally control material should reflect analyte levels at which clinical decisions are made. Currently this is true for pericardial, peritoneal and pleural fluids, but not for CSF.

The imprecision of the Diazyme assay (Diazyme, United States of America) at the proposed cut-off of 2.0 U/L is unknown. Data from our validation studies at the lower control level of 10.6 U/L showed a within-run standard deviation of 0.172 U/L, total standard deviation of 0.601 U/L, and the total coefficient of variation of 5.8%. As the allowable coefficient of variation was 7.0%, this performance was deemed to be acceptable. It is possible that the imprecision of the assay is poor at a cut-off of 2.0 U/L. This would require further investigation.

The retrospective analysis of clinical and laboratory data constituted a further limitation of this study. While every effort was made to find all data parameters relevant to the study, this was not always possible due to incomplete data in patient files and on the laboratory information system. This may have affected the categorisation process. Reflex testing of CSF ADA may have occurred. Many of the controls will have had a high pretest clinical probability of other diagnoses. In view of the fact that submission of insufficient CSF volume impacts on the sensitivity of TB culture, it is possible that microbiological confirmation of TBM was missed in some cases, as less than 10% of the 1490 patients who had a culture and ADA requested on a CSF specimen had more than one specimen submitted. As the majority of the population studied were HIV positive and for a quarter the HIV status was not known, these results cannot be extrapolated to non-HIV populations. This requires further investigation.

Conclusion

The authors cannot recommend CSF ADA as either a rule-in or a rule-out test. A clinical appropriate cut-off could not be determined, as at a cut-off of 2.0 U/L still 13 out of 92 cases of 'Confirmed TBM' were missed. Several pre-analytic and analytical factors affect interpretation of CSF ADA results. No definite conclusions can be reached regarding CSF ADA cut-off levels, without fully understanding these factors. The effect of sample integrity cannot be underestimated and there is a pressing need for standardisation of CSF ADA measurement. CSF culture remains the gold standard for the diagnosis of TBM. Its poor performance overall, however, makes it a problematic gold standard to which CSF ADA is compared to and a replacement is needed. The data from this study show that the CSF ADA result may potentially mislead clinicians in the diagnostic process. As such careful assessment and weighting of all the available evidence should prove more fruitful [17]. A future prospective multicentre study on a larger cohort, especially once the standardisation of CSF ADA measurement has improved, is advocated. In the meantime clinicians should be aware of the limitations of basing a diagnosis of TBM on a CSF ADA result.

Abbreviations

ADA: Adenosine deaminase; AUC: Area under the curve; CSF: Cerebrospinal fluid; ELISA: Enzyme-linked immunosorbent assay; HIV: Human Immunodeficiency virus; IQR: Interquartile range; IQRs: Interquartile ranges; PCR: Polymerase chain reaction; ROC: Receiver operating characteristic; TB: *Mycobacterium tuberculosis* complex; TBM: Tuberculous meningitis; WHO: World Health Organisation

Acknowledgements

The authors wish to acknowledge the contribution of Dr Hendrik Emanuel Van Deventer from Lancet Laboratories, South Africa, for his assistance with the statistical analysis of the data.

Funding

No funding was required for this study.

Author s contributions

JG conceived the research topic. PE performed the data mining, analysed and interpreted the data, performed a literature review and created the first draft of the manuscript. Both AD and JG assisted in the design and co-ordination of the study and assisted in revising the manuscript critically for important intellectual content. All authors read and approved the final manuscript.

Competing interests

All authors have no competing interests to declare.

Consent for publication

Not applicable.

Author details

[1]Department of Chemical Pathology, University of Witwatersrand and National Health Laboratory Service, Johannesburg, South Africa. [2]Department of Clinical Microbiology and Infectious Diseases, University of Witwatersrand and National Health Laboratory Service, Johannesburg, South Africa. [3]Department of Chemical Pathology and Department of Clinical Microbiology and Infectious Diseases, School of Pathology, Faculty of Health Sciences, University of Witwatersrand and National Health Laboratory Service, 7 York Road, Johannesburg, South Africa.

References

1. Mishra OP, Loiwal V, Ali Z, et al. Cerebrospinal fluid adenosine deaminase activity for the diagnosis of tuberculous meningitis in children. J Trop Pediatr. 1996;42:129–32.
2. Rana SV, Singhal RK, Singh K, et al. Adenosine deaminase levels in cerebrospinal fluid as a diagnostic test for tuberculous meningitis in children. Ind J Clin Biochem. 2004;19(2):5–9.
3. Pettersson T, Klockars M, Weber TH, et al. Diagnostic value of cerebrospinal fluid adenosine deaminase determination. Scand J Infect Dis. 1991;23:97–100.
4. Schutte C-M, Ungerer JPJ, du Plessis H, et al. Significance of cerebrospinal fluid adenosine deaminase isoenzymes in tuberculous (TB) meningitis. J Clin Lab Anal. 2001;15:236–8.
5. Corral I, Quereda C, Navas E, et al. Adenosine deaminase activity in cerebrospinal fluid of HIV-infected patients: limited value for diagnosis of tuberculous meningitis. Eur J Clin Microbiol Infect Dis. 2004;23:471–6.
6. Blake J, Berman P. The use of adenosine deaminase assays in the diagnosis of tuberculosis. S Afr Med J. 1982;62:19–21.
7. Ribera E, Martinez-Vasquez JM, Ocaña I, et al. Activity of adenosine deaminase in cerebrospinal fluid for the diagnosis and follow-up of tuberculous meningitis in adults. J Infect Dis. 1987;155(4):603–7.
8. Choi S-H, Kim YS, Bae I-G, et al. The possible role of cerebrospinal fluid adenosine deaminase activity in the diagnosis of tuberculous meningitis in adults. Clin Neurol Neurosurg. 2002;104:10–5.
9. Kaur A, Basha A, Ranjan M, et al. Poor diagnostic value of adenosine deaminase in pleural, peritoneal & cerebrospinal fluids in tuberculosis. Indian J Med Res. 1992;95:270–7.
10. Kashyap RS, Ramteke SP, Deshpande PS, et al. Comparison of an adenosine deaminase assay with ELISA for the diagnosis of tuberculous meningitis infection. Med Sci Monit. 2007;13(9):BR200–204.
11. Lópés-Cortés IF, Cruz-Ruiz M, Gómez-Mateos J, et al. Adenosine deaminase activity in the CSF of patients with aseptic meningitis: utility in the diagnosis of tuberculous meningitis or neurobrucellosis. Clin Infect Dis. 1995;20:525–30.
12. Oosthuizen HM, Ungerer JPJ, Bissbort SH. Kinetic determination of serum adenosine deaminase. Clin Chem. 1993;39(10):2182–5.
13. Maldarelli F. Diagnosis of HIV infection. In: Mandell GL, Bennett JE, Dolin R, editors. Principles and Practice of Infectious Diseases. London: Churchill Livingstone, 2005; pp 1516–20.
14. World Health Organization. Antiretroviral therapy for HIV infection in adults and adolescents. Available from: http://www.who.int/hiv/pub/arv/adult2010/en/index.html. Accessed 14 Nov 2011.
15. Dawson-Saunders B, Trapp RG, editors. Estimating and comparing means, Evaluating diagnostic procedures. In: Basic & Clinical Biostatistics. Appleton and Lange, 1994; pp 117–119, 243–245.
16. Akobeng AK. Understanding diagnostic tests 3: receiver operating characteristic curves. Acta Pediatr. 2007;96:644–7.
17. Marais S, Thwaites G, Schoeman JF, et al. Tuberculous meningitis: a uniform case definition for use in clinical research. Lancet Infect Dis. 2010;10:803–12.
18. Donald PR, Malan C, Van der Walt A, et al. The simultaneous determination of cerebrospinal fluid and plasma adenosine deaminase activity as a diagnostic aid in tuberculous meningitis. S Afr Med J. 1986;69:505–7.
19. Xu H-B, Jiang R-H, Sha W, et al. Diagnostic value of adenosine deaminase in cerebrospinal fluid for tuberculous meningitis: a meta-analysis. Int J Tuberc Lung Dis. 2010;14(11):1382–7.
20. Malan C, Donald PR, Golden M, et al. Adenosine deaminase levels in cerebrospinal fluid in the diagnosis of tuberculous meningitis. J Trop Med Hyg. 1984;87(1):33–40.
21. Coovadia YM, Dawood A, Ellis ME, et al. Evaluation of adenosine deaminase activity and antibody to Mycobacterium tuberculosis antigen 5 in cerebrospinal

fluid and the radioactive bromide partition test for the early detection of tuberculosis meningitis. Arc Dis Child. 1986;61:428–35.
22. Rohani MY, Cheong YM, Rani JM. The use of adenosine deaminase activity as a biochemical marker for the diagnosis of tuberculous meningitis. Malays J Pathol. 1995;17(2):67–71.
23. Donald PR, Malan C, Schoeman JF. Letter to the editor: Adenosine deaminase activity as a diagnostic aid in tuberculous meningitis. J Infect Dis. 1987;156(6):1040–1.
24. Feres MC, De Martino MC, Maldijian S, et al. Laboratorial validation of an automated assay for the determination of adenosine deaminase activity in pleural fluid and cerebrospinal fluid. J Bras Pneumol. 2008;34(12):1003–39.
25. Ungerer JPJ, Oosthuizen HM, Bissbort SH, et al. Serum adenosine deaminase: isoenzyme and diagnostic application. Clin Chem. 1992;38(7):1322–6.
26. Tuon FF, Higashino HR, Banks MI, et al. Adenosine deaminase and tuberculous meningitis – a systematic review with meta-analysis. Scand J Infect Dis. 2010;42:198–207.
27. Bota A, Gella F-J, Profilis C, et al. Production and certification of an enzyme reference material for adenosine deaminase 1 (BCR 647). Clin Chim Act. 2001;306:79–89.
28. Delacour H, Sauvanet C, Ceppa F, et al. Analytical performances of the Diazyme ADA assay on the Cobas® 6000 system. Clin Biochem. 2010;43:1468–71.

12

An outbreak of pneumococcal meningitis among older children (≥5 years) and adults after the implementation of an infant vaccination programme with the 13-valent pneumococcal conjugate vaccine in Ghana

Brenda Anna Kwambana-Adams[1†], Franklin Asiedu-Bekoe[2†], Badu Sarkodie[2], Osei Kuffour Afreh[3], George Khumalo Kuma[4], Godfred Owusu-Okyere[5], Ebenezer Foster-Nyarko[1], Sally-Ann Ohene[6], Charles Okot[6], Archibald Kwame Worwui[1], Catherine Okoi[1], Madikay Senghore[1], Jacob Kweku Otu[1], Chinelo Ebruke[1], Richard Bannerman[3], Kwame Amponsa-Achiano[2], David Opare[5], Gemma Kay[7], Timothy Letsa[3], Owen Kaluwa[6], Ebenezer Appiah-Denkyira[2], Victor Bampoe[8], Syed M. A. Zaman[9,10], Mark J. Pallen[7], Umberto D'Alessandro[9,10,11], Jason M. Mwenda[12] and Martin Antonio[1,7,10*]

Abstract

Background: An outbreak of pneumococcal meningitis among non-infant children and adults occurred in the Brong-Ahafo region of Ghana between December 2015 and April 2016 despite the recent nationwide implementation of a vaccination programme for infants with the 13-valent pneumococcal conjugate vaccine (PCV13).

Methods: Cerebrospinal fluid (CSF) specimens were collected from patients with suspected meningitis in the Brong-Ahafo region. CSF specimens were subjected to Gram staining, culture and rapid antigen testing. Quantitative PCR was performed to identify pneumococcus, meningococcus and *Haemophilus influenzae*. Latex agglutination and molecular serotyping were performed on samples. Antibiogram and whole genome sequencing were performed on pneumococcal isolates.

Results: Eight hundred eighty six patients were reported with suspected meningitis in the Brong-Ahafo region during the period of the outbreak. In the epicenter district, the prevalence was as high as 363 suspected cases per 100,000 people. Over 95 % of suspected cases occurred in non-infant children and adults, with a median age of 20 years. Bacterial meningitis was confirmed in just under a quarter of CSF specimens tested. Pneumococcus, meningococcus and Group B Streptococcus accounted for 77 %, 22 % and 1 % of confirmed cases respectively. The vast majority of serotyped pneumococci (80 %) belonged to serotype 1. Most of the pneumococcal isolates tested were susceptible to a broad range of antibiotics, with the exception of two pneumococcal serotype 1 strains that were resistant to both penicillin and trimethoprim-sulfamethoxazole. All sequenced pneumococcal serotype 1 strains belong to Sequence Type (ST) 303 in the hypervirulent ST217 clonal complex.
(Continued on next page)

* Correspondence: mantonio@mrc.gm
†Equal contributors
1Vaccines and Immunity Theme, The Medical Research Council Unit The Gambia, P.O Box 273, Banjul, Fajara, The Gambia
7Microbiology and Infection Unit, Warwick Medical School, Warwick, UK
Full list of author information is available at the end of the article

(Continued from previous page)

Conclusion: The occurrence of a pneumococcal serotype 1 meningitis outbreak three years after the introduction of PCV13 is alarming and calls for strengthening of meningitis surveillance and a re-evaluation of the current vaccination programme in high risk countries.

Keywords: Pneumococcus, Outbreak, Serotype 1, Ghana, Meningitis belt, West Africa, Meningitis, Pneumococcal conjugate vaccine (PCV)

Background

Acute bacterial meningitis is most commonly caused by *Neisseria meningitidis*, *Streptococcus pneumoniae* and *Haemophilus influenzae* Type b. In sub-Saharan Africa, there is a "meningitis belt" running from Ethiopia to Senegal where there is high seasonal incidence of bacterial meningitis. In West Africa, the highest incidence of bacterial meningitis occurs during the dry season (December to March) [1–3], with incidence rates in epidemics as high as 800 cases per 100,000 people [4, 5].

N. meningitidis, the meningococcus, is the leading cause of bacterial meningitis in West Africa after the first year of life, even in non-epidemic periods [1–3, 6, 7]. In the past, most West African meningococcal outbreaks were attributed to serogroup A [8]. However, the MenAfriVac™ vaccine, which protects against meningococcal serogroup A, has been rolled out in several countries in the meningitis belt. In Ghana, MenAfriVac™ vaccination campaigns conducted in 2012 covered the three northern regions within the meningitis belt [4].

Outbreaks of *S. pneumoniae*, the pneumococcus, were previously thought to be restricted to prisons, military camps and among people living in crowded conditions such as refugee camps [9–13]. However, in the early 2000s, large pneumococcal outbreaks were reported in a few West African countries including Ghana [3, 14–16]. A sustained increase in the cases of pneumococcal meningitis was reported in Northern Ghana between 2000 and 2003. The incidence of pneumococcal meningitis rose from ≤5 cases/100,000 people/year in 2000 to 15–26 cases/100,000 people/year at its peak [16]. Pneumococcal meningitis outbreaks were also reported in neighboring countries Burkina Faso, Togo and Niger around the same period [3, 14–16]. These West-African outbreaks have been characterised by high case-fatality rates (up to 40 %) and appear to mimic meningococcal meningitis outbreaks, with peaks in the hot dry season [3, 14, 16]. Pneumococci expressing the serotype 1 capsule dominated the West African pneumococcal meningitis outbreaks. Most of the strains belonged to the clonal complex dominated by Sequence Type (ST)217 [14, 16, 17].

The 13-valent pneumococcal polysaccharide-diphtheria CRM_{197} protein conjugate vaccine (PCV13) now part of the routine immunization programmes in many countries is particularly efficacious in infants. PCVs are thought to elicit mucosal immunity, possibly due to the induction of opsonizing IgA antibodies [18]. Widespread use of PCVs markedly reduces carriage of vaccine serotypes amongst both vaccinated and unvaccinated individuals [19–21]. PCVs are a remarkable public health success as they induce herd immunity and are associated with reductions in invasive pneumococcal disease globally [19–21]. PCV13 was introduced in the Ghana Expanded Programme on Immunisation (EPI) in April 2012.

The Brong Ahafo Region spans the central section of Ghana on the north–south axis and falls outside the meningitis belt, which is restricted to the northern region of the country. The WHO designated Regional Reference Laboratory (RRL) hosted at the Medical Research Council Unit The Gambia coordinates surveillance of invasive bacterial diseases across West Africa. The WHO RRL supported the Ghana Ministry of Health to confirm the causative pathogens and provided technical laboratory support teams at regional and district hospitals in the Brong Ahafo Region for bacteriologic processing of CSF specimens. The aim of this study was to confirm and characterise the pathogens that caused this unusual outbreak in Ghana.

Methods

Study area

The Brong-Ahafo Region is one of ten regions in Ghana and has a population of 2.4 million distributed in 27 districts. It has a bi-modal rainfall pattern with the major rainy season occurring between April and July and a minor rainy season between September and October. The dry season runs from November to March.

Patients

All cases of suspected meningitis in Brong Ahafo Region, which presented at private, mission, district and regional hospitals had a lumbar puncture performed. Suspected meningitis was defined as sudden onset of fever (>38.5 °C) and a combination of any of the following clinical symptoms: reduced level of consciousness, stiff neck, bulging fontanel, fit(s) if aged between six months and five years or partial seizures. When available, the CSF specimens were stored in Trans-isolate (T-I) media. The patients were treated with ceftriaxone or ampicillin.

Bacteriologic analysis of CSF specimens

CSF samples were initially processed at the health centers or hospitals where they were collected. However, when this was not possible, the processing was performed at the Regional Hospital, Sunyani. The primary method for the detection of pneumococcus, *Haemophilus influenzae* type b, meningococcus serogroups A, C, Y/W was the Pastorex meningitis kit (Biorad, UK), which was used following manufacturer's instructions.

For culture, 10 µl of un-centrifuged CSF was streaked onto Columbia blood agar (BA) and chocolate agar (CA) plates and incubated at 37 °C in 5 % CO_2 for 18–24 h (overnight). 1–2 drops of CSF were used to prepare a smear, air-dried and fixed by flooding with 95 % ethanol for 2 min or by passing through the flame for a few seconds. Gram stain was performed following WHO protocol [22].

Following overnight incubation, the CA and BA plates were examined for characteristic growth of pneumococcus, *H. influenzae*, meningococcus and other pathogens. Suspected pneumococcal colonies were confirmed and serotyped as previously described [23]. All suspected meningococcus or *H. influenzae* underwent biochemical confirmation using analytical profile index kits (API NH; Biomerieux, UK). Meningococcal serogroups were assessed by use of the Directigen™ meningitis combo kit (Oxoid Basingstoke, UK) following manufacturer's instructions. Pneumococcal isolates underwent antibiotic susceptibility testing by the disc and E-test diffusion methods for commonly prescribed antibiotics in the sub-region following CSLI guidelines [24]. Antibiotic activity in the CSF specimens was assessed by the disc diffusion antibiotic bioassay following the method described previously by Driscoll et al., (2012) [25]. All antibiotics were procured from Oxoid (Basingstoke, UK) and E-test strips from Biomerieux, UK.

The MRC Unit The Gambia, molecular microbiology laboratory submits to the external quality assurance programme of the UK National External Quality Assessment Service (http://www.ukneqas.org.uk) and is a World Health Organization (WHO) Regional Reference Laboratory for invasive bacterial pathogens.

Real time PCR detection and serotyping of pathogens

An aliquot of the CSF specimens was shipped to the WHO RRL hosted at MRCG in dry ice (−80 °C). Species-specific quantitative PCR (qPCR) assays for detection of pneumococcus, meningococcus and *H. influenzae* were conducted using the autolysin gene (*lytA*), the CU, Zn superoxide dismutase gene (*sodC*) and the protein D encoding gene (*hpd*) respectively as previously described [26–28]. *RNaseP* gene assay was performed on all CSF specimens to confirm samples of human origin and the integrity of the CSF specimens. Positivity for each of the targets was deduced using cycle threshold (CT) values. CTs of ≤36 were considered as positive.

Serogroup and serotype specific qPCR assays

Meningococcal serogrouping and *H. influenzae* serotyping were performed by direct qPCR as previously described [27]. Targets for the mentioned pathogens included *sacB, synD, synE, synG, xcbB, synF* genes for serogroups A, B, C, W, X, Y respectively. For *H. influenzae*, the following serotypes were screened: *acB* (Hia), *bcsB* (Hib), *ccsD* (Hic), *dscE* (Hid), *ecsH* (Hie) and *bexD* (Hif).

***Streptococcus pneumoniae* serotyping**

In preparation for nucleic acid extraction for pneumococcal serotyping, 200 µL of CSF was added to 50 µL of TE buffer containing 0.08 g/mL of lysozyme (Sigma-L-6876) and 150U/mL of mutanolysin (Sigma M-9901), and mixture was incubated for one hour at 37 °C. The remaining extraction procedures followed Qiagen DNA Mini kit (Qiagen, UK) manufacturer's instructions.

Purified DNA extracts were subjected to sequential triplex qPCR assay for detecting 21 pneumococcal capsular serotypes for the African scheme as previously described [29]. CSF specimens with CT values ≤32 were further subjected to conventional multiplex PCRs also described elsewhere [30, 31].

Whole-genome sequencing

Whole-genome sequencing was performed on nine purified pneumococcal isolates cultured from CSF specimens. All the isolates could not be sequenced due to cost considerations. Sequencing was performed on the illumina Miseq platform following a NexteraX library preparation step. Genomic data was analysed using the nullarbor pipeline (https://github.com/tseemann/nullarbor), which confirmed the species of the isolates, inferred MLST types, reported the presence of resistance genes and extracted a core genome. Draft genome assemblies for the nine outbreak strains were generated using spades (kmers: 21, 33, 55, 77, 99 and 127). To illustrate the phylogenetic relationship of the outbreak ST303 isolates, we included nine archived ST303 draft pneumococcal genome assemblies [32]. The assembled ST303 genomes from the pneumococcal outbreak strains and the draft genomes were compared against the P1031 pneumococcal reference genome; a pneumococcal historical isolate from Ghana [33]. Contigs were mapped against the reference and SNVs were called from the core genome using parsnp [34]. The pneumococcal genome sequences are available on the European Bioinformatics Institute (EBI) database under study accession PRJEB15437 at http://www.ebi.ac.uk/ena/data/view/PRJEB15437.

Data management

Demographic and clinical data of suspected cases were collected with designed case report forms and entered into Microsoft Excel and an EPI Info database tool.

Demographic and clinical data of the cases were extracted into a line list. The Excel data sets from the health facilities were imported and merged into a Microsoft Access database. Pathogen detection, serotyping and serogrouping data from qPCR and other methods were imported and merged with demographic and clinical data in the customized Microsoft Access database. Antibiotic and antibiogram data were also entered into the customized Microsoft Access database. Data analysis was carried out using GraphPad Prism, R statistics tool (version 3.2.4) for Windows and Microsoft Excel. The maps were generated using QGIS v1.0 software using Geographical Position System (GPS) coordinates from the US Geographical Survey (USGS) https://www.usgs.gov.

Results

The nationwide weekly incidence of meningitis rose from <5 cases/100,000 people in the 49th week of 2015 to 350 cases/100,000 people in the 7th week of 2016. Between 2 December 2015 (49th week) and 26 February 2016 (9th week), there were 886 suspected meningitis cases reported. A flow chart of the CSF specimens collected, tested and the outcomes are summarised in Fig. 1. Overall, 64 % (567/886) of CSF specimens were tested by rapid test, culture and/or qPCR. Meningitis was confirmed in 23.8 % (135/567). Pneumococcus, meningococcus and GBS accounted for 77 % (104/135), 22 % (30/135) and 1 % (1/135) of the confirmed cases of meningitis. One CSF was positive for both meningococcus and pneumococcus, an unusual finding probably due to contamination (Fig. 1).

The characteristics of the patients with suspected and confirmed meningitis are summarised in Table 1. The patients' median age was 20 years (IQR 13 and IQR 32) and the range was 9 months to 98 years. 15 to 29 year olds accounted for 40 % of the suspected and confirmed cases. Less than 5 % of the suspected and confirmed cases were among children less than 4 years old who would likely have received PCV13 (Table 1).

Although suspected meningitis patients were reported across the whole region, the epicenter of the outbreak was in four contiguous districts; Jaman North, Tain, Wenchi and Techiman municipal (Fig. 2a). There were 363 suspected meningitis cases per 100,000 people in Jaman North, more than double that reported in Tain with 156 per 100,000 people. Although Jaman North had the highest rate of suspected cases, Tain and Wenchi had the highest rates of confirmed cases. There were 25, 20, 11 and 10 confirmed cases per 100,000 people in Tain, Wenchi, Jaman North and Techiman Municipal, respectively (Fig. 2a/b). The number of confirmed cases declined after the 6th week of 2016, but those of suspected cases increased up to the 8th week of 2016 as shown in Additional file 1. The meningitis outbreak peaked at different weeks across the hardest hit districts (Additional file 1). Tain district crossed the epidemic threshold of 10 suspected cases per 100,000 population in week 53 of 2015 whereas Wenchi and Jaman North district crossed the epidemic threshold in weeks 3 and 6 of 2016 respectively (Additional file 1).

Pneumococcus was the sole or leading pathogen across all districts with the exception of Jaman North district where meningococcus was the dominant pathogen

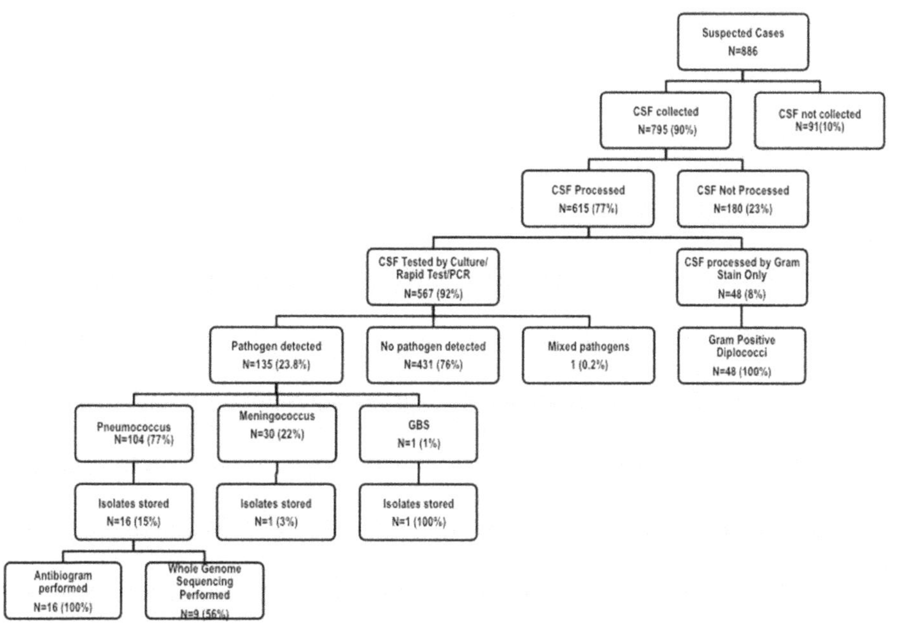

Fig. 1 Summary of CSF specimen collection and processing

Table 1 Patient characteristics and outcome

Characteristic	Category	Suspected Cases *n* (%)	Confirmed Cases *n* (%)	*S. Pneumoniae* *n* (%)	*N. Meningitidis* *n* (%)	*Group B Streptococcus* *n* (%)	*Mixed pathogen*
Gender	Female	458 (51.6)	55 (40.4)	43 (41.3)	10 (33.3)	1 (10)	1 (10)
	Male	348 (39.2)	54 (39.7)	42 (40.3)	12 (40.0)	0 (0)	0 (0)
	Unknown	80 (9.0)	27 (19.8)	19 (18.2)	8 (26.6)	0 (0)	0 (0)
Age	<1	11 (1.2)	2 (1.4)	2 (1.9)	0 (0)	0 (0)	0 (0)
	1–4	26 (2.9)	4 (2.9)	3 (2.8)	1 (3.3)	0 (0)	0 (0)
	5–14	174 (19.6)	35 (25.7)	30 (28.8)	4 (13.3)	1 (100)	0 (0)
	15–29	354 (39.9)	44 (32.3)	31 (29.8)	12 (4)	0 (0)	1 (100)
	30–59	203 (22.9)	19 (13.9)	16 (15.3)	3 (10)	0 (0)	0 (0)
	>60	37 (4.1)	5 (3.6)	3 (2.8)	2 (6.6)	0 (0)	0 (0)
	Unknown	81 (9.1)	27 (19.8)	19 (18.2)	8 (26.6)	0 (0)	0 (0)
	January	267 (30.1)	74 (54.4)	58 (55.7)	15 (5)	0 (0)	1 (100)
	February	499 (56.32)	30 (22.0)	22 (21.1)	7 (23.3)	1 (100)	0 (0)
	Unknown	100 (11.28)	27 (19.8)	19 (18.2)	8 (26.6)	0 (0)	0 (0)
Outcome	Alive	711 (80.2)	76 (55.8)	60 (57.6)	14 (46.6)	1 (10)	1 (100)
	Dead	75 (8.4)	33 (24.2)	25 (24.0)	8 (26.6)	0 (0)	0 (0)
	Unknown	100 (11.2)	27 (19.8)	19 (18.2)	8 (26.6)	0 (0)	0 (0)

accounting for 63 % (7/11) of confirmed cases (Fig. 2b). Pneumococcus was the leading pathogen from the 52nd week of 2015 to the 9th week of 2016 (Fig. 3a). Meningococcus was detected between weeks 2 and 7 of 2015. GBS was cultured from a CSF specimen in week 7 of 2015 (Fig. 3a).

The molecular and latex serotyping results by age group are summarised in Table 2. A tenth (10/104) of the pneumococci detected by PCR were either non-typeable by PCR or had a High Ct for molecular typing. Forty-five pneumococci could not be typed as the isolate and/or CSF was not available for serotyping. Serotype 1 accounted for 78 % (38/49) of the serotyped pneumococci. The distribution of the other serotypes was 12 % (6/49) serotype 12 F, 4 % (2/49) serotype 35B, 2 % (1/49) serotype of each, serotype 6A/6B, serotype 7 F and serotype 3. The only infant (10.8 month old) with confirmed pneumococcal meningitis had a serotype 35B infection, a non-PCV13 serotype. Serotype 1 was the only pneumococcal serotype detected among patients between four and 29 years old (Fig. 3d). In contrast, serotype 12 F, also a non-PCV13 serotype, was confirmed among cases aged ≥30 years. The serotype 12 F pneumococcal strains were detected across five districts including Tain in weeks 3 and 5 of 2015. The two serotype 35B strains were detected in Dormaa in week 8 of 2016 (Fig. 3c). Of the 20 meningococci that could be serotyped, 80 % (16/20) were serogroup W, 5 % (1/20) was a serogroup C and 15 % (3/20) could not be grouped by the real time PCR serotyping panel that includes serogroups A, B, C, W, X and Y.

A tenth (75/786) of the patients with suspected meningitis and a known outcome died. Among the confirmed cases, death was reported among 24 % (33/135) of the patients (Table 1). Amongst the deaths, the average length of time before reporting was 1.7 days and the average length of stay between admission and death was 2.3 days. The case fatality rates for confirmed meningococcal and pneumococcal meningitis were 36 % (8/22) and 29 % (25/85) respectively. The eight-year-old child with GBS meningitis survived.

Pneumococcal and meningococcal isolates were confirmed at the WHO RRL and underwent antibiotic susceptibility testing by disc diffusion and E-test [24]. Seventeen pneumococcal isolates from CSF were available for antimicrobial susceptibility testing by disc diffusion and E-test methods for commonly prescribed antibiotics in the subregion following CSLI guidelines [24]. The antibiogram of the isolates, serotype and the basic patient characteristics are summarised in Additional file 2. All the pneumococcal isolates tested were fully susceptible to ceftriaxone, vancomycin, chloramphenicol, clindamycin, erythromycin and rifampin. In contrast, 76 % (13/17) of the strains were resistant or had intermediate resistance to trimethoprim-sulfamethoxazole. Over 80 % (14/17) of the isolates were resistant to tetracycline. Resistance to penicillin was found in two isolates, both serotype 1 strains. These two serotype 1 strains were also resistant to trimethoprim-sulfamethoxazole and tetracycline. Both serotype 35B strains were fully susceptible to all the antibiotics screened. Antimicrobial activity in the CSF specimens was assessed by the disc diffusion antibiotic bioassay. Antimicrobial activity was detected in 1.5 % (5/325) of

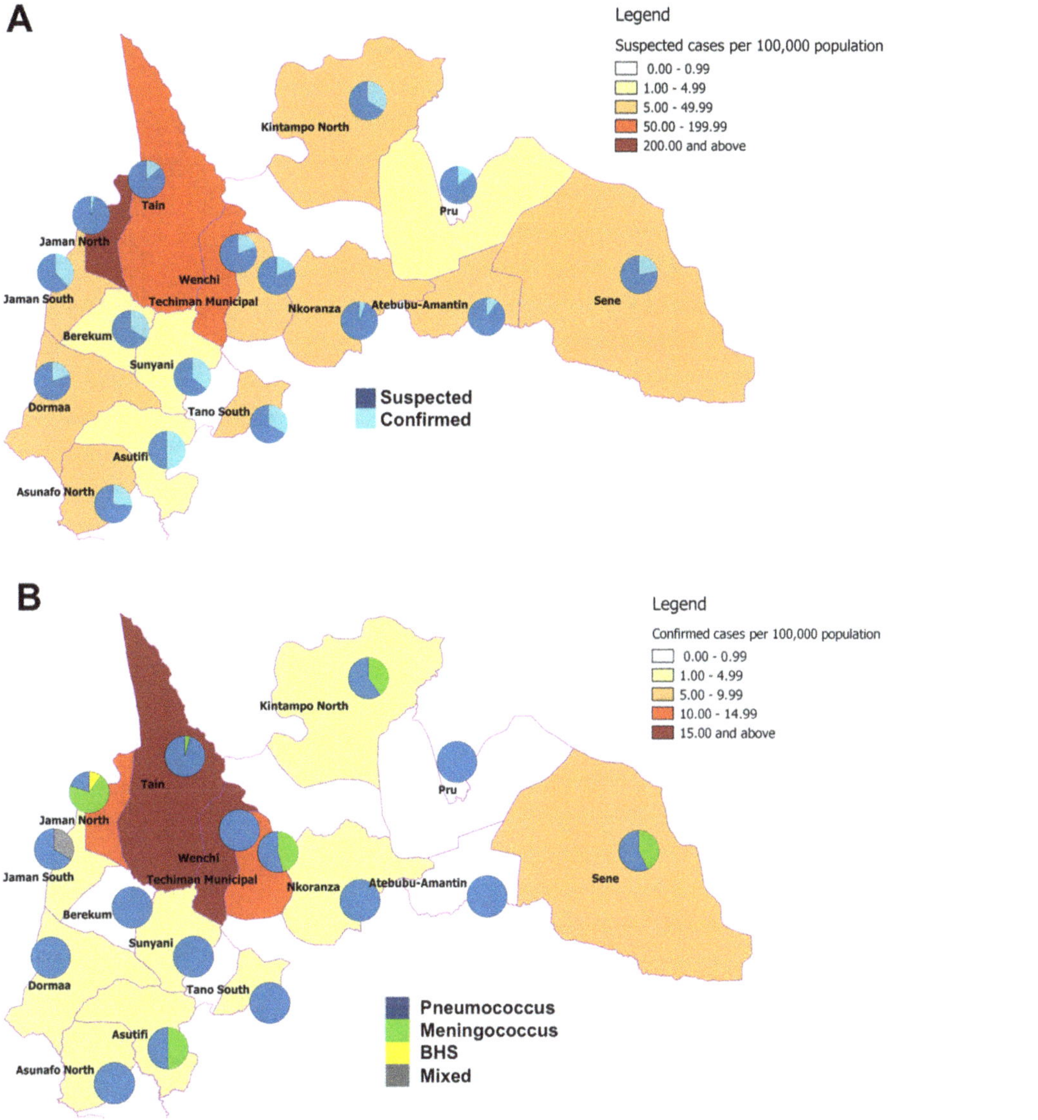

Fig. 2 The geographical distribution of the suspected and confirmed meningitis cases in Brong Ahafo region. The districts are shaded by suspected meningitis per 100,000 population and the pie charts representing the proportion of confirmed cases (**a**). The districts are shaded by the confirmed cases per 100,000 population and the pie charts represent the distribution of pathogens (**b**). The maps were generated using QGIS v1.0 software using Geographical Position System (GPS) coordinates from the US Geographical Survey (USGS) https://www.usgs.gov

the CSF specimens tested. A pathogen was detected in 2 of the 5 CSF specimens with antimicrobial activity.

Whole genome sequencing was performed on nine randomly selected pneumococcal isolates. The predominant lineage was ST303 ($n = 7$) found among serotype 1 isolates. The serotype 3 and 7 F strains belonged to ST700 and ST2833 lineages respectively. The phylogenetic tree of our outbreak strains showed that the ST303 isolates formed two separate clusters (Fig. 4a). To illustrate the diversity of ST303 within the outbreak, the phylogeny was reconstructed from the ST303 outbreak strains and other previously sequenced ST303 pneumococcal genomes (Fig. 4b). Four outbreak isolates (BAR_GH_2016_10, 13, 14 and 17) clustered on a clade characterized by a long branch from the closest relatives and short branches within the clade. The average pairwise distance between strains on this branch was 18 core genome SNVs. BAR_GH_2016_16 bore similarity to a cluster of ST303 previously isolated from Togo, a neighboring country, east of Ghana. BAR_GH_2016_7 and 18 presented as outgroups in our phylogeny without any marked identity to other isolates.

Discussion

To our knowledge, this is the first large pneumococcal meningitis outbreak to occur in Ghana since the early 2000s and the first report of a pneumococcal meningitis

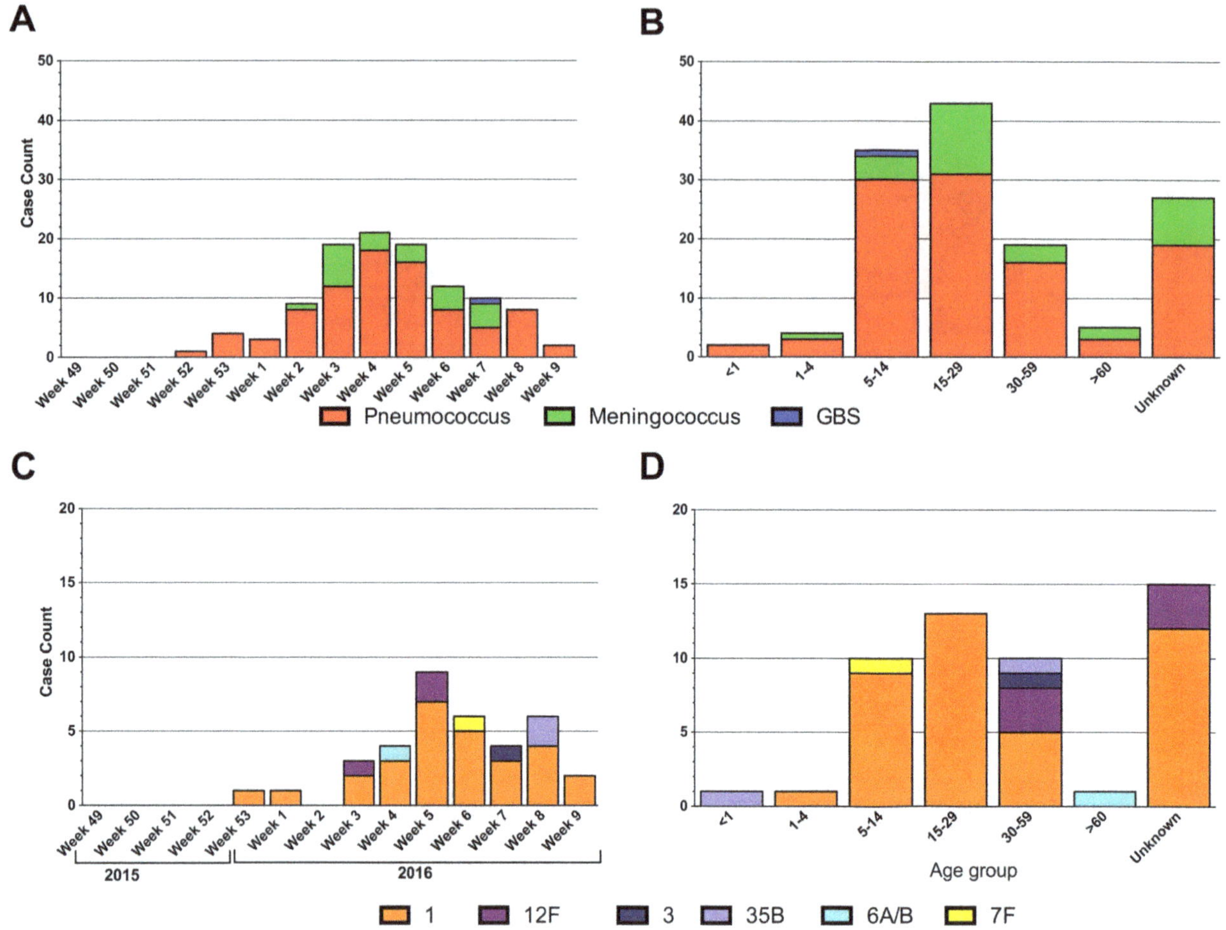

Fig. 3 The distribution of pathogens by week and age. The distribution of pathogens by week (**a**) and age (**b**). The distribution of pneumococcal serotypes by week (**c**) and age (**d**)

outbreak outside of the Northern regions of Ghana. [16]. Between 2004 and 2013, there were on average 600 cases of suspected and confirmed meningitis reported per year in Ghana [35]. However, at least 886 cases of suspected meningitis, probable and confirmed meningitis had been reported in Brong Ahafo Region alone by the 9th week of 2016. Although pneumococcal meningitis affected individuals of all ages, nearly 60 % of the cases were among individuals between 5 and 29 years old. Nearly 80 % of the confirmed pneumococcal meningitis cases were attributed to serotype 1. Whole genome sequencing of pneumococcal isolates showed that the serotype

Table 2 Distribution of pneumococcal serotypes which caused meningitis by age group

Age Group	1	12 F	3	35B	6A/6B	7 F	[a]High Ct value	[b]Nontypeable	[c]Not serotyped	Total
<1	0	0	0	1	0	0	0	1	0	2
1–4	1	0	0	0	0	0	0	1	1	3
5–14	8	0	0	0	0	1	0	1	20	30
15–29	12	0	0	0	0	0	0	2	17	31
30–59	5	3	1	1	0	0	0	0	6	16
>60	0	0	0	0	1	0	1	0	1	3
Unknown	12	3	0	0	0	0	2	2	0	19
Grand Total	38	6	1	2	1	1	3	7	45	104

[a]These CSF had a Ct value >32 and <36 for pneumococcal detection which is above the threshold for molecular serotyping
[b]The pneumococci could not be serotyped using molecular techniques which detect a limited panel of serotypes
[c]The CSF specimens and isolates were not available for serotyping

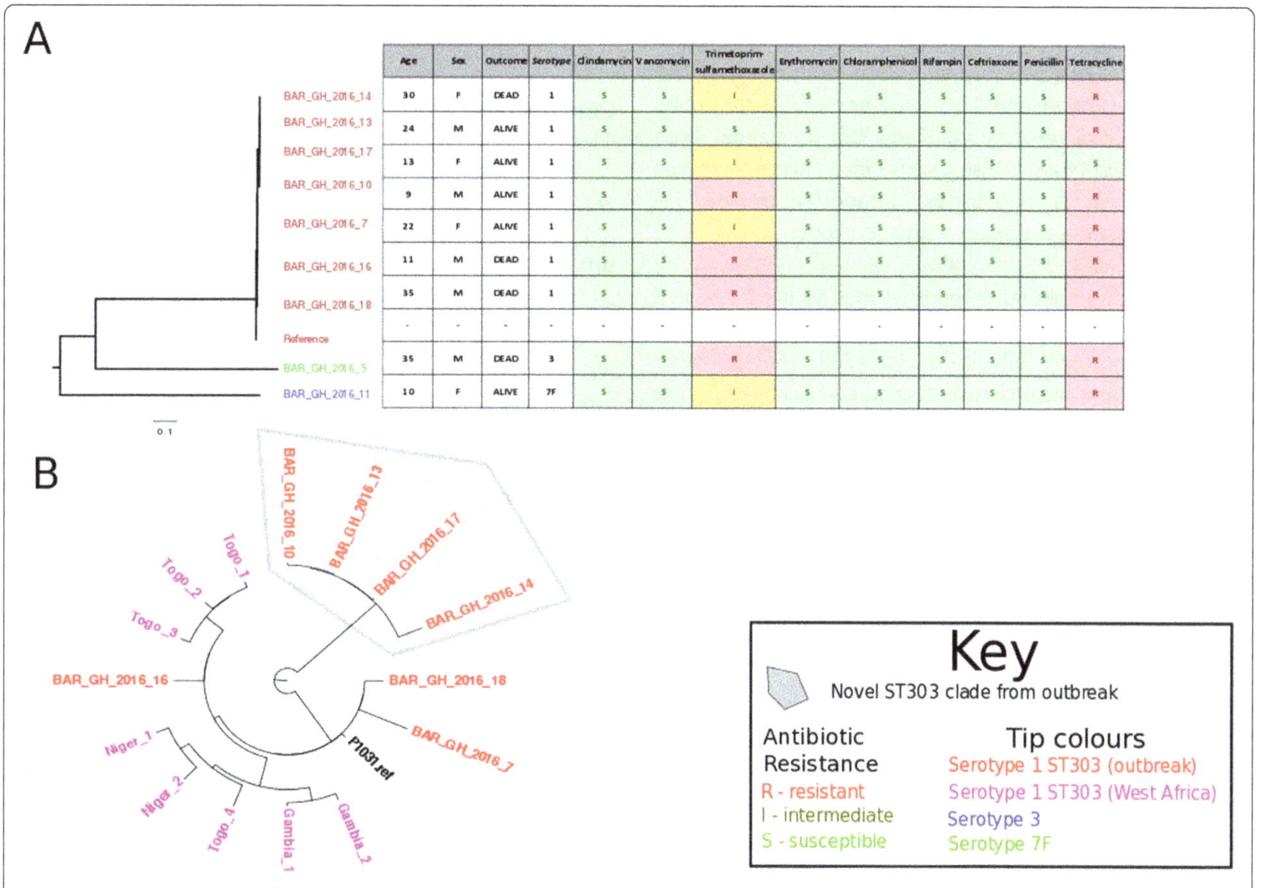

	Age	Sex	Outcome	Serotype	Clindamycin	Vancomycin	Trimetoprim-sulfamethoxazole	Erythromycin	Chloramphenicol	Rifampin	Ceftriaxone	Penicillin	Tetracycline
BAR_GH_2016_14	30	F	DEAD	1	S	S	I	S	S	S	S	S	R
BAR_GH_2016_13	24	M	ALIVE	1	S	S	S	S	S	S	S	S	R
BAR_GH_2016_17	13	F	ALIVE	1	S	S	I	S	S	S	S	S	S
BAR_GH_2016_10	9	M	ALIVE	1	S	S	R	S	S	S	S	S	R
BAR_GH_2016_7	22	F	ALIVE	1	S	S	I	S	S	S	S	S	R
BAR_GH_2016_16	11	M	DEAD	1	S	S	R	S	S	S	S	S	R
BAR_GH_2016_18	35	M	DEAD	1	S	S	R	S	S	S	S	S	R
Reference	-	-	-	-	-	-	-	-	-	-	-	-	-
BAR_GH_2016_5	35	M	DEAD	3	S	S	R	S	S	S	S	S	R
BAR_GH_2016_11	10	F	ALIVE	7F	S	S	I	S	S	S	S	S	R

Fig. 4 Phylogenetic analysis of outbreak strains. Phylogenetic tree of outbreak strains with antibiogram and patient data (**a**). Phylogenetic analysis of serotype 1 outbreak ST303 strains and historical West African ST303 strains. A novel clade of ST303 serotype distinct from the historic West African ST303 strains is evident (**b**)

1 strains from the outbreak belonged to the hypervirulent ST217 clonal complex [14, 33]. Although the increasingly important role of pneumococcus in meningitis outbreaks has been reported previously [14, 16, 17], the occurrence of a pneumococcal meningitis outbreak outside the meningitis belt post PCV13 introduction is alarming and highlights the need for vigilant monitoring of pneumococcal invasive disease in Ghana.

Implemented pneumococcal vaccination strategies in Ghana and across Africa almost exclusively target infants. The huge burden of invasive pneumococcal disease among children less than 5 years old globally, together with cost considerations and the lack of data on the burden of disease in other age categories, probably led to policies that protect the youngest and most vulnerable. PCV13 was introduced in Ghana in 2012 and includes serotype 1, which is probably why less than 5 % of pneumococcal meningitis cases were among children less than five years old. In northern Ghana, between 1998 and 2003 prior to the introduction of PCV into the expanded programme of immunization (EPI), the highest incidence of pneumococcal meningitis was found among infants with an annual incidence of 43 cases per 100,000 population [16]. Likewise in neighboring Burkina Faso and Togo between 2002 and 2006, 36 % of pneumococcal meningitis cases were among children less than 5 years old prior to the introduction of pneumococcal conjugate vaccines [3].

PCVs induce herd immunity, markedly reducing vaccine serotype carriage and invasive pneumococcal disease amongst both vaccinated and unvaccinated individuals [36]. However, the high prevalence of pneumococcal serotype 1 meningitis among older children (≥5 years) and adults heralds the need to revisit the current policy and to include all age groups in high-risk populations. Kenya has recorded success with an extensive catch up campaign with PCV-10 for all children less than five years old; there was a 66 % decline in carriage of vaccine serotypes in individuals older than 5 years [37]. If the cost of rolling out PCV13 across all age groups is considered an obstacle, the possibility of implementing a pneumococcal serotype 1 monovalent conjugate vaccine following the model used for meningococcus could be explored. However, it is important to note that the national PCV13 coverage in Ghana was only 41 % and 68 % in 2012 and 2013, respectively, which may be inadequate to induce herd immunity. Although PCV13 coverage rose to 85 % in 2014, maintenance of this coverage and close monitoring of vaccine serotype carriage and disease are needed. Furthermore, the occurrence of serotype 12 F and 35B meningitis, both non-PCV13 serotypes, is also a cause for concern. Serotype 12 F in particular is emerging as an important cause of invasive pneumococcal disease with the propensity to cause outbreaks [38–40].

Leimkugel and colleagues reported that ST303 accounted for 55 % of the serotype 1 strains responsible for a meningitis outbreak in northern Ghana in 2001–2003. All the other serotype 1 strains were clonally related and belonged to the ST217 clonal complex [16]. Likewise, closely related serotype 1 lineages belonging to the ST217 clonal complex were the predominant strains in the highly lethal meningitis epidemic between 2003 and 2004 in Burkina Faso, which borders northern Ghana [14]. All seven serotype 1 strains sequenced in the 2015–2016 Ghana meningitis outbreak belonged to ST303 and at least four are very likely to be the product of a recent clonal expansion within ST303. These strains, which belong to a unique clade, are likely to have diverged from the other previously sequenced ST303 lineages, including strain P1031 from a previous meningitis outbreak in Ghana [16].

All the pneumococcal isolates were fully susceptible to chloramphenicol and ceftriaxone. The recommended treatment for pneumococcal meningitis is vancomycin and a third generation cephalosporin (ceftriaxone and cefotaxime) or rifampin. Similarly, the recommended antimicrobial therapy for meningococcal meningitis is ceftriaxone or cefotaxime although penicillin G, ampicillin and chloramphenicol are also effective treatments [41]. It is reassuring that all the pneumococcal isolates tested were fully susceptible to ceftriaxone and chloramphenicol. Two isolates were resistant to three antibiotics, penicillin G, trimethoprim-sulfamethoxazole and tetracycline. The only meningococcal isolate available for antimicrobial susceptibility testing showed intermediate resistance to chloramphenicol. However, more isolates would have to be tested to confirm the prevalence of reduced susceptibility within the population.

This study has shown that pneumococcal outbreaks caused by closely related strains can reoccur within West Africa. Although the factors that drive pneumococcal meningitis outbreaks are not well understood, it is likely that environmental factors play an important role. As with meningococcal meningitis outbreaks, the highest incidence occurs during the dry season (December to March) [1–3] in West African countries. Greenwood has suggested that the hot dry conditions damage the mucosal defences increasing vulnerability to invasive pneumococcal and meningococcal disease [42]. Although this is a plausible contributing factor, there are likely to be other environmental and biological determinants of pneumococcal meningitis outbreaks that need to be investigated.

Conclusions

The results reported here are of great public health importance and summarised as follows: 1) Pneumococcus continues to be of increasing importance in meningitis outbreaks, even outside the meningitis belt; 2) In a post-PCV13 era, pneumococcal serotype 1 still has the propensity to cause large outbreak; 3) Non-vaccine serotypes such as serotype 12 F can be important causes of meningitis during outbreaks. The reoccurrence of pneumococcal serotype 1meningitis outbreaks in the sub-region highlights the need for a monovalent vaccine targeted to older non-infant children and adults in high-risk populations. Clear guidelines on the prevention, control and treatment of pneumococcal meningitis outbreaks need to be developed for West Africa. Meningitis surveillance and monitoring is needed even in regions that do not typically experience outbreaks as well as a careful review of the geographical areas previously considered to be at high risk for meningitis outbreaks within the West African sub-region.

Acknowledgements

We would like to acknowledge the Ministry of Health, Ghana and the clinicians, nurses, physician assistants, disease surveillance officers, biomedical scientists and data managers who managed patient care, collected the clinical and demographic data and processed the CSF specimens. We would also like to thank the National Public Health Laboratory, which coordinated the laboratory efforts during the outbreak including shipment of the CSF specimens to the WHO RRL at MRCG. The WHO Country Office, Ghana and the WHO Africa Regional Office funded and supported the RRL MRC technical mission in Ghana. The MRCG hosts the WHO RRL and provided the platform to perform molecular processing of the samples. Special thanks also go to all the members of the research molecular microbiology group at MCRG who contributed to this work. We acknowledge the Pneumococcal African Genomics Consortium (PAGe) who sequenced and assembled the ST303 draft genomes included in this analysis. This work benefited from use of the MRC Cloud Infrastructure for Microbial Bioinformatics (CLIMB).

Funding

This work was funded by the Medical Research Council Unit The Gambia, Ministry of Health Ghana, WHO Country Office Ghana and WHO Africa Regional Office.

Authors' contributions

BAKA, FAB, EF, CO, JMM, MJP, SMZ, UDA and MA drafted the manuscript. GK, GOO, EF, CE, DO, RB and JKO processed CSF specimens by Gram Stain, rapid test and culture in Ghana. MA and CO conducted molecular analysis of CSF specimens at the RRL hosted at MRC. MJP, GK and MS performed whole genome sequencing of the isolates, assembled and analysed the genomes. FAB, OKA, KAA, TL, BS, EAD, VB led and coordinated the outbreak response. Data management and data analysis were performed by KAA, BAKA and AKW. SAO, CO and OK contributed to drafting the manuscript and supported Ghana MOH with the outbreak response and facilitated the technical team from RRL at MRCG while they were in Ghana. All authors have read and approved the manuscript for submission.

Competing interests

The authors declare that they have no competing interests.

Declarations

The authors have nothing to declare.

Author details

[1]Vaccines and Immunity Theme, The Medical Research Council Unit The Gambia, P.O Box 273, Banjul, Fajara, The Gambia. [2]Ghana Health Service, Accra, Ghana. [3]Brong Ahafo Regional Health Directorate, Sunyani, Brong Ahafo, Ghana. [4]Regional Hospital Sunyani, Sunyani, Brong Ahafo Region, Ghana. [5]National Public Health Reference Laboratory, Ghana Health Service, Accra, Ghana. [6]WHO Country Office Ghana, Accra, Ghana. [7]Microbiology and Infection Unit, Warwick Medical School, Warwick, UK. [8]Ministry of Health, Accra, Ghana. [9]Disease Control and Elimination Theme, Medical Research Council Unit The Gambia, Fajara, The Gambia. [10]London School of Hygiene and Tropical Medicine, London, UK. [11]Institute of Tropical Medicine, Antwerp, Belgium. [12]WHO Regional Office for Africa, Brazzaville, Republic of Congo.

References

1. Parent du Chatelet I, Traore Y, Gessner BD, Antignac A, Naccro B, Njanpop-Lafourcade BM, Ouedraogo MS, Tiendrebeogo SR, Varon E, Taha MK. Bacterial meningitis in Burkina Faso: surveillance using field-based polymerase chain reaction testing. Clin Infect Dis. 2005;40(1):17–25.
2. Campagne G, Schuchat A, Djibo S, Ousseini A, Cisse L, Chippaux JP. Epidemiology of bacterial meningitis in Niamey, Niger, 1981–96. Bull World Health Organ. 1999;77(6):499–508.
3. Traore Y, Tameklo TA, Njanpop-Lafourcade BM, Lourd M, Yaro S, Niamba D, Drabo A, Mueller JE, Koeck JL, Gessner BD. Incidence, seasonality, age distribution, and mortality of pneumococcal meningitis in Burkina Faso and Togo. Clin Infect Dis. 2009;48 Suppl 2:S181–9.
4. LaForce FM, Okwo-Bele JM. Eliminating epidemic Group A meningococcal meningitis in Africa through a new vaccine. Health Aff (Millwood). 2011; 30(6):1049–57.
5. Marc LaForce F, Ravenscroft N, Djingarey M, Viviani S. Epidemic meningitis due to Group A Neisseria meningitidis in the African meningitis belt: a persistent problem with an imminent solution. Vaccine. 2009;27 Suppl 2:B13–9.
6. Delrieu I, Yaro S, Tamekloe TA, Njanpop-Lafourcade BM, Tall H, Jaillard P, Ouedraogo MS, Badziklou K, Sanou O, Drabo A, et al. Emergence of epidemic Neisseria meningitidis serogroup X meningitis in Togo and Burkina Faso. PLoS One. 2011;6(5):e19513.
7. Gessner BD, Mueller JE, Yaro S. African meningitis belt pneumococcal disease epidemiology indicates a need for an effective serotype 1 containing vaccine, including for older children and adults. BMC Infect Dis. 2010;10:22.
8. al-Gahtani YM, el Bushra HE, al-Qarawi SM, al-Zubaidi AA, Fontaine RE. Epidemiological investigation of an outbreak of meningococcal meningitis in Makkah (Mecca), Saudi Arabia, 1992. Epidemiol Infect. 1995;115(3):399–409.
9. Dawood FS, Ambrose JF, Russell BP, Hawksworth AW, Winchell JM, Glass N, Thurman K, Soltis MA, McDonough E, Warner AK, et al. Outbreak of pneumonia in the setting of fatal pneumococcal meningitis among US Army trainees: potential role of Chlamydia pneumoniae infection. BMC Infect Dis. 2011;11:157.
10. DeMaria Jr A, Browne K, Berk SL, Sherwood EJ, McCabe WR. An outbreak of type 1 pneumococcal pneumonia in a men's shelter. Jama. 1980; 244(13):1446–9.
11. Nuorti JP, Butler JC, Crutcher JM, Guevara R, Welch D, Holder P, Elliott JA. An outbreak of multidrug-resistant pneumococcal pneumonia and bacteremia among unvaccinated nursing home residents. N Engl J Med. 1998;338(26):1861–8.
12. Tan CG, Ostrawski S, Bresnitz EA. A preventable outbreak of pneumococcal pneumonia among unvaccinated nursing home residents in New Jersey during 2001. Infect Control Hosp Epidemiol. 2003;24(11):848–52.
13. Mercat A, Nguyen J, Dautzenberg B. An outbreak of pneumococcal pneumonia in two men's shelters. Chest. 1991;99(1):147–51.
14. Yaro S, Lourd M, Traore Y, Njanpop-Lafourcade BM, Sawadogo A, Sangare L, Hien A, Ouedraogo MS, Sanou O, Parent du Chatelet I, et al. Epidemiological and molecular characteristics of a highly lethal pneumococcal meningitis epidemic in Burkina Faso. Clin Infect Dis. 2006; 43(6):693–700.
15. A Study of the Meningococcus. British medical journal 1929, 1(3552):210–211.
16. Leimkugel J, Adams Forgor A, Gagneux S, Pfluger V, Flierl C, Awine E, Naegeli M, Dangy JP, Smith T, Hodgson A, et al. An outbreak of serotype 1 Streptococcus pneumoniae meningitis in northern Ghana with features that are characteristic of Neisseria meningitidis meningitis epidemics. J infect dis. 2005;192(2):192–9.
17. Antonio M, Hakeem I, Awine T, Secka O, Sankareh K, Nsekpong D, Lahai G, Akisanya A, Egere U, Enwere G, et al. Seasonality and outbreak of a predominant Streptococcus pneumoniae serotype 1 clone from The Gambia: expansion of ST217 hypervirulent clonal complex in West Africa. BMC Microbiol. 2008;8:198.
18. Pletz MW, Maus U, Krug N, Welte T, Lode H. Pneumococcal vaccines: mechanism of action, impact on epidemiology and adaption of the species. Int J Antimicrob Agents. 2008;32(3):199–206.
19. Millar EV, Watt JP, Bronsdon MA, Dallas J, Reid R, Santosham M, O'Brien KL. Indirect effect of 7-valent pneumococcal conjugate vaccine on pneumococcal colonization among unvaccinated household members. Clin Infect Dis. 2008; 47(8):989–96.
20. Moore MR, Hyde TB, Hennessy TW, Parks DJ, Reasonover AL, Harker-Jones M, Gove J, Bruden DL, Rudolph K, Parkinson A, et al. Impact of a conjugate vaccine on community-wide carriage of nonsusceptible Streptococcus pneumoniae in Alaska. J infect dis. 2004;190(11):2031–8.
21. O'Brien KL, Dagan R. The potential indirect effect of conjugate pneumococcal vaccines. Vaccine. 2003;21(17–18):1815–25.
22. WHO: Bacterial meningitis (including Haemophilus influenzae type b (Hib), Neisseria meningitidis, and Streptococcus pneumoniae). 2015.
23. Hill PC, Akisanya A, Sankareh K, Cheung YB, Saaka M, Lahai G, Greenwood BM, Adegbola RA. Nasopharyngeal carriage of Streptococcus pneumoniae in Gambian villagers. Clin Infect Dis. 2006;43(6):673–9.
24. Performance Standards for Antimicrobial Susceptibility Testing. Twenty-Fourth Information Supplement (M100-S24); January 2014.
25. Driscoll AJ, Bhat N, Karron RA, O'Brien KL, Murdoch DR. Disk diffusion bioassays for the detection of antibiotic activity in body fluids: applications for the Pneumonia Etiology Research for Child Health project. Clin Infect Dis. 2012;54 Suppl 2:S159–64.
26. Messmer TO, Sampson JS, Stinson A, Wong B, Carlone GM, Facklam RR. Comparison of four polymerase chain reaction assays for specificity in the identification of Streptococcus pneumoniae. Diagn Microbiol Infect Dis. 2004;49(4):249–54.
27 Vuong J, Collard JM, Whaley MJ, Bassira I, Seidou I, Diarra S, Ouedraogo RT, Kambire D, Taylor Jr TH, Sacchi C, et al. Development of Real-Time PCR Methods for the Detection of Bacterial Meningitis Pathogens without DNA Extraction. PLoS One. 2016;11(2):e0147765.
28 Janson H, Ruan M, Forsgren A. Limited diversity of the protein D gene (hpd) among encapsulated and nonencapsulated Haemophilus influenzae strains. Infect Immun. 1993;61(11):4546–52.
29 Pimenta FC, Roundtree A, Soysal A, Bakir M, du Plessis M, Wolter N, von Gottberg A, McGee L, Carvalho Mda G, Beall B. Sequential triplex real-time PCR assay for detecting 21 pneumococcal capsular serotypes that account for a high global disease burden. J Clin Microbiol. 2013;51(2):647–52.
30 Pai R, Gertz RE, Beall B. Sequential multiplex PCR approach for determining capsular serotypes of Streptococcus pneumoniae isolates. J Clin Microbiol. 2006;44(1):124–31.
31 Dias CA, Teixeira LM, Carvalho Mda G, Beall B. Sequential multiplex PCR for determining capsular serotypes of pneumococci recovered from Brazilian children. J Med Microbiol. 2007;56(Pt 9):1185–8.
32 Cornick JE, Chaguza C, Harris SR, Yalcin F, Senghore M, Kiran AM, Govindpershad S, Ousmane S, Plessis MD, Pluschke G, et al. Region-specific diversification of the highly virulent serotype 1 Streptococcus pneumoniae. Microbial Genomics. 2015;1(2):1–13.
33 Williams TM, Loman NJ, Ebruke C, Musher DM, Adegbola RA, Pallen MJ, Weinstock GM, Antonio M. Genome analysis of a highly virulent serotype 1 strain of Streptococcus pneumoniae from West Africa. PLoS One. 2012;7(10):e26742.
34 Treangen TJ, Ondov BD, Koren S, Phillippy AM. The Harvest suite for rapid core-genome alignment and visualization of thousands of intraspecific microbial genomes. Genome Biol. 2014;15(11):524.
35 Lingani C, Bergeron-Caron C, Stuart JM, Fernandez K, Djingarey MH, Ronveaux O, Schnitzler JC, Perea WA. Meningococcal Meningitis Surveillance in the

African Meningitis Belt, 2004–2013. Clin Infect Dis. 2015;61 Suppl 5:S410–5.
36 Fitzwater SP, Chandran A, Santosham M, Johnson HL. The worldwide impact of the seven-valent pneumococcal conjugate vaccine. Pediatr Infect Dis J. 2012;31(5):501–8.
37 Feazel LM, Santorico SA, Robertson CE, Bashraheil M, Scott JA, Frank DN, Hammitt LL. Effects of Vaccination with 10-Valent Pneumococcal Non-Typeable Haemophilus influenza Protein D Conjugate Vaccine (PHiD-CV) on the Nasopharyngeal Microbiome of Kenyan Toddlers. PLoS One. 2015; 10(6):e0128064.
38 Del Amo E, Esteva C, Hernandez-Bou S, Galles C, Navarro M, Sauca G, Diaz A, Gassiot P, Marti C, Larrosa N, et al. Serotypes and Clonal Diversity of Streptococcus pneumoniae Causing Invasive Disease in the Era of PCV13 in Catalonia. Spain PloS one. 2016;11(3):e0151125.
39 Janoir C, Lepoutre A, Gutmann L, Varon E. Insight Into Resistance Phenotypes of Emergent Non 13-valent Pneumococcal Conjugate Vaccine Type Pneumococci Isolated From Invasive Disease After 13-valent Pneumococcal Conjugate Vaccine Implementation in France. Open forum infect dis. 2016;3(1):ofw020.
40 Deng X, Peirano G, Schillberg E, Mazzulli T, Gray-Owen SD, Wylie JL, Robinson DA, Mahmud SM, Pillai DR. Whole-Genome Sequencing Reveals the Origin and Rapid Evolution of an Emerging Outbreak Strain of Streptococcus pneumoniae 12 F. Clin Infect Dis. 2016;62(9):1126–32.
41 Tunkel AR, Hartman BJ, Kaplan SL, Kaufman BA, Roos KL, Scheld WM, Whitley RJ. Practice guidelines for the management of bacterial meningitis. Clin Infect Dis. 2004;39(9):1267–84.
42 Greenwood B. Pneumococcal meningitis epidemics in Africa. Clin Infect Dis. 2006;43(6):701–3.

13

Tuberculous meningitis is a major cause of mortality and morbidity in adults with central nervous system infections in Kota Kinabalu, Sabah, Malaysia

Heng Gee Lee[1], Timothy William[1,2], Jayaram Menon[1], Anna P. Ralph[3], Eng Eong Ooi[4], Yan'an Hou[4], October Sessions[4] and Tsin Wen Yeo[3,5,6*]

Abstract

Background: Central nervous system (CNS) infections are a significant contributor to morbidity and mortality globally. However, most published studies have been conducted in developed countries where the epidemiology and aetiology differ significantly from less developed areas. Additionally, there may be regional differences due to variation in the socio-economic levels, public health services and vaccination policies. Currently, no prospective studies have been conducted in Sabah, East Malaysia to define the epidemiology and aetiology of CNS infections. A better understanding of these is essential for the development of local guidelines for diagnosis and management.

Methods: We conducted a prospective observational cohort study in patients aged 12 years and older with suspected central nervous system infections at Queen Elizabeth Hospital, Kota Kinabalu, Sabah, Malaysia between February 2012 and March 2013. Cerebrospinal fluid was sent for microscopy, biochemistry, bacterial and mycobacterial cultures, *Mycobacterium tuberculosis* polymerase chain reaction (PCR), and multiplex and MassCode PCR for various viral and bacterial pathogens.

Results: A total of 84 patients with clinically suspected meningitis and encephalitis were enrolled. An aetiological agent was confirmed in 37/84 (44 %) of the patients. The most common diagnoses were tuberculous meningitis (TBM) (41/84, 48.8 %) and cryptococcal meningoencephalitis (14/84, 16.6 %). *Mycobacterium tuberculosis* was confirmed in 13/41 (31.7 %) clinically diagnosed TBM patients by cerebrospinal fluid PCR or culture. The acute case fatality rate during hospital admission was 16/84 (19 %) in all patients, 4/43 (9 %) in non-TBM, and 12/41 (29 %) in TBM patients respectively ($p = 0.02$).

Conclusion: TBM is the most common cause of CNS infection in patients aged 12 years or older in Kota Kinabalu, Sabah, Malaysia and is associated with high mortality and morbidity. Further studies are required to improve the management and outcome of TBM.

Keywords: Central nervous system infections, Tuberculous meningitis, Meningitis, Encephalitis, Meningo-encephalitis

* Correspondence: yeotsinwen@ntu.edu.sg
[3]Menzies School of Health Research, Darwin, Australia
[5]Lee Kong Chian School of Medicine, Nanyang Technological University, Singapore, Singapore
Full list of author information is available at the end of the article

Background

Central nervous system (CNS) infections including meningitis and encephalitis result in significant morbidity and mortality in hospitalized patients [1–6]. The worldwide incidence and reported aetiology of CNS infections vary according to age, geographical region, economic status, vaccination policies and diagnostic capacity.

Prospective studies in various countries conducted to define the aetiology of CNS infections have shown contrasting results [1–6]. In an encephalitis study in England, infections (42 %) were the leading aetiology, followed by undetermined (37 %) and immune-mediated causes (21 %) [3]. Among those with infectious encephalitis, herpes simplex virus (19 %), varicella zoster virus (5 %) and *Mycobacterium tuberculosis* (MTB) (5 %) were the most common diagnoses [3]. In the California Encephalitis Project, the frequency of autoimmune N-methyl-D-aspartate receptor (anti-NMDAR) encephalitis was four times that of viral aetiologies in a cohort of young individuals [7]. In Vietnam, viral encephalitis and meningitis accounted for 34 % of adult CNS infections, with dengue (11 %), enteroviruses (10 %) and herpes simplex (11 %) being the most commonly identified pathogens, while tuberculous meningitis (TBM) accounted for 14 % of cases [5]. *Streptococcus pneumoniae* and *Neisseria meningitides* are the most common pathogens of bacterial meningitis in developed countries, however *Streptococcus suis*, a zoonotic pathogens from pigs, is the most common cause in Vietnam [4, 5]. Taken together, these data suggest that local data are required to develop clinically relevant guidelines

In Malaysia, only confirmed cases of viral encephalitis are notifiable while meningitis is not, requiring prospective studies to detail the epidemiology of CNS infections. In Sarawak, East Malaysia, paediatric studies of CNS Japanese encephalitis and human enterovirus 71 infections have been undertaken [8, 9]. However, no prospective studies have been conducted in Malaysian Borneo, to define the epidemiology and aetiology of meningitis and encephalitis in adults. In anticipation of future development of local clinical guidelines, we conducted a prospective hospital-based study to evaluate the aetiology and epidemiology of CNS infections in Kota Kinabalu, Sabah, Malaysia.

Methods

Study site and design

This was a prospective observational cohort study conducted at Queen Elizabeth Hospital, Kota Kinabalu, Sabah, East Malaysia, an adult tertiary care hospital with a catchment population of over 1 million. We screened all inpatients with suspected meningitis or encephalitis from February 2012 till March 2013. Research clinicians used a standardised data sheet to collect demographic data, epidemiological information, clinical history, vital signs, physical observations, biochemical and microbiological data, imaging reports, treatment, outcome, and final diagnosis. The research team followed up patients regularly until discharge or death. All patients were managed according to Malaysian Ministry of Health guidelines. For TBM, in addition to anti-tubercular medication, this included dexamethasone 0.3–0.4 mg/kg/day for week 1, 0.2–0.3 mg/kg/day for week 2, 0.1–0.2 mg/kg/day for week 3 and 0.1 mg/kg/day for week 4, followed by 4 weeks of dexamethasone decreasing by 1 mg each week. Childhood vaccinations for potential CNS pathogens in Sabah, Malaysia include diphtheria-pertussis-tetanus, measles-mumps-rubella, polio, Bacillus Calmette-Guerin (BCG) and *Haemophilus influenza type B* vaccine. In Malaysia, HIV screening is performed only for pathogens and infections associated with HIV including *Mycobaterium tuberculosis, Cryptococcus* species and syphilis but is not routine.

Definitions of clinical syndromes and outcome

Meningitis was defined as cerebrospinal fluid (CSF) pleocytosis (≥5 WBC/μL) plus two or more of the following: i) fever or history of fever (≥38^{0}C), ii) neck stiffness, iii) headache, and was further classified as acute if symptoms were present ≤ 7 days or chronic if longer.

Encephalitis was defined as encephalopathy (altered level of consciousness, lethargy, irritability, and change in behaviour or personality) longer than 24 h with two or more of the following: i) fever or history of fever (≥38^{0}C), ii) CSF pleocytosis (≥5 WBC/μL), iii) seizures or focal neurological findings, iv) abnormal neuroimaging consistent with encephalitis or v) abnormal electroencephalogram findings compatible with encephalitis. Patients with neck stiffness and encephalitis were defined as meningoencephalitis. A published consensus case definition was used to classify TBM into confirmed, probable and possible cases [10].

Criteria for exclusion were non-infectious CNS disorders due to hypoxic, vascular, toxic and metabolic causes, patients with CNS disorders lasting less than 24 h, and patients with malaria diagnosed on microscopy. Patients with an immune mediated post-infectious aetiology such as acute disseminated encephalomyelitis (ADEM) were enrolled as these often were associated with a parainfectious aetiology. We used the modified Rankin score (0 Asymptomatic, 1 Symptomatic; but no significant disability, and able to carry out all usual activities and duties, 2 Mild disability; able to function without assistance but unable to perform all previous activities, 3 Moderate disability; walk without assistance but needs help for some activities, 4 Moderately severe disability; unable to walk without assistance and attend to bodily functions, 5 Severe disability; bedridden and requiring constant care, 6 Death) to categorize the neurological status of the study subjects at the time of discharge from the hospital.

Laboratory and microbiological study procedure

Blood and CSF samples collected as part of clinical care were used for routine and research investigations. Blood was sent for bacterial cultures, malaria screening by microscopy, rapid plasma reagin (RPR) and HIV testing if indicated as mentioned above. In addition to this, a convalescent blood, nasopharyngeal and throat swab, and rectal swab were obtained if indicated. Routine CSF testing involved (i) Gram stain for bacteria, (ii) Ziehl-Nielsen stain for mycobacteria, (iii) India ink stain and cryptococcal antigen for cryptococcus, (iv) bacterial culture, (v) glucose and total protein, and (vi) total and differential white cell count. For suspected TBM cases, 1-6 ml of CSF was sent for MTB PCR and/or culture at the Sabah State Public Health Laboratory. Anti-NMDAR antibodies were measured with a semi-quantitative indirect fluorescent antibody method at a local laboratory. CSF analysis for Japanese encephalitis IgM was performed at the Malaysian National Public Health Laboratory at Sungai Buloh, Peninsular Malaysia.

Molecular testing procedures

A standardised and stratified approach was used with first line testing on CSF samples using RT-PCR in a research laboratory for viral pathogens as detailed in Table 1. Negative results were followed by second line testing using the MassCode (Agilent) platform.

In brief, nucleic acid from CSF was extracted using the QIAmp Viral RNA mini kit. Complementary DNA synthesis, PCR and purification of amplicons were done using Agilent's MassCode reagents. MassCode is a form of multiplex PCR, which utilizes a 'tag' with a distinct molecular mass conjugated directly to PCR primers [11]. Upon amplification of a pathogen sequence, these masses are then incorporated into the resulting amplicons. Masses are then cleaved off the amplicons and identified via mass spectrometry. This methodology allows for rapid and simultaneous screening against large panels of known pathogens using minimal amount of sample [12, 13]. The list of pathogens tested for using this method are detailed in Table 1.

Statistical analysis

Patients were classified according to clinical syndrome and the final aetiological diagnosis. Continuous variables were summarized as medians and range and differences between groups were analysed using Kruskal-Wallis test. Categorical variables were summarized as numbers and percentages and differences between groups compared using chi-squared or Fisher's exact test. All analyses were performed using Stata version 12 (StataCorp, College Station, Texas, USA). A two-sided value of $p < 0.05$ was considered significant.

Ethics statement

The study was approved by the Medical Research Sub-Committee of the Malaysian Ministry of Health (Reference NMRR-11-623-9629) and Menzies School of Health Research, Australia (Reference 2011-1636). All data were anonymised prior to analysis. Informed consent was obtained from patients or available relatives if their neurological condition did not allow them to. Informed consent was additionally obtained from these patients upon recovery.

Results

Baseline characteristics

There were 92 patients screened for the study and eight were excluded with alternative diagnoses (1 septic encephalopathy, one hypoxic encephalopathy, one cerebellar tumour, two acute psychosis, one cerebrovascular accident, one pneumonia, one suspected prion disease). The median age was 32.5 (range 13–67) years, 60 (71 %) were male, 15(18 %) HIV positive, and 55 (65 %) had no significant past medical history. Of the HIV patients, 11 had CD4 counts of <50/ml, 1 had 50/ml, and three had between 100–200/ml. Patients were from 18 of 23 districts in Sabah; 34/84 (40.5 %) were from the Kota

Table 1 Molecular Tests Conducted on CSF Samples

	Viral pathogens	Bacterial pathogens
First Level Tests Done for CSF samples	(i) herpes simplex virus 1 and 2, (ii) varicella zoster virus, (iii) enterovirus, (iv) Japanese encephalitis virus, (v) dengue virus, (vi) nipah virus, (vii) cytomegalovirus, (viii) West Nile virus, and (ix) bunyavirus	Not Done
Second Level Test Done for CSF samples	cytomegalovirus, Epstein Barr virus, La Crosse Virus, mumps, varicella zoster virus, measles,, human herpes virus 6, rabies, LCMV, California encephalitis group (Bunyavirus), Human Alphavirus group (Eastern, Western, Venezualan EEV), Bartonella, Flavivirus group, Enterovirus group,, St. Louis Encephalitis virus and West Nile Virus	*Haemophilus influenza, Listeria monocytogenes, Mycoplasma pneumoniae, Streptococcus pneumoniae, Staphylococcus aureus, Streptococcus agalactiae, Neisseria meningitis, Rickettsia, Leptospira, Borrelia, Legionella pneumoniae, Mycobacterium tuberculosis*

Kinabalu district and 63/84 (75 %) from the urban West Coast Division of Sabah. 68/84 (81 %) patients were Malaysian; with 22/84 (26.2 %) and 13/84 (15.5 %) from the majority Kadazan-Dusun and Bajau ethnic groups respectively.

Clinical syndromes and aetiological diagnosis

Patients were categorized into the following clinical syndromes; acute meningitis ($n = 10$: viral = 2, bacterial = 1, fungal = 4, unidentified = 3), chronic meningitis ($n = 9$: all *Cryptococcus sp*), meningoencephalitis ($n = 12$: viral = 1, fungal = 1, parasitic = 1, neurosyphilis = 2, unidentified = 7), encephalitis ($n = 12$: viral = 2, parasitic = 3, autoimmune encephalitis = 1, ADEM = 1, unidentified = 5), confirmed tuberculous meningitis ($n = 13$), probable tuberculous meningitis ($n = 20$), and possible tuberculous meningitis ($n = 8$) (Table 2). The demographic details, vital signs, laboratory results and cerebrospinal fluid results of these patients are summarized in Table 2.

A confirmed aetiological diagnosis was made in 37 of 84 (44 %) patients, with *Mycobacterium tuberculosis* (13/84, 15.5 %) the most common confirmed pathogen (Table 3). In the 43 patients who did not have confirmed, probable or possible TBM, the following aetiologies were: viral ($n = 5$, (3 enterovirus, 1 Epstein Barr virus, 1 Japanese encephalitis), bacterial ($n = 1$, *Streptococcus pneumonia*), fungal ($n = 14$, all *Cryptococcus species*), parasitic ($n = 4$, (3 *Toxoplasma* sp, 1 *Naegleria fowleri*), neurosyphilis ($n = 2$), anti-NMDAR encephalitis ($n = 1$) and acute disseminated encephalomyelitis (ADEM) ($n = 1$), while 15 remained unidentified (Table 3). No cases of herpes simplex virus meningitis or encephalitis were diagnosed.

TBM was the clinical diagnosis in 41/84 (48.8 %) of cases with CSF sent for MTB culture and PCR in 59 patients. Of those with clinical TBM, 13 of 41 (32 %) were confirmed by MTB PCR and four of this 13 were additionally MTB culture-positive (overall culture-positive rate 4/41 (9.8 %); none were culture-positive but PCR

Table 2 Demographic, vitals signs, laboratory and cerebrospinal fluid results on enrolment

	Tuberculous meningitis	Acute meningitis	Chronic meningitis	Encephalitis	Meningoencephalitis	*P* values
Number	41	10	9	12	12	
Demographic results						
Age; years, (median, range)	31 (13–64)	33 (15–65)	36.5 (22–67)	38 (16–57)	36 (14–62)	$p = 0.8$
Males; (number, percentage)	31 (75.6 %)	6 (66.6 %)	7 (77.7 %)	9 (75 %)	6 (50 %)	$p = 0.4$
Fever History (number, percentage)	32 (78 %)	9 (100 %)	7 (77.8 %)	10 (83.3 %)	8 (66.6 %)	$p = 0.4$
Days of fever before presentation (median, range)	14 (3–90)	3 (1–19)	35 (7–90)	5 (2–21)	4 (2–10)	$p < 0.001$
Headache	33 (80.5 %)	8 (88.9 %)	8 (88.9 %)	8 (66.6 %)	7 (63.6 %)	$p = 0.6$
Coma (GCS < 11)	12 (29.2 %)	2 (22.2 %)	0 (0 %)	4 (33.3 %)	3 (25 %)	$p = 0.4$
HIV Positive (number, percentage)	4 (9.8 %)	3 (33.3 %)	4 (44.4 %)	2 (16.6 %)	3 (27.7 %)	$p = 0.3$
Vitals signs and laboratory results						
Pulse Rate; median (range), (beats/min)	85 (55–155)	101 (50–160)	88 (68–108)	101 (65–140)	99 (60–162)	$p = 0.2$
Temperature; mean (range) (degrees Celsius)	37.8 (36–40)	38.5 (36.5–39)	37.6 (36.2–38.2)	38 (36.6–40.8)	36.8 (36.8–39.3)	$p = 0.4$
White blood cell count; mean (range), $\times 10^3/\mu L$	10.3 (4.3–25.3)	10.8 (6–30.3)	9.8 (4.3–13)	15.2 (4.1 to 24.9)	10 (4–22.2)	$p = 0.3$
Hemoglobin; mean (range), (g/dl)	12.4 (8.1–16.8)	13.4 (7.4–15.9)	12.1 (8–16.4)	12 (8.2–15.9)	12.1 (8.8–15.3)	$p = 0.8$
Platelet; mean (range), $\times 10^9/L$	314 (83–582)	251 (86–296)	274 (212–443)	193 (58–767)	299 (61–470)	$p = 0.1$
Lumbar Puncture Results						
Opening Pressure (cm H_2O)	21 (8–65)	6 (4–27)	17 (4–40)	15 (8–40)	15 (3–34)	$p = 0.2$
Total White Cell Count	60 (0–1160)	95 (20–220)	40 (5–1050)	50 (8–615)	30 (0–305)	$p = 0.4$
Neutrophil (Percentage)	5 (0–92)	20 (5–89)	30 (0–99)	10 (0–100)	4 (0–30)	$p = 0.09$
>50 % Neutrophils (number, percentage)	7 (17.1 %)	2 (22.2 %)	3 (33.3 %)	5 (41.7 %)	6 (50 %)	$p = 0.04$
Glucose (mmol/L)	2 (0.2-4.6)	3 (0.1-6)	1.7 (0.2-3)	3.8 (0.5-6.2)	4 (2-5)	$p = 0.7$
CSF:blood glucose ratio	0.26 (0.09–0.51)	0.45 (0.05–0.87)	0.17 (0.1–0.31)	0.55 (0.06–0.83)	0.64 (0.32–0.8)	$p < 0.001$
CSF:blood glucose ratio <50 % (number, percentage)	37 (90.2)	5 (55.5)	8 (88.8)	4 (33.3)	2 (18.2)	$p = 0.03$
Total Protein g/L	1.6 (0.3–7.1)	1.3 (0.5–4.2)	1.2 (0.7–3.8)	0.9 (0.4–8.3)	0.95 (0.3–1.6)	$p = 0.06$

$P < .05$ by analysis of variance, the Kruskal-Wallis tests, χ^2 test or Fisher's exact test comparing the groups

Table 3 Classification and causes of CNS infections

Aetiology	Total (%)
Infectious Cause	n=67 (80%)
Mycobacterium tuberculosis (Confirmed, probable and possible)	41 (50 %)
Cryptococcus sp	14 (15 %)
Treponema pallidum	2 (2 %)
Toxoplasma gondii	3 (4 %)
Japanese Encephalitis virus	1 (1 %)
Epstein–Barr virus	1 (1 %)
Naegleria fowleri	1 (1 %)
Enterovirus	3
Streptococcus pneumoniae	1
Immune-mediated cause	n = 2 (2 %)
ADEM	1 (1 %)
NMDAR Encephalitis	1 (1 %)
Unidentified	n = 15 (23 %)
Total	n = 84

negative and no non-TBM patient was PCR or culture positive for MTB. The remaining 18/41 (43.9 %) patients had probable TBM and 11/41 (26.8 %) possible TBM using the consensus case definition [10]. Four of 41 (9.8 %) patients with TBM had HIV and 37 (90.5 %) were HIV negative and apparently immunocompetent (Table 4).

Cryptococcal meningoencephalitis was the second commonest CNS infection (14/84, 16.6 %) diagnosed by cryptococcal antigen detection, with fungal culture and speciation unavailable. In this group, 9/14 (64 %) patients had HIV or other immunodeficiencies while 5 had no apparent immunodeficiency (Table 4). There were two cases (2.4 %) of confirmed neurosyphilis, three cases (3.6 %) of probable cerebral toxoplasmosis in HIV patients, three patients with enterovirus infection and one case (1.2 %) each of confirmed Japanese encephalitis (CSF Japanese encephalitis IgM positive) and Epstein-Barr virus meningitis. There was a case of probable primary amoebic meningoencephalitis (PAM) due to *Naegleria fowleri* diagnosed by CSF wet mount examination. Besides infectious aetiologies, we diagnosed one case each of acute disseminated encephalomyelitis (ADEM) and anti-N-methyl D-aspartate receptor (anti-NMDAR) encephalitis. There were 15 patients with no aetiological diagnosis after initial microbiological testing and who did not have a clinical diagnosis of TBM. In these patients, cerebrospinal fluid was available for extended molecular testing, but no additional aetiological agent was identified. The use of the MassCode platform did not result in the detection of any new pathogen not previously diagnosed.

Table 4 Causes of CNS infections in immunocompetent versus immunocompromised patients

Aetiology	Immunocompetent[a] *n* = 64 (76 %)	Immunocompromised[b] *n* = 20 (24 %)	Total *n* = 84
Mycobacterium tuberculosis	37	4	41
Cryptococcus sp	5	9	14
Toxoplasma gondii	-	3	3
Treponema pallidum	1	1	2
Japanese Encephalitis virus	1	-	1
Epstein–Barr virus	1	-	1
Naegleria fowleri	1	-	1
ADEM	1	-	1
NMDAR Encephalitis	1	-	1
Unidentified	12	3	15

[a]Includes cases for whom immune status was unknown
[b]Reasons for immunocompromised status: 15 HIV positive; 3 on steroid therapy; 1 post bone marrow transplant; 1 post splenectomy

Outcome

The overall acute case fatality rate was 19 % (16/84) during hospital admission. Additionally, 4 % (3/84), 15 % (13/84) and 20 % (17/84) had severe, moderately severe, or moderate neurological disability respectively on discharge. Five percent (4/84) had slight or no significant disability and 37 % (31/84) made a full recovery. The duration of hospital stay was prolonged in all categories, with a median of 28 days (range 4–59) in acute meningitis, 33 days (range 22–80) for chronic meningitis, 22 days (range 12-72) for encephalitis and 24 days (range 1-280) for confirmed, probable and possible tuberculous meningitis.

The outcome from TBM was significantly worse than non-tuberculous causes, with respective mortality rates of 29 % (12/41) versus 9 % (4/43) ($p = 0.02$), and severe or moderately-severe neurological deficits of 27 % (11/41) versus 11 % (5/43) ($p = 0.04$). All TBM patients received corticosteroids and anti-tubercular medications. In TBM patients, there was no significant difference in the median time to start of specific anti-tubercular medication in the patients who died or were severely disabled (2.5 days (range 0–4)) compared to those who had a good outcome (2 days (range 1–3)). In the TBM patients who died, nine were within 30 days; eight from presumed hydrocephalus and extensive cerebral infarctions, and one from multiple tuberculomas with brainstem herniation, while 3 others expired at 52, 63 and 140 days after admission. In patients with cryptococcal meningitis, 14 % (2/14) patients had a fatal outcome while 21 % (3/14) were severely disabled. In the 15 patients without TBM and no aetiological agent identified, there were two deaths (13.3 %), while 12 (80 %) made a full or good recovery. The other two patients with a fatal outcome included one with Japanese encephalitis and another with HIV and toxoplasmosis.

Discussion

In this prospective study of adult CNS infection in a tertiary hospital in Kota Kinabalu, Sabah, East Malaysia, an aetiological diagnosis was confirmed in 44 % of patients. Whether classified according to clinical syndrome or a confirmed aetiology, tuberculous meningitis (TBM) was the most common diagnosis, accounting for almost 50 % of CNS infections. Compared to other diagnoses, TBM was associated with a significantly higher proportion of death and severe neurological disability. TB is well-recognized as a major problem in East Malaysia, but rates of drug resistance and HIV in the community are fortunately low [14, 15]. For all categories of central nervous system infections, the duration of hospital stay was also fairly long, probably reflecting the time for neurological sequelae to resolve or stabilize. The aetiological agents identified in this study contrast with those previously described in developed countries including England, USA and France, where viral infections and autoimmune encephalitis were the major diagnoses [1–3]. These differences may not be surprising due to geographic, climatic and economic differences. However, our results also differ compared to studies conducted from the South and East Asian countries of Nepal and Vietnam [4–6], highlighting the importance of local data.

The diagnosis of TBM remains challenging despite availability of new diagnostic tools [16]. In this cohort, only 32 % of patients clinically classified as TBM according to a consensus criteria had a microbiological diagnosis. All were confirmed by MTB PCR with a smaller proportion also culture-positive, while no patient had CSF acid-fast bacilli observed by microscopy using the Ziehl-Neelsen stain. These and other published results suggest novel diagnostic methods with increased sensitivity are required to further improve the diagnosis of TBM [16]. Over half of TB meningitis patients had either a fatal outcome or severe neurological deficits despite institution of anti-tubercular therapy and steroids; a finding similar to other studies [17]. A recent large well-powered study of intensified dose rifampicin for TBM did not result in an improvement in outcome [18], and adjunctive agents will be required to improve the poor outcome.

Cryptococcal sp. was the major cause of CNS infection in immunocompromised patients (Table 4), emphasising the importance of testing for Cryptococcus in this group using serum/CSF cryptococcal antigen and/or Indian ink. However, 5/14 patients diagnosed with cryptococcal meningoencephalitis were immunocompetent. *Cryptococcus gatti* and *Cryptococcus neoformans var grubii* CNS infections are well-recognized in apparently immunocompetent hosts and have been reported in Vietnam and Malaysia [19–21]. However local microbiological facilities were not able to differentiate the cryptococcal species and we did not comprehensively exclude obscure forms of immunosuppression. We speculate that some of these cases were likely to be *Cryptococcus gatti.* This has clinical importance since longer treatment durations of up to 18 months and worse neurological outcomes are reported in *Cryptococcus gatti* infections [19, 20]. Similar to previous studies, cryptococcal meningitis was associated with a poor outcome with approximately one third of diagnosed patients dead or disabled.

In non-TB, non-cryptococcal meningitis, the proportion of microbiologically confirmed diagnoses was low. Only one patient had a bacterial pathogen isolated from CSF by culture, which may be due to the high rate of outpatient antibiotic use. Bacterial PCR may be more sensitive in detecting pathogens after antibiotic use, but no additional bacterial pathogens were detected using this, and more studies are needed to further evaluate the utility in this setting. The availability of viral PCR allowed us to confirm a viral diagnosis in several patients. Finally, clinicians need to be aware of rare but serious causes of CNS infection and inflammation in Sabah, Malaysia. Identification of single patients with ADEM, anti-NMDAR encephalitis and primary amoebic meningoencephalitis highlight the broad spectrum of aetiologies requiring consideration. This is of more than academic importance as the treatment strategies are radically different. The patients with ADEM and anti-NMDAR encephalitis were managed by immunomodulation using steroids in the former, and intravenous immunoglobulins and steroids in the latter. The patient with amoebic meningoencephalitis survived after receiving a combination of amphotericin B, fluconazole and rifampicin. Despite the use of modern molecular methods, almost 60 per cent of the aetiological agents responsible for central nervous infections in our study remained unidentified. This is comparable to previously-mentioned studies conducted in England, France, USA and Vietnam. However, non-identification of a confirmed pathogen was not associated with increased mortality compared to TBM or the fatality rates observed in the aforementioned studies.

Conclusion

Tuberculous meningitis was the most common diagnosis in a prospective study of CNS infections in an adult tertiary hospital in Sabah, East Malaysia, and was associated with high rates of death and severe neurological disability. Central nervous system involvement is the most serious complication of *Mycobacterium tuberculosis* infection, and further research is required to improve the diagnosis and outcome of this devastating disease.

Abbreviations

ADEM, acute disseminated encephalomyelitis; CNS, central nervous system; CSF, cerebrospinal fluid; HIV, human immunodeficiency virus; MTB, *mycobacterium tuberculosis;* NMDAR, N-methyl D-aspartate; PCR, polymerase chain reaction; TBM, tuberculous meningitis

Acknowledgments

We thank Dr Julie Granerod for her advice on the design of the study and Professor Nick Anstey for general advice on the study. We also like to thank Makmal Kesihatan Awam Kota Kinabalu, Sabah for performing the TB PCR and TB cultures. We thank the Director General of Health, Malaysian Ministry of Health for permission to publish this manuscript.

Funding

The study was funded by the Malaysian Ministry of Health. The funding body did not have any role in the conduct of the study, or writing of the manuscript.

Authors' contributions

HGL, TW, JM, APR, TWY designed and conducted the study. EEO, OS and YH did the CSF assays PCR and MassCode assays. HGL and TWY performed the statistical analysis. All authors contributed towards writing of the final manuscript and have read and approved it.

Competing interests

The authors declare that they have no competing interests.

Consent for publication

Not applicable.

Author details

[1]Department of Medicine, The Infectious Disease Unit, Queen Elizabeth Hospital, Kota Kinabalu, Sabah, Malaysia. [2]Jesselton Medical Centre, Kota Kinabalu, Sabah, Malaysia. [3]Menzies School of Health Research, Darwin, Australia. [4]Program in Emerging Infectious Diseases, Duke-NUS Graduate Medical School, Singapore, Singapore. [5]Lee Kong Chian School of Medicine, Nanyang Technological University, Singapore, Singapore. [6]Communicable Disease Centre, Institute of Infectious Diseases and Epidemiology, Tan Tock Seng Hospital, Singapore, Singapore.

References

1. Glaser CA, Gilliam S, Schnurr D, Forghani B, Honarmand S, Khetsuriani N, Fischer M, Cossen CK, Anderson LJ, California Encephalitis Project. In search of encephalitis etiologies: diagnostic challenges in the California Encephalitis Project, 1998-2000. Clin Infect Dis. 2003;36(6):731–42.
2. Mailles A, Stahl JP, Steering C, Investigators G. Infectious encephalitis in france in 2007: a national prospective study. Clin Infect Dis. 2009;49(12): 1838–47.
3. Granerod J, Ambrose HE, Davies NW, Clewley JP, Walsh AL, Morgan D, Cunningham R, Zuckerman M, Mutton KJ, Solomon T, et al. Causes of encephalitis and differences in their clinical presentations in England: a multicentre, population-based prospective study. Lancet Infect Dis. 2010; 10(12):835–44.
4. Taylor WR, Nguyen K, Nguyen D, Nguyen H, Horby P, Nguyen HL, Lien T, Tran G, Tran N, Nguyen HM, et al. The spectrum of central nervous system infections in an adult referral hospital in Hanoi, Vietnam. PLoS Os. 2012;7(8): e42099.
5. Ho Dang Trung N, Le Thi Phuong T, Wolbers M, Nguyen Van Minh H, Nguyen Thanh V, Van MP, Thieu NT, Van TL, Song DT, Thi PL, et al. Aetiologies of central nervous system infection in Viet Nam: a prospective provincial hospital-based descriptive surveillance study. PLoS ONE. 2012;7(5): e37825.
6. Giri A, Arjyal A, Koirala S, Karkey A, Dongol S, Thapa SD, Shilpakar O, Shrestha R, van Tan L, Thi Thuy Chinh BN, et al. Aetiologies of central nervous system infections in adults in Kathmandu, Nepal: a prospective hospital-based study. Sci Rep. 2013;3:2382.
7. Gable MS, Sheriff H, Dalmau J, Tilley DH, Glaser CA. The frequency of autoimmune N-methyl-D-aspartate receptor encephalitis surpasses that of individual viral etiologies in young individuals enrolled in the California Encephalitis Project. Clin Infect Dis. 2012;54(7):899–904.
8. Ooi MH, Wong SC, Podin Y, Akin W, del Sel S, Mohan A, Chieng CH, Perera D, Clear D, Wong D, et al. Human enterovirus 71 disease in Sarawak, Malaysia: a prospective clinical, virological, and molecular epidemiological study. Clin Infect Dis. 2007;44(5):646–56.
9. Ooi MH, Lewthwaite P, Lai BF, Mohan A, Clear D, Lim L, Krishnan S, Preston T, Chieng CH, Tio PH, et al. The epidemiology, clinical features, and long-term prognosis of Japanese encephalitis in Central Sarawak, Malaysia, 1997–2005. Clin Infect Dis. 2008;47(4):458–68.
10. Marais S, Thwaites G, Schoeman JF, Torok ME, Misra UK, Prasad K, Donald PR, Wilkinson RJ, Marais BJ, et al. Tuberculous meningitis: a uniform case definition for use in clinical research. Lancet Infect Dis. 2010;10(11):803–12.
11. Briese T, Palacios G, Kokoris M, Jabado O, Liu Z, Renwick N, Kapoor V, Casas I, Pozo F, Limberger R, et al. Diagnostic system for rapid and sensitive differential detection of pathogens. Emerg Infect Dis. 2005;11(2):310–3.
12. Palacios G, Briese T, Kapoor V, Jabado O, Liu Z, Venter M, Zhai J, Renwick N, Grolla A, Geisbert TW, et al. MassTag polymerase chain reaction for differential diagnosis of viral hemorrhagic fever. Emerg Infect Dis. 2006;12(4): 692–5.
13. Lamson D, Renwick N, Kapoor V, Liu Z, Palacios G, Ju J, Dean A, St George K, Briese T, Lipkin WI, et al. MassTag polymerase-chain-reaction detection of respiratory pathogens, including a new rhinovirus genotype, that caused influenza-like illness in New York State during 2004-2005. J Infect Dis. 2006; 194(10):1398–402.
14. Rashid Ali MR, Parameswaran U, William T, Bird E, Wilkes CS, Lee WK, Yeo TW, Anstey NM, Ralph AP. A prospective study of tuberculosis drug susceptibility in sabah, malaysia, and an algorithm for management of isoniazid resistance. J Trop Med. 2015;2015:261925.
15. William T, Parameswaran U, Lee WK, Yeo TW, Anstey NM, Ralph AP. Pulmonary tuberculosis in outpatients in Sabah, Malaysia: advanced disease but low incidence of HIV co-infection. BMC Infect Dis. 2015;15:32.
16. Ho J, Marais BJ, Gilbert GL, Ralph AP. Diagnosing tuberculous meningitis - have we made any progress? Trop Med Int Health. 2013; 18(6):783–93.
17. Thwaites GE, Nguyen DB, Nguyen HD, Hoang TQ, Do TT, Nguyen TC, Nguyen QH, Nguyen TT, Nguyen NH, Nguyen TN, et al. Dexamethasone for the treatment of tuberculous meningitis in adolescents and adults. New Engl J Med. 2004;351(17):1741–51.
18. Heemskerk AD, Bang ND, Mai NT, Chau TT, Phu NH, Loc PP, Chau NV, Hien TT, Dung NH, Lan NT, et al. Intensified Antituberculosis Therapy in Adults with Tuberculous Meningitis. New Engl J Med. 2016;374(2):124–34.

19. Franco-Paredes C, Womack T, Bohlmeyer T, Sellers B, Hays A, Patel K, Lizarazo J, Lockhart SR, Siddiqui W, Marr KA. Management of Cryptococcus gattii meningoencephalitis. Lancet Infect Dis. 2015;15(3):348–55.
20. Chen SC, Meyer W, Sorrell TC. Cryptococcus gattii infections. Clin Microbiol Rev. 2014;27(4):980–1024.
21. Chau TT, Mai NH, Phu NH, Nghia HD, Chuong LV, Sinh DX, Duong VA, Diep PT, Campbell JI, Baker S, et al. A prospective descriptive study of cryptococcal meningitis in HIV uninfected patients in Vietnam - high prevalence of Cryptococcus neoformans var grubii in the absence of underlying disease. BMC Infect Dis. 2010;10:199.

14

Characteristics and outcomes of cryptococcal meningitis in HIV seronegative children in Beijing, China, 2002–2013

Ling-yun Guo[1,2], Lin-lin Liu[1], Yue Liu[3], Tian-ming Chen[1], Shao-ying Li[1], Yong-hong Yang[2*†] and Gang Liu[1*†]

Abstract

Background: Data regarding HIV-seronegative pediatric patients with cryptococcal meningitis (CM) have been very limited.

Methods: We retrospectively reviewed non-HIV-infected in patients with CM from January 2002 through December 2013 in Beijing Children's Hospital. Records of the all patients were obtained and compared.

Results: The 34 children had a median age of 5.6 years. Most of the patients were male (67.6 %). Only 23.5 % of the cases had identifiable underlying diseases. The sensitivity of the CSF cryptococcal antigen, India ink smear and CSF culture in our study were 81.5, 85.3 and 82.4 %, respectively. And the sensitivity of combinations of these tests was 91.2 %. Out of the 34 patients, 16 (47.1 %) had other organs involvement in addition to the brain. The main abnormal features via magnetic resonance imaging (MRI) were Virchow-Robin space dilatation (44.4 %), hydrocephalus (38.9 %), gelatinous pseudocysts (33.3 %), brain atrophy (33.3 %), meningeal enhancement (27.8 %) and local lesions (27.8 %). In total, 64.7 % of the patients were successfully treated at discharge, whereas treatment failed in 35.3 % of the patients.

Conclusions: Cryptococcal meningitis is an infrequent disease with a high fatality rate in children in China. The majority of patients were apparently healthy. Clinicians should consider cryptococcal infection as a potential pathogen of pediatric meningitis. Cryptococcal antigen, India ink smear and culture tests are recommended for diagnosis.

Background

Cryptococcal meningitis (CM) is the most common fungal infection of the central nervous system and has a high morbidity and mortality. Globally, approximately 957,900 cases of CM occur annually, resulting in 624,700 deaths within 3 months after infection [1]. Many large studies have been conducted in adults, but few studies have been dedicated to pediatric patients. On the basis of these limited data, the incidence of cryptococcosis in children was 0.016–100 cases/100,000 children [2]. The average annual incidence of CM was found to be 0.43/100,000 in China [3]. Reported pediatric patients only account for 2 % of all cryptococcal cases [4] but could potentially result in higher morbidity and mortality [5]. Furthermore, the average annual incidence of CM is less frequent especially in non-HIV (human immunodeficiency virus) pediatric population [1–3, 6–9]. Human immunodeficiency virus (HIV) infection is a main risk factor and accounts for 95 % of CM cases in middle- and low-income countries and 80 % of CM cases in high-income countries [7, 8]. However, the majority of adult patients with CM in China are apparently healthy (66.9 %) [9].

Data regarding predisposed and normal in children have been very limited. Here, we present a single-center study of CM in non-HIV-infected pediatric patients with a comprehensive analysis of clinical features and outcomes.

* Correspondence: yyh628628@sina.com; liugangbch@sina.com
†Equal contributors
[2]Key Laboratory of Major Diseases in Children and National Key Discipline of Pediatrics (Capital Medical University), Ministry of Education, National Clinical Research Centre for Respiratory Diseases, Beijing Key Laboratory of Pediatric Respiratory Infection Diseases, Beijing Pediatric Research Institute, Beijing Children's Hospital, Capital Medical University, Beijing, China
[1]Department of Infectious Diseases, Beijing Children's Hospital, Capital Medical University, Beijing, China
Full list of author information is available at the end of the article

Methods

Study population

We retrospectively reviewed non-HIV-infected in patients with CM from January 2002 through December 2013 in Beijing Children's Hospital (a 970-bed tertiary health care hospital), China. Records of all of the patients with CM during a 12-year period were obtained. Demographic data, underlying diseases, clinical features in the patients' history, laboratory findings, cranial imaging, antifungal treatments and outcomes were analyzed.

Definitions

Diagnosis of cryptococcal meningitis

A definite diagnosis of CM was determined if the patient met at least one of the following criteria [10]; (1) positive culture of *Cryptococcus* from cerebrospinal fluid (CSF), (2) positive India ink smear of CSF centrifuged sediment for *Cryptococcus*, or (3) positive cryptococcal antigen findings in the CSF and/or in the blood.

Cryptococcal antigen assay

The Immy Latex-Crypto Antigens (Immuno-Mycologics, Inc.) were used to perform the antigen assay.

Normal and predisposed hosts

Patients with one or more predisposing factors, such as underlying diseases (nephrotic syndrome, Henoch-Schon leinpurpura, juvenile rheumatoid arthritis, pyothorax, lung tuberculosis, X-linked agammaglobulinemia (XLA), hepatitis B virus infection, or congenital heart disease), were classified as predisposed hosts. Patients with no identifiable underlying diseases were classified as previously healthy hosts.

The severity of fever

A low degree of fever indicates a temperature between 37.4 and 38 °C; a moderate degree of fever indicates a temperature between 38 and 39 °C; and a high degree of fever indicates a temperature more than 39 °C.

Outcomes

Major outcomes could be in-hospital all-cause mortality and mortality at 6-months; and minor outcomes are CSF sterilization rate after the induction phase, the proportion of neurologicalsequelae (hearing and visual impairment) after the onset of disease and the length of hospitalization. Long-term outcomes were assessed via telephone at the end point of follow-up.

Statistical analysis

Mean and standard deviations (SDs) are shown when distributions were confirmed normal; median and interquartile range (IQRs) are reported otherwise. The categorical variables were compared using the Chi-square test or Fischer's exact test, as appropriate. Continuous variables within two groups were compared using the independent t-test for parametric data and the Mann-Whitney U test for non-parametric data. P values <0.05 were considered statistically significant. All of the statistical analyses were conducted using SPSS 17.0 (SPSS Inc., USA).

Results

Overall, 34 HIV-negative children with CM were enrolled in this study.

Baseline characteristics of the patients

The median onset age was 5.6 (range 1.6, 12.6) years and 88.2 % of the children were more than three years old. Twenty-three patients were male (67.6 %) and from a rural area (76.5 %). The male/female ratio was 2.09:1. Half of the patients (50 %) obtained the disease in the summer (June-August) during the 12-year period. Nearly half of the patients (44.1 %) had contact history with birds before the onset of illness. All of the children were Han people. The patients were from 10 provinces and districts of China; the largest subset of the population came from Hebei province. The numbers of cases were evenly distributed over the 12-year period with four cases every year apart from 2012 when there were eight cases (Fig. 1).

The median time from symptom onset to diagnosis was 30 (interquartile range 17, 54) days. In six cases (17.6 %), symptoms appeared less than two weeks before the diagnosis of CM, whereas in 23 patients (67.6 %), symptoms appeared between two weeks to two months prior to diagnosis. The other five patients (14.7 %) displayed symptoms more than two months prior to diagnosis. Of the participants, 70.6 % (24 cases) of the children were misdiagnosed as having other diseases before admission to our study, with tuberculosis (11/24, 45.8 %) accounting for the majority of these other diagnoses.

Predisposing factors

All of the children were confirmed to be non-HIV infected by negative serum HIV antibodies. Only 8 cases (23.5 %) had identifiable underlying diseases. The following immunocompromising conditions were found in one of each of those eight cases: nephrotic syndrome, Henoch-Schonleinpurpura, juvenile rheumatoid arthritis, pyothorax, lung tuberculosis, X-linked agammaglobulinemia (XLA), hepatitis B virus infection, or congenital heart disease. The remaining 26 (76.5 %) patients were apparently healthy with basically normal levels of immunoglobulins and T cell subsets (CD4+ Tcells and CD8+ T cells). The CD4+ T lymphocyte count of all the patients were more than $500/mm^3$.

Signs and symptoms

All of the patients had fever, which was the most common symptom, with 5.9 % (2 cases) presenting a low degree,

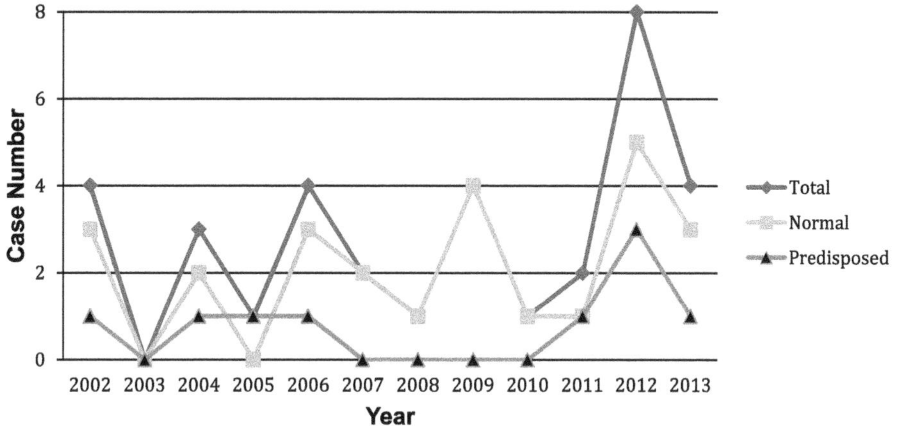

Fig. 1 Number of cryptococcal meningitis cases diagnosed per year. The number of cases diagnosed remained constant each year except for 2012

35.3 % (12 cases) presenting a moderate degree, and 58.8 % (20 cases) presenting a high degree. Other common clinical manifestations included nausea (22 cases, 64.7 %), headache (21 cases, 61.8 %), vomiting (21 cases, 61.8 %), meningeal signs (18 cases, 52.9 %) and neck stiffness (16 cases, 47.1 %). Eleven patients (32.4 %) presented with altered mental status, consciousness or fundus changes. Cranial nerve palsies were observed in 10 (29.4 %) cases involving the optic nerve, oculomotor nerve and facial nerve. Ten cases (29.4 %) experienced seizures, including five patients who had grand mal seizures. Five patients (14.7 %) presented limb weakness.

Laboratory data

Blood findings

The median white blood cell (WBC) count in the blood was 10.5 (interquartile range 8.6, 14.9) × 10^9/L with a predominance of neutrophils. 52.2 % of the patients had eosinophilia with the median eosinophil 1.07 (interquartile range 0.3, 1.24) × 10^9/L. The median CRP was 15.6 mg/L with a maximum of 150 mg/L (inflammation was evaluated with a test that measured levels in excess of 8 mg/L). The erythrocyte sedimentation rate (ESR) was 46.5 ± 30.2 mm/h, and 18/29 (62.1 %) of the patients had elevated IgE levels. There were not any other clinical features of these in the children with eosinophilia and raised IgE, like recurrent boils, rashes etc., indicating that there was no suspected Hyperimmunoglobulin E Syndrome (Job's syndrome) patients.

Cerebrospinal fluid (CSF) findings

All of the patients underwent lumbar puncture. 27/34 (79.4 %) had the medical records of CSF opening pressure .55.6 % (15/27) of the patients had high CSF opening pressure (>200 mmH2O) and the other 12 patients had normal CSF opening pressure. 8/15 (53.3 %) had the values records, 75 % (6/8) of the patients > 300 mmH_2O, the other two patients' values were between 200 ~ 300 mmH_2O. The median WBC count in the CSF was 31 (interquartile range 9, 100) × 10^6/L, with 67.6 % (23 cases) having pleocytosis. The median CSF glucose concentration was 2.38 ± 1.41 mmol/L, and 67.6 % (23 cases) had below normal levels (2.8 mmol/L). Seven of the 34 (20.6 %) patients had the ratio of CSF to plasma glucose at the meantime, and 42.9 % (3/7) of those patients had a CSF: glucose ratio that was less than 50 % of their plasma. The median CSF protein concentration was 585 (interquartile range 361, 860) mg/L, with 64.7 % (22 cases) having above normal levels (450 mg/L).

Neuroradiological manifestation

Eighteen and 17 cases underwent cranial MRI or CT scans, respectively. All of the patients had abnormal results. Among these, the main radiological features via MRI were Virchow-Robin space dilatation (8/18, 44.4 %), hydrocephalus (7/18, 38.9 %), gelatinous pseudocysts (6/18, 33.3 %), brain atrophy (6/18, 33.3 %), meningeal enhancement (5/18, 27.8 %) and local lesions (5/18, 27.8 %). Common sites of Virchow-Robin space dilatation and gelatinous pseudocysts were the basal ganglia region and corona zone. The MRI scans also detected two cases of granuloma. We found that 90 % of the patients (9/10) had abnormal results as detected by magnetic resonance venography (MRV), mostly as transverse sinus and sigmoid sinus slim or discontinuous imaging. The vast majority of the patients obtained normal magnetic resonance angiography (MRA) results, whereas only two cases had a thinner middle cerebral artery. In contrast to MRI, common abnormal results for CT scans were hydrocephalus (9/17, 52.9 %) and brain atrophy (11/17, 64.7 %) without Virchow-Robin space dilatation and gelatinous pseudocysts.

Electroencephalogram
In 12 cases, the patients underwent an electroencephalogram test, and seven cases (58.3 %) had abnormal results with varying slow wave levels.

Pathogen findings
The sensitivity of the CSF cryptococcal antigen, India ink smear and CSF culture in our study were 81.5, 85.3 and 82.4 %, respectively. And the sensitivity of combinations of these three tests was 91.2 %. Of these, 88.2 % (30/34) of cases obtained positive results in the first three lumbar punctures. One patient obtained positive results in the ninth lumbar punctures. We had three patients who had all negative results of these three pathogen tests in the CSF, but had positive results antigens for Cryptococcus in the blood (Table 1).

Other organs involvement
Sixteen of the 34 patients (47.1 %) had other organs involvement in addition to the brain. All but one patient had lung involvement. Other organs included the liver, spleen, lymph node, renal and bone marrow. Infections were diagnosed in two patients by mesentery lymph node histopathology and sputum sampling, respectively.

Initial antifungal therapy and outcomes
Four initial antifungal regimens were prescribed to the patients. A combination of amphotericin B and fluconazole, with or without flucytosine for 12 cases accounted for the first regimen, followed by fluconazole with or without flucytosine for 10 cases, and amphotericin B for five cases. Seven more patients were administered other treatments including amphotericin B colloidal dispersion, itraconazole, voriconazole, and others. Amphotericin B was given intrathecally to 11 patients (32.4 %) during hospitalization. Ventricular drainage or lumbar drainage was performed in two cases (5.9 %). Three patients (8.8 %) were transferred to the pediatric intensive care unit because of disease deterioration; two of these patients experienced mechanical ventilation. Two cases (5.9 %) experienced cerebral herniation during the hospitalization, three cases (8.8 %) had renal injury and 16 cases (47.1 %) had hypokalemia. In those patients who took amphotericin B therapy, 85.7 % of patients had anemia, 44.4 % had elevated aminotransferase and 15.4 % had neutropenia. There was no patient died in the hospital. Of all of the patients, 22 (64.7 %) obtained a successful outcome at discharge; half of those patients had a complete response, and the other half had a partial response. However, 12 cases (35.3 %) experienced failure results, with six cases having stable or progressive status at the time of discharge. CSF sterilization rate after the induction phase was 13.6 % (3/22). Fifteen patients under went followed up for a median time of two years. Seven patients (46.7 %) had a poor outcome at the endpoint, five of these patients (33.3 %) died, and two (13.3 %) were left with an altered mental status and visual impairment. Eight patients (53.3 %) recovered with no complications. No patients progressed to epilepsy. Compared to the survival group and the death group, the patients in death group were more likely to have neck stiffness (100 vs. 30 %, $P < 0.05$). The patients in survival group had higher ESR and eosinophil than patients in death group. There were no significant differences in baseline characteristics such as age, area, contact history, time to diagnosis, hospitalization, daily cost and CSF tests (Table 2).

Table 1 Pathogen findings of cryptococcal meningitis in CSF

Times	Antigen (%) ($n = 27$)	India ink smear (%) ($N = 34$)	Culture (%) ($N = 34$)	Combination (%) ($N = 34$)
1st	20 (74.1)	9 (26.5)	11 (32.4)	26 (76.5)
2nd	22 (81.5)	20 (58.9)	16 (47.1)	29 (85.3)
3rd	22 (81.5)	23 (67.6)	22 (64.7)	30 (88.2)
>3rd	22 (81.5)	29 (85.3)	28 (82.4)	31 (91.2)
Negative	5 (18.5)	5 (14.7)	6 (17.6)	3 (8.8)
Total	27 (100)	34 (100)	34 (100)	34 (100)

Comparison between normal and predisposed hosts
There were 26 (76.5 %) normal host patients and eight (23.5 %) cases in the predisposed host group. The patients in the two hosts groups showed no significant differences in baseline characteristics such as age, area, contact history, time to diagnosis, hospitalization, daily cost and prognosis both at discharge and follow-up. In terms of manifestations, compared to normal hosts, the patients who had underlying diseases were more prone to having an altered mental status (62.5 vs. 19.2 %, $P < 0.05$) and seizures (62.5 vs. 15.4 %, $P < 0.05$). The patients in the normal hosts group had a higher ESR than patients in the predisposed hosts group. Other routine CSF and chemistry tests as well as blood findings had similar results in the two host groups (Table 3).

Discussion
The central nervous system is the main involved area in cryptococcosis disease both in pediatric and adults' population. Data showed that there was 83.4 % of central nervous system involvement in 8769 cases of cryptococcosis in China from 1985 to 2010 [11] and 87.1 % of the pediatric cases had central nervous system involvement in China [4]. However, this is less frequent pediatric cases reported, particularly in non-HIV patients [1–3, 6–9]. Reported pediatric patients only account for 2 % of all cryptococcal-cases [4] but could potentially result in higher morbidity and mortality rates [5].

In our study, 67.6 % of the patients were boys. This is similar to other hospital-based reports of CM in both

Table 2 Comparison between the survival group and the death group ($N = 15$)

	Survival group (%) ($n = 10$)	Death group (%) ($n = 5$)	P
Age (year)	6 (4–10)	8 (5–10)	0.624
Sex (Male:Female)	3:2	1:4	0.282
Area (rural)	6 (60)	5 (100)	0.231
Contacting history	5 (50)	2 (40)	1.000
Predisposed hosts	4 (40)	2 (40)	1.000
Time to diagnosis (day)	28 ± 13	24 ± 20	0.732
Hospitalization (day)	53 ± 28	25 ± 23	0.084
Daily cost (RMB)	1258 (685–2502)	1304 (1187–2321)	0.540
Manifestations			
Fever	39.3 (38.6–39.8)	38.5 (38.5–39.2)	0.156
Headache	5 (50)	4 (80)	0.580
Vomiting	6 (60)	5 (100)	0.231
Altered mental status	1 (10)	3 (60)	0.077
Seizure	3 (30)	4 (80)	0.119
Vision damage	3 (30)	2 (40)	1.000
Neck stiffness	3 (30)	5 (100)	0.026*
Fundus abnormality	2 (25)	2 (100)	0.133
CSF			
CSF WBC ($\times10^6$/L)	24.5 (7.5–91.0)	16.0 (2.0–69.0)	0.581
Glu (mmol/L)	2.82 (1.88–3.76)	2.80 (1.54–5.40)	0.903
Pro (mg/L)	523 (333–856)	361(170–1492)	0.806
Blood			
WBC ($\times10^9$/L)	10.4 (8.6–18.2)	10.7 (9.0–12.1)	0.806
CRP (mg/L)	29.8 (7.8–41.6)	11.9 (1.7–54.5)	0.315
ESR (mm/h)	51 (44–76)	24 (16–31)	0.042*
EO ($\times10^9$/L)	1.37 (0.55–2.81)	0.2 (0.07–1.05)	0.040*

*$P < 0.05$

Table 3 Comparison between the predisposed hosts and normal hosts ($N = 34$)

	Normal hosts (%) ($n = 26$)	Predisposed hosts (%) ($n = 8$)	P
Age (year)	5 (3–9)	7 (4–10)	0.900
Sex (Male: Female)	19:7	1:1	0.388
Area (rural)	21 (80.8)	5 (62.5)	0.355
Contacting history	10 (38.5)	5 (62.5)	0.417
Time to diagnosis (day)	30 (20–56)	25 (13–56)	0.759
Hospitalization (day)	41 ± 25	53 ± 44	0.352
Daily cost (RMB)	846 (567–1615)	1080 (621–1080)	0.138
Disseminated cryptococcosis	14 (53.8)	2 (25.0)	0.233
Manifestations			
Fever	39.2 ± 0.7	38.9 ± 0.8	0.242
Headache	14 (53.8)	7 (87.5)	0.116
Vomiting	14 (53.8)	7 (87.5)	0.116
Altered mental status	5 (19.2)	5 (62.5)	0.031*
Seizure	4 (15.4)	5 (62.5)	0.017*
Vision damage	4 (15.4)	4 (50.0)	0.066
Neck stiffness	13 (50.0)	5 (62.5)	0.693
Blood			
WBC ($\times10^9$/L)	12.4 (8.6–16.3)	10.2 (8.8–11.3)	0.274
CRP (mg/L)	11.9 (0–63.5)	16 (0–30.9)	0.592
ESR (mm/h)	50 (26–79)	10 (1–52)	0.037*
EO ($\times10^9$/L)	0.72 (0.31–1.77)	0.38 (0.2–1.24)	0.504
CSF			
WBC ($\times10^6$/L)	32 (10–113)	25 (7–102)	0.313
Glu (mmol/L)	2.24 ± 1.23	2.80 ± 1.92	0.332
Pro (mg/L)	625 (436–890)	660 (386–938)	0.528
Prognosis			
Success at discharge	16 (61.5)	6 (75.0)	0.618
Success at follow-up	4/10 (40.0)	3/5 (60.0)	0.608

*$P < 0.05$

adults and children with male predominance [2, 3, 12–17]. Why there is a male predominance in patients with CM is an interesting question requiring further evaluation. In our series, most of the patients were from rural areas with a history of contacting birds. Guo Jiahua reported that 73.9 and 73.26 % of infected children were from rural areas and had a history of avian contact in Shi Jiazhuang, China [3]. Similar results were also obtained in a population-based study in Australia and New Zealand [18]. The reason for this phenomenon is unknown but may partly be due to increased environmental exposure.

The median age of the infected children was approximately 5.6 years old in the current study, and only three cases were younger than two years of age consistent with prior studies of CM in non-HIV children [2, 3, 15, 18]. Only 3 % of the cases in the reported literature and 9.5 % of new patients are younger than 2 years [19]. This finding could be explained by the increase in the mobility and independence of children, resulting in increased environmental exposure.

In our study, 52.2 and 62.1 % of the patients had an eosinophilia or elevated IgE level, respectively. There were not any other clinical features of these in the children with eosinophilia and raised IgE, indicating that there was no suspected Hyperimmunoglobulin E Syndrome. Although eosinophilia has been reported in HIV-negative cryptococcal infection patients, it is still relatively rare [11, 20–23]. Yamaguchi reported a 23-year-old patient was diagnosed as disseminated cryptococcosis including meningitis with very marked eosinophilia (75 %). And the eosinophilia was successfully alleviated by treatment for cryptococcal meningitis [24]. In addition, infections presenting with elevated

IgE have been associated with a high risk of systemic cryptococcal dissemination, including meningitis [25, 26]. Th_2-dominant immune status has been reported to cause increases in serum IgE, as well as susceptibility to cryptococcal infections [27].

In terms of clinical symptoms and signs, in the current study, fever was the most frequent symptom, followed by nausea, vomiting, headaches, meningeal signs, neck stiffness, altered mental status and consciousness, seizure and cranial nerve palsies. Visual and hearing impairment were less common. These results were similar to those described in the literature [3, 9, 15, 18]. Pleocytosis, elevated CSF proteins, and decreased CSF glucose levels were also common. Such findings are also consistent with previous reports of cryptococcosis in non-HIV-infected children by Guo and Zhu [3, 15, 18].

Notably, 70.6 % of the children were diagnosed as having other diseases before admission in our study, with tuberculosis accounting for the most frequent misdiagnosis. It is unexpected that up to 70–100 % of CM patients experienced misdiagnosis in previous studies, mostly as tuberculosis-associated diseases [15]. CM is an important differential diagnosis with tuberculosis. Moreover, it takes a long time to diagnose this disease. Thus, the tests for pathogen detection play an important role in helping doctors make a definite diagnosis. The high sensitivity of combinations with variety cryptococcal tests in our study is encouraging. The sensitivity of the CSF cryptococcal antigen, India ink smear and CSF culture in our study were 81.5, 85.3 and 82.4 %, respectively. Apparently, the India ink stain, culture and cryptococcal antigen tests should be performed in children suspected to have CM, even those with normal cerebrospinal fluid and biochemical test results.

Consistent with other studies, CM patients had poor outcomes with a longer hospitalization duration despite multi-antifungal treatments [3, 15]. 35.2 % of the patients had no response at discharge and 33.3 % died during the follow-up time. Therefore, CM in pediatric populations remains a large challenge for pediatricians.

The proportion of immunocompetent patients with CM varies among non-HIV-infected patients in different regions and countries regardless of the age. Studies from the U.S., France, and Thailand reported a relatively small rate (17–35 %) of cryptococcosis occurring in patients with an apparently healthy condition [8, 14, 28]. However, a significantly higher rate of cryptococcosis was reported in immunocompetent individuals in China. In our study, only 8 cases (23.5 %) had identifiable underlying diseases, and the remaining 26 (76.5 %) patients were apparently healthy with basically normal levels of CDs and immunoglobulins. This is consistent with other studies. For example, among the 154 CM cases reported at Huashan Hospital, Shanghai, 66.9 % cases were identified in immunocompetent individuals [9]. Similarly, 68 % of CM cases were reported in immunocompetent individuals in another study performed at Changzheng Hospital, Shanghai [29]. In terms of the 23 HIV-negative children with CM in Shi Jiazhuang, China, only 26.1 % of the cases had underlying diseases. A population-based study reported that 61.9 % of cryptococcosis cases were from immunocompetent individuals in Taiwan [30]. Furthermore, studies from other Asian countries where Chinese is the predominant ethnic group reported similar results. In a study on HIV-uninfected patients with CM in Vietnam, 81 % (57 patients) had no clear predisposing factor [31]. Taken together, these reports suggest that cryptococcosis predominantly occurs in immunocompetent hosts in the Chinese ethnic population, which may be more susceptible to cryptococcal infections than other ethnic groups. The reason for this phenomenon is not well known. Ou et al. [32] performed a study regarding the association between mannose-binding lectin (MBL) polymorphisms and the development of CM in non-HIV Chinese patients. The authors found that the genotypes underlying deficient MBL production were associated with CM in the Chinese Han ethnicity, particularly in immunocompetent patients, suggesting that MBL deficiency is a genetic predisposition to CM. Another investigation revealed that FccRIIB polymorphisms are an important genetic factor contributing to CM in HIV-uninfected Chinese individuals [33].

To our knowledge, the present study is one of the largest case series of CM in non-HIV pediatric patients around world. However, this study has some limitations. It was a single center, hospital-based retrospective design, which introduces the possibility of unrecognized biases, a high dropout rate and incomplete data collection including CSF pressure measurements, EO etc. Because of cryptococcal meningitis in non-HIV pediatric population being relatively rare, we had a small sample in the study and the small number of deaths precluding multivariate analysis of factors influencing mortality. We had no data regarding pathogen serotype or molecular type. Thus, we would like to use our central nervous system follow-up system to perform more prospective studies in the future. Further multicenter studies are necessary to enrich the generalizability of CM in children.

Conclusions

CM is an infrequent disease with a high fatality rate in children in China. The majority of patients were apparently healthy. Clinicians should consider cryptococcal infection as a potential pathogen of pediatric meningitis. Cryptococcal antigen, India ink smear and culture tests are recommended.

Abbreviations

AmB: Amphotericin B deoxycholate; CM: Cryptococcal meningitis; CSF: Cerebrospinal fluid; ESR: Erythrocyte sedimentation rate; FC: Flucytosine; Flu: Fluconazole; HIV: Human immunodeficiency virus; MBL: Mannose-binding lectin; MRA: Magnetic resonance angiography; MRI: Magnetic resonance imaging; MRV: Magnetic resonance venography; WBC: White blood cell; XLA: X-linked agammaglobulinemia

Acknowledgments

The Beijing Municipal Administration of Hospitals Incubating Program (Grant No. PX2016035) and the Beijing Health System Top Level Health Technical Personnel Training Plan (No. 2015-3-082) financially supported this study. We would like to thank the Medical Records and Statistics Room, Beijing Children's Hospital, which provided hospital discharge data.

Funding

This work was supported by the Beijing Municipal Administration of Hospitals Incubating Program (No. PX2016035) and the Beijing Health System Top Level Health Technical Personnel Training Plan (No. 2015-3-082). The funders had no role in study design, data collection and analysis, decision to publish, or preparation of the manuscript.

Authors' contributions

All of the authors had access to the full dataset (including the statistical reports and tables) and take responsibility for the integrity of the data and the accuracy of the data analysis. LG, YYH, GLY, LLL, LY and LSY conceived and designed the study. LG, GLY, LLL, LY and CTM collected the data and designed the analysis. LG, YYH, GLY, LLL and LY interpreted the data. GLY and LLL wrote the first draft of the paper. LG, YYH, GLY and LLL reviewed and approved the final report.

Competing interests

The authors declare that they have no competing interests.

Consent for publication

Not applicable.

Author details

[1]Department of Infectious Diseases, Beijing Children's Hospital, Capital Medical University, Beijing, China. [2]Key Laboratory of Major Diseases in Children and National Key Discipline of Pediatrics (Capital Medical University), Ministry of Education, National Clinical Research Centre for Respiratory Diseases, Beijing Key Laboratory of Pediatric Respiratory Infection Diseases, Beijing Pediatric Research Institute, Beijing Children's Hospital, Capital Medical University, Beijing, China. [3]Department of Radiology, Beijing Children's Hospital, Capital Medical University, Beijing, China.

References

1. Park BJ, Wannemuehler KA, Marston BJ, Govender N, Pappas PG, Chiller TM. Estimation of the current global burden of cryptococcal meningitis among persons living with HIV/AIDS. AIDS. 2009;23:525–30. doi:10.1097/QAD.0b013e328322ffac.
2. Lizarazo J, Escandon P, Agudelo CI, Castaneda E. Cryptococcosis in Colombian children and literature review. Mem Inst Oswaldo Cruz. 2014; 109(6):797–804. doi:10.1590/0074-0276130537.
3. Guo J, Zhou J, Zhang S, Zhang X, Li J, Sun Y, Qi S. A case-control study of risk factors for HIV-negative children with cryptococcal meningitis in Shi Jiazhuang, China. BMC Infect Dis. 2012;12:376. doi:10.1186/1471-2334-12-376.
4. Liao WQ, Wen H. Clinical Cryptococcosis. Shelton: People's Medical Publishing House; 2013. p. 255.
5. Speed BR, Kaldor J. Rarity of cryptococcal infection in children. Pediatr Infect Dis J. 1997;16:536–7. doi:10.1097/00006454-199705000-00024.
6. Sloan D, Parris V. Cryptococcal meningitis: epidemiology and therapeutic options. Clin Epidemiol. 2014;6:169–82. doi:10.2147/CLEP.S38850.
7. Leal AL, Faganello J, Fuentefria AM, Boldo JT, Bassanesi MC, Vainstein MH. Epidemiological profile of cryptococcal meningitis patients in Rio Grande do Sul, Brazil. Mycopathologia. 2008;166:71–175. doi:10.1007/s11046-008-9123-2.
8. Pyrgos V, Seitz AE, Steiner CA, Prevots DR, Williamson PR. Epidemiology of cryptococcal meningitis in the US: 1997–2009. PLoS One. 2013;8:e56269. doi:10.1371/journal.pone.0056269.
9. Zhu LP, Wu JQ, Xu B, Ou XT, Zhang QQ, Weng XH. Cryptococcal meningitis in non-HIV-infected patients in a Chinese tertiary care hospital, 1997–2007. Med Mycol. 2010;48:570–9. doi:10.3109/13693780903437876.
10. De PB, Walsh TJ, Donnelly JP, Stevens DA, Edwards JE, Calandra T, et al. Revised definitions of invasive fungal disease from the European Organization for Research and Treatment of Cancer/Invasive Fungal Infections Cooperative Group and the National Institute of Allergy and Infectious Diseases Mycoses Study Group (EORTC/MSG) Consensus Group. Clin Infect Dis. 2008;46(12):1813–21. doi:10.1086/588660.
11. Chen YC, Fubin C, Chen JH, Wei FL, Xu N, Yang MH, et al. Cryptococcosis in China (1985–2010): review of cases from Chinese database. Mycopathologia. 2012;173:329–35. doi:10.1007/s11046-011-9471-1.
12. Mirza SA, Phelan M, Rimland D, Graviss E, Hamill R, Brandt ME, et al. The changing epidemiology of cryptococcosis: an update from population-based active surveillance in 2 large metropolitan areas, 1992–2000. Clin Infect Dis. 2003;36:789–94. doi:10.1086/368091.
13. Zonios DI, Falloon J, Huang CY, Chaitt D, Bennett JE. Cryptococcosis and Idiopathic CD4 Lymphocytopenia. Medicine (Baltimore). 2007;86:78–92.
14. Pappas PG, Perfect JR, Cloud GA, Larsen RA, Pankey GA, Lancaster DJ, et al. Cryptococcosis in human immunodeficiency virus-negative patients in the era of effective azole therapy. Clin Infect Dis. 2001;33:690–9. doi:10.1086/322597.
15. Zhu YJ, Chen JH, Xu N, Wang XJ, Wen H, Liao WQ, et al. Cryptococcal meningitis in immunocompetent children. Mycoses. 2012;55:168–71. doi:10.1111/j.1439-0507.2011.02063.x.
16. Gonzalez CE, Shetty D, Lewis LL, Mueller BU, Pizzo PA, Walsh TJ. Cryptococcosis in human immunodeficiency virus-infected children. Pediatr Infect Dis. 1996;15:796–800. doi:10.1097/00006454-199609000-00012.
17. Chen S, Sorrell T, Nimmo G, Speed B, Currie B, Ellis D, et al. Epidemiology and host- and variety-dependent characteristics of infection due to Cryptococcus neoformans in Australia and New Zealand. Australasian Cryptococcal Study Group. Clin Infect Dis. 2000;31:499–508. doi:10.1086/313992.
18. Huang KY, Huang YC, Hung IJ, Lin TY. Cryptococcosis in nonhuman immunodeficiency virus-infected children. Pediatr Neurol. 2010;42:267–70. doi:10.1016/j.pediatrneurol.2009.10.015.
19. Goldman DL, Khine H, Abadi J, Lindenberg DJ, Pirofski L, Niang R, et al. Serologic evidence for cryptococcus neoformans infection in early childhood. Pediatrics. 2001;107:66. doi:10.1542/peds.107.5.e66.
20. Marwaha RK, Trehan A, Jayashree K, Vasishta RK. Hypereosinophilia in disseminated cryptococcal disease. Pediatr Infect Dis J. 1995;14:1102–3.
21. Starr JC, Che H, Montgomery J. Cryptococcal pneumonia simulating chronic eosinophilic pneumonia. South Med J. 1995;88:845–6.
22. Tanaka H, Urase F, Hasegawa K, Tsubaki K, Irimajiri K, Horiuchi A, et al. Sarcoidosis with severe eosinophlia due to Cryptococcus infection. Rinsho Ketsueki. 1988;29:208–13.
23. Xin B, Zhu YF, Wang XH, Yu H, Zeng M, Lu Y, et al. Clinical features and prognosis of disseminated cryptococcosis in 8 children. Chin J Evid Based Pediatr. 2015;10(4):281–6.
24. Yamaguchi H, Komase Y, Ikehara M, Yamamoto T, Shinagawa TJ. Disseminated cryptococcal infection with eosinophilia in a healthy person. Infect Chemother. 2008;14(4):319–24. doi:10.1007/s10156-008-0618-z.
25. Stone BD, Wheeler JG. Disseminated cryptoccocal infection in a patient with hyperimmunoglobulinemia E syndrome. J Pediatr. 1990;117:92–5.
26. Garty BZ, Wolach B. Cryptoccocal meningitis in a child with hyperimmunoglobulin E syndrome. Pediatr Allergy Immunol. 1995;6:175–7.
27. Traynor TR, Kuziel WA, Toews GB, Huffnagle GB. CCR2 expression determines T1 versus T2 polarization during pulmonary Cryptococcusneoformansinfection. J Immunol. 2000;164:2021–7.

28. Kiertiburanakul S, Wirojtananugoon S, Pracharktam R, Sungkanuparph S. Cryptococcosis in human immunodeficiency virus-negative patients. Int J Infect Dis. 2006;10:72–8. doi:10.1016/j.ijid.2004.12.004.
29. Chen J, Varma A, Diaz MR, Litvintseva AP, Wollenberg KK, Kwon-Chung KJ. Cryptococcus neoformans strains and infection in apparently immunocompetent patients, China. Emerg Infect Dis. 2008;14:755–62. doi: 10.3201/eid1405.071312.
30. Chen YY, Lai CH. Nationwide population-based epidemiologic study of cryptococcal meningitis in Taiwan. Neuroepidemiology. 2011;36:79–84. doi: 10.1159/000323390.
31. Chau TT, Mai NH, Phu NH, Nghia HD, Chuong LV, Sinh DX, et al. A prospective descriptive study of cryptococcal meningitis in HIV uninfected patients in Vietnam – high prevalence of Cryptococcus neoformans var grubii in the absence of underlying disease. BMC Infect Dis. 2010;10:199. doi:10.1186/1471-2334-10-199.
32. Ou XT, Wu JQ, Zhu LP, Guan M, Xu B, Hu XP, et al. Genotypes coding for mannose-binding lectin deficiency correlated with cryptococcal meningitis in HIV-uninfected Chinese patients. J Infect Dis. 2011;203:1686–91. doi:10.1093/infdis/jir152.
33. Hu XP, Wu JQ, Zhu LP, Wang X, Xu B, Wang RY, et al. Association of Fcgamma receptor IIB polymorphism with cryptococcal meningitis in HIV-uninfected Chinese patients. PLoS One. 2012;7:e42439. doi:10.1371/journal.pone.0042439.

15

Time to antibiotic therapy and outcome in bacterial meningitis

Jacob Bodilsen[1,2*], Michael Dalager-Pedersen[1], Henrik Carl Schønheyder[3,4] and Henrik Nielsen[1,4]

Abstract

Background: Community-acquired bacterial meningitis (CABM) is a life-threatening disease and timing of antibiotic therapy remains crucial. We aimed to analyse the impact of antibiotic timing on the outcome of CABM in a contemporary cohort.

Methods: We conducted a population-based cohort study based on chart reviews of all adult cases (>16 years of age) of CABM in North Denmark from 1998 to 2014 excluding patients given pre-hospital parenteral antibiotics. We used modified Poisson regression analyses to compute the adjusted risk ratio (adj. RR) with 95 % confidence intervals (CIs) for in-hospital mortality and unfavourable outcome at discharge by time after arrival to hospital to adequate antibiotic therapy.

Results: We identified 195 adults with CABM of whom 173 patients were eligible for further analyses. The median door-to-antibiotic time was 2.0 h (interquartile range (IQR) 1.0–5.5). We observed increased adjusted risk ratios for in-hospital mortality of 1.6 (95 % CI 0.8–3.2) and an unfavourable outcome at discharge of 1.5 (95 % CI 1.0–2.2, $p = 0.03$) when treatment delays exceeded 6 h versus treatment within 2 h of admission. These findings corresponded to adjusted risk ratios of in-hospital mortality of 1.1 per hour of delay (95 % CI 0.8–1.5) and an unfavourable outcome at discharge of 1.1 per hour of delay (95 % CI 1.0–1.3) within the first 6 h of admission. Some patients (31 %) were diagnosed after admission and had more delays in antibiotic therapy and correspondingly increased in-hospital mortality (30 vs 14 %, $p = 0.01$) and unfavourable outcome (62 vs 37 %, $p = 0.002$).

Conclusions: Delay in antibiotic therapy was associated with unfavourable outcome at discharge.

Keywords: Bacterial meningitis, Antibiotic therapy, Outcome

Background

Community-acquired bacterial meningitis (CABM) is a devastating disease with substantial morbidity and mortality despite treatment with modern antibiotics, advanced intensive care and adjuvant dexamethasone treatment [1, 2]. Thus far, attempts to further improve outcome, including supplemental treatment with glycerol and induced hypothermia, have failed [3–6].

Therefore, timing of initiation of antibiotic therapy in CABM and potential consequences of delays remains a topic of major interest. Some studies addressing door-to-antibiotic time have had inconclusive results, but most reports suggest more unfavourable outcomes with delayed antibiotic administration [7–12]. However, the two most cited studies were based on study populations from 1990-2002 and 2002–2004, respectively, and they consisted of relatively small cohorts in the era prior to standard use of adjuvant dexamethasone therapy [11, 12]. To our understanding, these studies did not account for whether any patients were treated with parenteral antibiotics before admission, which has been associated with a high mortality elsewhere [13, 14]. Moreover, these studies did not specify if patients were diagnosed at admission to the emergency department or later. This could confound analyses of delays in antibiotic therapy and outcome as these patients may have increased

* Correspondence: Jacob.bodilsen@rn.dk
[1]Department of Infectious Diseases, Aalborg University Hospital, Mølleparkvej 4, 9100 Aalborg, Denmark
[2]Department of Medicine, Vendsyssel Hospital, Hjørring, Denmark
Full list of author information is available at the end of the article

mortality and morbidity due to other reasons, e.g. predominance of different bacterial aetiologies, impaired immunological response, comorbidity etc. Therefore, timing of antibiotic therapy and outcome needs further clarification in a contemporary cohort.

We conducted a retrospective study of adult patients with CABM in North Denmark over the last 17 years with the aim of examining time to antibiotic therapy and outcome.

Methods

Setting

We carried out a population-based cohort study in patients with CABM from 1 January 1998 to 31 December 2014 in North Denmark Region. The catchment population was approximately 500,000 in 1998 and approximately 580,000 in 2014 [15]. In Denmark, primary health-care and hospital care are tax-paid and free of charge. A unique personal identification number is provided to all residents at birth or immigration and is used for all health-care contacts.

Owing to health administrative reforms, the number of hospitals providing acute care for patients decreased from nine in 1998 to five in 2014. The Department of Clinical Microbiology at Aalborg University Hospital was the sole provider of microbiological diagnostics for every hospital in the region throughout the entire study period. This department also kept records of specimens sent for supplementary analyses at Statens Serum Institut, Copenhagen.

Since 1998 local guidelines recommended intravenous penicillin G (supplemented with gentamicin in patients aged above 40 years) as empiric treatment for CABM and since 2003 adjuvant dexamethasone was added. In 2009, the advised antibiotic regimen was replaced by the combination of penicillin G and cefotaxime to all adults according to national Danish guidelines. Throughout the study period, cerebrospinal fluid isolates of *Streptococcus pneumoniae* and *Neisseria meningitidis* in Denmark have retained wildtype sensitivity to penicillin (94.7 and >99 % of isolates, respectively), and high-level resistant isolates of pneumococci have been rare [16, 17].

Study population

The laboratory information system (ADBakt, Autonik, Sweden) at the Department of Clinical Microbiology, Aalborg University Hospital, was used to identify cases of CABM in North Denmark Region. All patients aged over 16 years were included if they had a clinical presentation strongly suggestive of CABM, including signs such as neck stiffness, petechiae, headache, fever, confusion, or impaired level of consciousness, and at least one of the following:

1. Positive CSF culture
2. Positive blood culture and more than >10 leukocytes × 10^6/L in the CSF [18].
3. Presence of bacteria in Gram stain of CSF
4. Non-culture detection of bacteria in CSF by either bacterial antigen test or 16S rRNA gene amplification.

If a patient fulfilled multiple criteria, only the strongest criterion was noted (1>2>3>4). Patients with concomitant infections, e.g. endocarditis or spondylodiscitis, were included if their initial main presentation was characteristic of meningitis and they fulfilled one of the above inclusion criteria.

Exclusion criteria were: cerebral abscess, hospital-acquired bacterial meningitis as defined by the Centers for Disease Control [19], an implanted neurosurgical device, or cases where an exact time of antibiotic treatment or the clinical records could not be retrieved.

Data sources

The main author reviewed all patient records. Time of arrival at hospital was retrieved from ambulance charts or, secondarily, from registrations made by secretaries or nurses at admission to the Emergency Department. Detailed information on patient history, pre-hospital antibiotic treatment, clinical findings, preliminary diagnoses at admission and outcome were obtained from the ambulance, nurses' and doctors' charts. When available, letters of referral from general practitioners and ambulance records were checked for remarks indicating suspicion of bacterial meningitis. Electronic records systems were used to obtain timing and results of diagnostic tests, i.e. blood tests (Labka I and Labka II, CSC, USA), microbiological samples (ADBakt) and cranial imaging (Easyviz, Karos Health, Denmark). For patients admitted to an intensive care unit (ICU), observation charts of vital signs and medical treatment were examined.

Sources for time of antibiotic therapy included doctors', nurses' and ICU charts, emergency triage notes, and manual medication administration records. These also included the electronic medication administration systems Theriak (TM Software, Iceland) from 2004 to 2012 and Opus (CSC, USA) from 2012 onwards.

Time to antibiotic therapy

To obtain the time to antibiotic therapy, we prioritised nurses' signatures for antibiotic administration on triage forms or on nurses' charts or in medication administration systems – paper and electronic – unless an exact time of treatment was specified elsewhere, e.g. in the doctors' charts. Time to antibiotic therapy was calculated as time from arrival at hospital to administration of first dose of antibiotic therapy providing coverage for the specific bacterial aetiology and antibiogram in the given patient in dosages recommended for treating bacterial meningitis.

Patient data

The criterion 'diagnosed with meningitis at referral to hospital' was defined as when the referral letter from the general practitioner or the ambulance records mentioned suspicion of bacterial meningitis. The criterion 'diagnosed with bacterial meningitis at admission' denotes patients listed above and/or where meningitis was mentioned in the admission records. This also included cases that had a lumbar puncture performed or planned at admission and patients started on antibiotic therapy for bacterial meningitis. All other cases were regarded as diagnosed later.

Baseline data were collected for the day of admission in all patients. Symptoms or clinical findings were categorised as not present if they were not mentioned in the medical records. Adjuvant dexamethasone was registered if it was administered (10 mg four times daily for 4 days) within 1 h of intravenous antibiotic treatment. We categorised disseminated intravascular coagulation (DIC) at admission as thrombocytopenia (platelet count below 150×10^9/L) and an activated plasmatic coagulation profile and/or petechiae or ecchymoses with systemic complications. An exact Glasgow Coma Scale (GCS) score at admission was reported in about two-thirds of the records, and if not reported, a categorical classification was made based on observations in the patients' records (GCS < 9, GCS 9–12, GCS > 12). Impaired mental status was noted if the patient had any level of reduced consciousness not explained by previous comorbidity. The duration of hospitalisation was registered from the day of admission to the day of discharge or transfer to a rehabilitation unit.

Outcome

Outcome was graded according to the Glasgow Outcome Scale (GOS) at discharge [20]. The scores and their corresponding conditions are as follows: 1, death; 2, a vegetative state (unable to interact with the environment); 3, severe sequelae and dependency upon others in daily life; 4, moderate sequelae but retainment of the capability of independent living; and 5, no – or only minor – sequelae. A score of 5 was considered favourable and 1–4 as unfavourable.

Statistical analysis

Categorical data were analysed using Fisher's exact test or the χ^2 test, and continuous data were analysed using the Mann–Whitney *U*-test. A two-tailed *p*-value <0.05 was considered significant. Because odds ratio are difficult to interpret when events are common, we computed the risk and risk ratio for the primary outcomes in-hospital mortality and unfavourable outcome at discharge by time to adequate antibiotic therapy [21]. To compute the adjusted risk ratios (adj. RRs) with 95 % confidence intervals (95 % CIs), we used modified Poisson regression analyses [22]. Due to the number of events we could only adjust for age >65 years, GCS score at admission (GCS < 13), and presence of hypotension (systolic blood pressure <90 mmHg) in analyses of in-hospital mortality (33 events) with further adjustment for bacterial aetiology (*S. pneumoniae* yes/no) and adjunctive dexamethasone treatment in analyses of unfavourable outcome at discharge (77 events). In regression analyses, we omitted patients who had been treated with parenteral beta-lactams prior to admission.

We used Stata 11.2 (StataCorp., College Station, TX) for all analyses.

Results

We identified 195 adult cases of CABM during the study period. In six cases we could not identify an accurate time of the first adequate dose of antibiotics and in two cases the patient records could not be retrieved. Another patient had died at home and was diagnosed by a forensic autopsy. Prior to admission 13 patients had been treated by the referring general practitioners with intramuscular benzylpenicillin 3.0 g on suspicion of bacterial meningitis, seven (53 %) of whom died (Additional file 1: Table S1). Therefore, 22 patients were excluded, with 173 patients remaining for further analysis of time to antibiotic therapy.

Baseline characteristics of the patients are presented in Table 1 and the bacterial aetiologies are shown in Additional file 2: Table S2. Examining all 173 patients, the median time to antibiotic therapy was 2.0 h (IQR 1.0–5.5). We observed that increased time to antibiotic therapy was associated with in-hospital mortality (Fig. 1a, $p = 0.04$) and unfavourable outcome at discharge (Fig. 1b, $p = 0.01$), reaching statistical significance when treatment delays exceeded 6 h compared with patients treated within 2 h of admission. Adjusted risk ratios of in-hospital mortality and an unfavourable outcome at discharge were 1.6 (95 % CI 0.8–3.2) and 1.5 (95 % CI 1.0–2.2, $p = 0.03$), respectively, in patients treated more than 6 h after admission, using patients treated within 2 h as reference (Table 2). These findings corresponded to an adjusted risk ratio of in-hospital mortality of 1.1 per hour of delay (95 % CI 0.8–1.5) and an unfavourable outcome at discharge of 1.1 per hour of delay (95 % CI 1.0–1.3) during the first 6 h of admission.

Comparing patients diagnosed immediately at admission with patients diagnosed after admission, we found a median time to antibiotic therapy of 1.3 h (interquartile range (IQR) 0.8–2.7) vs 8.5 h (IQR 3.9–24.5) ($p < 0.001$), and correspondingly in-hospital mortality of 14 vs. 30 %

Table 1 Baseline characteristics at admission of patients with community-acquired bacterial meningitis excluding patients treated with pre-hospital parenteral antibiotics

Patient characteristic at admission ($n = 173$)	Total cohort
Age (years)	58 (45–70)
Male	84 (49)
Comorbidity[a]	62/173 (36)
Diagnosis of meningitis suspected at referral to hospital	35/173 (20)
Diagnosed with meningitis at admission to hospital	120/173 (69)
Duration of symptoms (days) ($n = 164$)	2 (2–5)
Headache	96/119 (81)
Nausea/vomiting	87/102 (85)
Petechiae/echimoses	40/135 (30)
Neck stiffness	113/160 (71)
Focal neurological deficit[b]	29/130 (22)
New-onset seizures	17/173 (10)
Meningitis triad (neck stiffness, fever, impaired mental status)	78/173 (45)
Temperature (°C) ($n = 169$)	38.9 (38.0–39.9)
Blood pressure, systolic (mmHg) ($n = 157$)	138 (119–159)
Pulse rate (bpm) ($n = 156$)	99 (87–116)
Glasgow Coma Score	
12–15	82 (47)
9–12	61 (35)
<9	30 (17)
C-reactive protein (mg/L) ($n = 170$)	211 (110–298)
Blood leukocytes (10^9/L) ($n = 171$)	17 (11–24)
Disseminated intravascular coagulopathy	31/173 (18)
CSF	
Leukocytes (10^6/L) ($n = 164$)	1925 (204–6081)
Erythrocytes (10^6/L) ($n = 164$)	145 (18–593)
CSF-glucose (mmol/L) ($n = 163$)	0.9 (0.1–3.1)
CSF/blood glucose ratio ($n = 163$)	0.1 (0.01–0.4)
CSF protein (g/L) ($n = 166$)	3.7 (1.9–7.9)
Aetiology	
S. pneumoniae	96/173 (55)
N. meningitidis	36/173 (21)
Other	41/173 (24)
Antibiotics for sepsis given before meningitis was diagnosed	11/173 (6)
Time to antibiotic therapy for meningitis (h, $n = 173$)	2.0 (1.0–5.5)
Dexamethasone treatment[c]	55/116 (47)
Cranial imaging before lumbar puncture	60/173 (35)
Cranial imaging during hospitalisation	134/173 (77)
Intensive care unit admission	104/173 (60)
Unfavourable outcome (GOS 1–4)	77/173 (45)
Mortality	33/173 (19)

Binary variables are listed as n/N (%) and continuous variables as medians (IQR). [a]Alcoholism, asplenia, cancer, cirrhosis, congenital or acquired immunodeficiency including HIV, diabetes mellitus, heart failure (ejection fraction <40 %) and renal impairment (serum creatinine >130 μmol/L). [b]Paraesthesia, motor or cranial nerve paresis. [c]Patients included after implementation of adjunctive dexamethasone treatment in 2002

($p = 0.01$) and an unfavourable outcome at discharge of 37 vs. 62 % ($p = 0.002$).

Similarly, patients presenting without the meningitis triad (fever, neck stiffness, altered mental status) had longer door-to-antibiotic time (median 3.1 vs. 1.3 h, $p < 0.001$), but no substantial differences in in-hospital mortality (16 vs. 23 %, $p = 0.3$) and unfavourable outcome (41 vs. 49 %, $p = 0.4$).

Cranial imaging before lumbar puncture was more frequent in patients diagnosed after admission (58 vs. 24 %, $p < 0.001$) and was associated with a substantial treatment delay (median door-to-antibiotics 3.1 vs. 1.5 h, $p = 0.01$). A trend towards increased in-hospital mortality (26 vs 16 %, $p = 0.1$) and unfavourable outcome at discharge (51 vs. 41 %, $p = 0.3$) was also found.

Antibiotic delay of more than 2 h after admission in patients with a pre-hospital diagnosis of meningitis ($n = 35$) showed a trend towards increased mortality (RR 1.4; 95 % CI 0.1–14.6) and unfavourable outcome at discharge (RR 1.2; 95 % CI 0.4–3.9). Further details on treatment and outcome according to time of day of admission, bacterial aetiology and duration of symptoms are available in Additional file 3: Table S3.

Discussion

In this contemporary population-based cohort study of CABM, we observed a median time to antibiotic therapy of 2.0 h after admission. We found a 10 % increase of in-hospital mortality and risk for unfavourable outcomes at discharge with each hour of delay for the first 6 h of admission (of note the increase was non-linear for unfavourable outcome). Antibiotic delays of more than 6 h resulted in a 50–60 % relative increase in in-hospital mortality and unfavourable outcome at discharge when compared with patients receiving adequate antibiotic therapy within 2 h of admission, although statistical significance was not reached in adjusted analyses regarding in-hospital mortality. When compared to patients diagnosed with CABM on admission, patients diagnosed after admission had increased time to antibiotics (8.5 vs. 1.3 h, $p < 0.001$) and mortality (30 vs. 14 %, $p = 0.01$).

The median time to adequate antibiotic therapy in our study was faster than that reported by Proulx et al. (3.8 h)

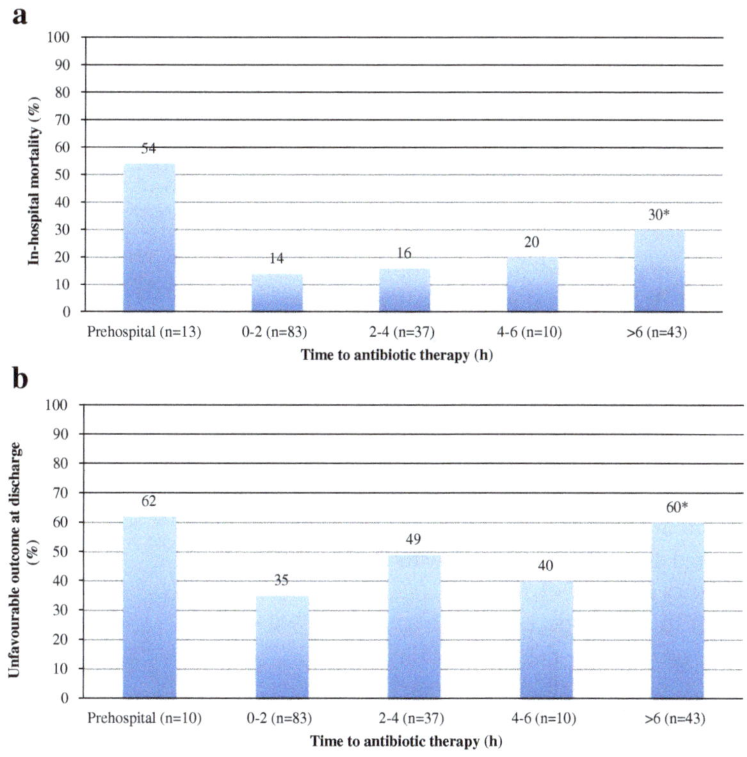

Fig. 1 **a** Time to antibiotic therapy and in-hospital mortality in community-acquired bacterial meningitis. **P*-value <0.05 compared with patients treated 0–2 h from admission. **b** Time to antibiotic therapy and unfavourable outcome at discharge in community-acquired bacterial meningitis. **P*-value <0.05 compared with patients treated 0–2 h from admission

[11] but comparable to observations in another Danish study by Køster-Rasmussen et al. (2.0 h) [12]. Proulx et al. observed increased case fatality (OR 8.4, 95 % CI 1.7–40.9) when treatment delays exceeded 6 h after admission, but without any sign of increased mortality with less delay. Our study consistently showed an increased in-hospital mortality and unfavourable outcome with step-wise delays in time to antibiotic therapy underscoring the biological rationale of the association. Similar to our study, Køster-Rasmussen et al. also found increased unfavourable outcomes with treatment delays (OR 1.1 per hour of delay) in adjusted analyses, but without any report on effect on mortality. Both studies were based on less contemporary cohorts, included fewer adult cases (118 and 125 cases, respectively), and did not specify if patients were given pre-hospital parenteral antibiotics. Furthermore, these studies did not account for time of diagnosis of CABM, which had a substantial effect on antibiotic timing and outcome in our study.

A recently published prospective Swedish observational study with 609 adult cases from 2005 to 2012 also found a median time to antibiotic treatment of 2 h after admission and an improved survival after an amendment of national guidelines limiting the indications for cranial

Table 2 Time to adequate antibiotic therapy and risk ratios for in-hospital mortality and unfavourable outcome at discharge among patients with community-acquired bacterial meningitis

Adequate antibiotic therapy initiated	Risk ratio for in-hospital mortality (95 % CI)		Risk ratio for unfavourable outcome (95 % CI)	
	Crude	Adjusted[a]	Crude	Adjusted[b]
0–2 h after admission	Ref.	Ref.	Ref.	Ref.
2–4 h after admission	1.1 (0.5–2.8)	1.2 (0.5–2.7)	1.4 (0.9–2.2)	1.5 (0.9–2.2)
4–6 h after admission	1.4 (0.4–5.3)	1.4 (0.5–3.6)	1.1 (0.5–2.6)	1.1 (0.6–2.2)
>6 h after admission	2.1 (1.0–4.2)*	1.6 (0.8–3.2)	1.7 (1.2–2.5)*	1.5 (1.0–2.2)*

*$p < 0.05$. CI indicates confidence interval. [a]Adjusted for age >65 years, Glasgow Coma Score <13 and arterial systolic hypotension (<90 mmHg) at admission. [b]Adjusted for age >65 years, Glasgow Coma Score <13, arterial systolic hypotension (<90 mmHg), bacterial aetiology (*S. pneumoniae* yes/no) and adjunctive dexamethasone treatment (yes/no)

imaging before lumbar puncture [23]. However, information was incomplete regarding time of diagnosis and disease severity (e.g. occurrence of seizures, signs of systemic compromise, and CSF leukocyte count). The study also included a few patients without a proven diagnosis of meningitis, and the completeness of patient inclusion varied during the study period (increasing from 60 to 80 %) [23].

Our study has both strengths and limitations when examining time to antibiotic therapy and outcome of CABM. The population-based design and the inclusion of uniquely identifiable adults limited selection bias, and the validity of the diagnoses was ensured by rigorous inclusion criteria comprising clinical description, CSF findings and microbiological diagnostics. Moreover, we only included cases with an exact time of antibiotic treatment listed in the charts, although we cannot exclude random error (e.g. inaccurate signing off of antibiotic administration by nurses). We also accounted for patients treated with pre-hospital parenteral antibiotics and time of diagnosis.

Several limitations inherent to a retrospective observational study exist, including incomplete data of certain clinical characteristics (e.g. time to antibiotic therapy and GCS score at admission in some patients). We may also have missed a small number of blood-culture negative cases admitted at other departments without a lumbar puncture performed during admission. Differential misclassification in timing of antibiotic therapy may also be present because patients diagnosed immediately at admission more often had an exact point of time documented in their records compared with patients with more uncharacteristic presentations diagnosed later during admission. Moreover, data on time to antibiotic therapy were derived from different data sources without a fixed prioritised order.

Patients diagnosed after admission experienced treatment delay and increased in-hospital mortality and unfavourable outcome at discharge. Patients without typical signs of CABM at admission also had treatment delay, but in this group we found no clear differences in mortality and unfavourable outcome. Still, as the prognosis for these patients remain poor, a high index of suspicion of CABM seems prudent even in patients without all the typical signs of CNS infection.

Duration of disease may be crucially linked to disease severity and thereby outcome, but categorisation of prodromal disease and onset of meningitis is almost impossible in clinical settings, and even more so in retrospective studies. Therefore, we cannot exclude residual confounding although we reported data on disease duration exactly as stated in the medical records. Moreover, we did not see differences in outcome according to duration of symptoms for >24 or <24 h.

Conclusion

In conclusion, delayed initiation of antibiotic therapy for bacterial meningitis is associated with increased in-hospital mortality and an unfavourable outcome at discharge.

Abbreviations

CABM, community-acquired bacterial meningitis; CIs, confidence intervals; CSF, cerebrospinal fluid; GCS, Glasgow coma scale; GOS, Glasgow outcome score; ICU, intensive care unit; IQR, interquartile ranges; OR, odds ratios; RR, risk ratios

Funding

We did not receive any funding for this study.

Authors' contributions

All authors (JB, MDP, HCS, HN) participated in the design of the study and drafting of the manuscript. JB gathered all the data and MDP did the statistical analyses. All authors read and approved the final manuscript.

Competing interests

Dr. Schønheyder reports a patent for a pneumococcal vaccine adjuvant, US 20120052088AI.

Author details

[1]Department of Infectious Diseases, Aalborg University Hospital, Mølleparkvej 4, 9100 Aalborg, Denmark. [2]Department of Medicine, Vendsyssel Hospital, Hjørring, Denmark. [3]Department of Clinical Microbiology, Aalborg University Hospital, Aalborg, Denmark. [4]Department of Clinical Medicine, Aalborg University, Aalborg, Denmark.

References

1. Swartz MN. Bacterial meningitis–a view of the past 90 years. N Engl J Med. 2004;351:1826–8.
2. Kasanmoentalib ES, Brouwer MC, van de Beek D. Update on bacterial meningitis: epidemiology, trials and genetic association studies. Curr Opin Neurol. 2013;26:282–8.
3. Pelkonen T, Roine I, Cruzeiro ML, Pitkäranta A, Kataja M, Peltola H. Slow initial β-lactam infusion and oral paracetamol to treat childhood bacterial meningitis: a randomised, controlled trial. Lancet Infect Dis. 2011;11:613–21.
4. Molyneux EM, Kawaza K, Phiri A, Chimalizeni Y, Mankhambo L, Schwalbe E, Kataja M, Pensulo P, Chilton L, Peltola H. Glycerol and acetaminophen as adjuvant therapy did not affect the outcome of bacterial meningitis in Malawian children. Pediatr Infect Dis J. 2014;33:214–6.
5. Ajdukiewicz KMA, Cartwright KEC, Scarborough MS, Mwambene JBMDM, Goodson PGDM, Molyneux MEMDM, Zijlstra EEZ, French NF, Whitty CJW, Lalloo DGL. Glycerol adjuvant therapy in adults with bacterial meningitis in a high HIV seroprevalence setting in Malawi: a double-blind, randomised controlled trial. Lancet Infect Dis. 2011;11:293–300.
6. Mourvillier B, Tubach F, Tubach F, van de Beek D, Garot D, Garot D, Pichon N, Pichon N, Georges H, Georges H, Lefevre LM, Lefevre LM, Bollaert P-E, Bollaert P-E, Boulain T, Boulain T, Luis D, Luis D, Cariou A, Cariou A, Girardie P, Girardie P, Chelha R, Chelha R, Megarbane B, Megarbane B, Delahaye A, Delahaye A, Chalumeau-Lemoine L, Chalumeau-Lemoine L, et al. Induced hypothermia in severe bacterial meningitis: a randomized clinical trial. JAMA. 2013;310:2174–83.
7. Bryan CS, Reynolds KL, Crout L. Promptness of antibiotic therapy in acute bacterial meningitis. Ann Emerg Med. 1986;15:544–7.
8. Talan DA, Guterman JJ, Overturf GD, Singer C, Hoffman JR, Lambert B.

Analysis of emergency department management of suspected bacterial meningitis. Ann Emerg Med. 1989;18:856–62.
9. Talan DA, Zibulewsky J. Relationship of clinical presentation to time to antibiotics for the emergency department management of suspected bacterial meningitis. Ann Emerg Med. 1993;22:1733–8.
10. Aronin SI, Peduzzi P, Quagliarello VJ. Community-acquired bacterial meningitis: risk stratification for adverse clinical outcome and effect of antibiotic timing. Ann Intern Med. 1998;129:862–9.
11. Proulx N, Fréchette D, Toye B, Chan J, Kravcik S. Delays in the administration of antibiotics are associated with mortality from adult acute bacterial meningitis. QJM. 2005;98:291–8.
12. Køster-Rasmussen R, Korshin A, Meyer CN. Antibiotic treatment delay and outcome in acute bacterial meningitis. J Infect. 2008;57:449–54.
13. Sørensen HT, Nielsen GL, Schønheyder HC, Steffensen FH, Hansen I, Sabroe S, Dahlerup JF, Hamburger H, Olsen J. Outcome of pre-hospital antibiotic treatment of meningococcal disease. J Clin Epidemiol. 1998;51:717–21.
14. Harnden A, Ninis N, Thompson M, Perera R, Levin M, Mant D, Mayon-White R. Parenteral penicillin for children with meningococcal disease before hospital admission: case-control study. BMJ. 2006;332:1295–8.
15. StatBank Denmark. http://www.statbank.dk/statbank5a/default.asp?w=1440. Accessed October 15th 2015
16. Lind I, Berthelsen L. Epidemiology of meningococcal disease in Denmark 1974–1999: contribution of the laboratory surveillance system. Epidemiol Infect. 2005;133:205–15.
17. Agersø Y, Hald T, Helwigh B, Høg BB. DANMAP 2013: Use of antimicrobial agents and occurrence of antimicrobial resistance in bacteria from food animals, food and humans in Denmark. 2013. Accessible at www.danmap.org. Accessed on May 20th 2015.
18. McMillan DA, Lin CY, Aronin SI, Quagliarello VJ. Community-acquired bacterial meningitis in adults: categorization of causes and timing of death. Clin Infect Dis. 2001;33:969–75.
19. Garner JS, Jarvis WR, Emori TG, Horan TC, Hughes JM. CDC definitions for nosocomial infections, 1988. Am J Infect Control. 1988;16:128–40.
20. Teasdale GM, Pettigrew LE, Wilson JT, Murray G, Jennett B. Analyzing outcome of treatment of severe head injury: a review and update on advancing the use of the Glasgow Outcome Scale. J Neurotrauma. 1998;15:587–97.
21. Sackett DL, Deeks JJ, Altman DG. Down with odds ratios! Evid Based Med. 1996;1:164–6.
22. Cummings P. Methods for estimating adjusted risk ratios. Stata J. 2009;9:175–96.
23. Glimåker M, Johansson B, Grindborg Ö, Bottai M, Lindquist L, Sjölin J. Adult bacterial meningitis: earlier treatment and improved outcome following guideline revision promoting prompt lumbar puncture. Clin Infect Dis. 2015;60:1162–9.

16

Cost-effectiveness of CRAG-LFA screening for cryptococcal meningitis among people living with HIV in Uganda

Anu Ramachandran[1], Yukari Manabe[1,2], Radha Rajasingham[3] and Maunank Shah[1*]

Abstract

Background: Cryptococcal meningitis (CM) constitutes a significant source of mortality in resource-limited regions. Cryptococcal antigen (CRAG) can be detected in the blood before onset of meningitis. We sought to determine the cost-effectiveness of implementing CRAG screening using the recently developed CRAG lateral flow assay in Uganda compared to current practice without screening.

Methods: A decision-analytic model was constructed to compare two strategies for cryptococcal prevention among people living with HIV with CD4 < 100 in Uganda: No cryptococcal screening vs. CRAG screening with WHO-recommended preemptive treatment for CRAG-positive patients. The model was constructed to reflect primary HIV clinics in Uganda, with a cohort of HIV-infected patients with CD4 < 100 cells/uL. Primary outcomes were expected costs, DALYs, and incremental cost-effectiveness ratios (ICERs). We evaluated varying levels of programmatic implementation in secondary analysis.

Results: CRAG screening was considered highly cost-effective and was associated with an ICER of $6.14 per DALY averted compared to no screening (95% uncertainty range: $-20.32 to $36.47). Overall, implementation of CRAG screening was projected to cost $1.52 more per person, and was projected to result in a 40% relative reduction in cryptococcal-associated mortality. In probabilistic sensitivity analysis, CRAG screening was cost-effective in 100% of scenarios and cost saving (ie cheaper and more effective than no screening) in 30% of scenarios. Secondary analysis projected a total cost of $651,454 for 100% implementation of screening nationally, while averting 1228 deaths compared to no screening.

Conclusion: CRAG screening for PLWH with low CD4 represents excellent value for money with the potential to prevent cryptococcal morbidity and mortality in Uganda.

Background

Cryptococcal meningitis (CM) constitutes a significant source of global morbidity and mortality for people living with HIV (PLWH), particularly in resource limited settings [1]. Nearly 1 million cases of cryptococcal disease with 625,000 deaths are estimated to occur annually, surpassing tuberculosis and other opportunistic infections in some highly prevalent areas [1]. Of these, the vast majority of cases occur in sub-Saharan Africa, where CM is the cause of 10–44% of HIV-associated deaths [1–4]. New cost-effective approaches for prevention, detection and treatment of cryptococcal disease are needed.

Several factors contribute to high cryptococcal morbidity and mortality, including difficulty with accurate diagnosis and complicated disease management consisting of hospitalization, serial lumbar punctures, and expensive treatments that are difficult to access such as amphotericin and flucytosine, both with significant side effects [5, 6]. CM mortality remains high in both resourced (9–38%) and resource-limited settings (30–59%) despite increasing access to ART, likely due to late presentation [7, 8]. Universal primary prophylaxis (UPP) with fluconazole has not demonstrated a clear mortality reduction and incurs significant costs and side effects [7, 9, 10]. Strategies that

* Correspondence: mshah28@jhmi.edu
[1]Johns Hopkins University School of Medicine, 725 N. Wolfe St. PCTB building-224, Baltimore, MD 21205, USA
Full list of author information is available at the end of the article

allow targeted early interventions to identify those at greatest risk for cryptococcal disease are thus warranted.

To this end, cryptococcal antigen (CRAG) screening of immunosuppressed HIV-infected (CD4 < 100 cells/μL) allows early identification of individuals with cryptococcal infection or those at risk for increased mortality. In 2011, the cryptococcal antigen Lateral Flow Assay (IMMY CrAg LFA, Norman, OK, 2011), was developed. This is a rapid dipstick test, approved by the Food and Drug Administration, with a very high sensitivity and specificity for detecting cryptococcal glucuronylmannan in serum [11–16]. CRAG LFA is heat-stable, inexpensive (estimated $2.50 per test), and requires minimal training for optimal use in resource-limited settings. Several studies have demonstrated its effectiveness in detecting cryptococcal antigenemia and diagnosing cryptococcal disease [17, 18].

CRAG is detectable in the blood 3 weeks before onset of meningitis, and is an independent predictor of meningitis and death [19–23]. CRAG screening targeting those HIV-infected with a CD4 count <100 cells/uL is now recommended by the WHO, and several national HIV guidelines [24]. For those who are CRAG positive, preemptive treatment with fluconazole (800 mg for 2 weeks, followed by 400 mg for 8 weeks) reduces mortality [25].

Despite the WHO recommendations, implementation and scale-up of CRAG screening remains limited in Sub-Saharan Africa. Fewer than 30% of eligible patients receive screening, partly due to concerns regarding cost and feasibility of incorporation into routine HIV care [26]. Previous economic evaluations from middle-income settings have suggested that incorporating CRAG-LFA screening into HIV care may be cost-effective at current willingness to pay thresholds [27]. There is a lack of data from low-income settings in Sub-Saharan Africa where disease burden is highest [28–30]. Meya et al. previously assessed costs of CRAG screening using a latex agglutination assay ($16 per test) in Uganda as part of a cohort study; however, the cost-effectiveness of population-level implementation was not evaluated [28]. The impact of preemptive treatment, relapse, or loss to follow-up on the cost-effectiveness of CRAG screening has not been modeled, and an economic analysis of the impact and cost of scaling up current screening protocols is important for guiding policy decisions. Furthermore, alternative implementation algorithms including intensified diagnostic evaluation of all CRAG-positive patients or full CM treatment for all CRAG-positive patients may improve morbidity and mortality for patients with sub-clinical CM disease. Current recommendations do not have provisions for such intensified diagnostics, and have not evaluated their cost-effectiveness.

We thus sought to evaluate the costs and cost-effectiveness of implementing CRAG screening for PLWH with advanced immunosuppression (including preemptive treatment for those CRAG positive) compared to current practice in Uganda. Additionally, we sought to explore the health-system costs of CRAG screening at various levels of programmatic implementation as well as alternative algorithms for screening.

Methods

We conducted a cost-effectiveness analysis from a health-systems perspective using a decision-analytic model (Fig. 1) with a target population of HIV-infected, ART-naïve Ugandan patients with a baseline CD4 < 100 cells/μL. We used a 1-year time-frame for the intervention, and evaluated outcomes from cryptococcal disease over a 5-year period. Disability-adjusted life years (DALYs) were analyzed across a lifetime horizon of the cohort representing PLWH on ART. The model was developed and analyzed using TreeAge software (TreeAge Software Inc., Williamstown, MA, USA).

Decision-Tree Model

Two practices for PLWH with CD4 < 100 cells/uL were compared: No screening vs universal CRAG screening followed by preemptive treatment for those CRAG positive.

In both model arms, patients were stratified by prevalence of baseline CM disease and cryptococcal antigenemia, based on currently available data from published literature [20, 25, 28, 29] (Table 1). All patients in both model arms were initiated on ART per current guidelines in Uganda. Regardless of CRAG screening strategy, all patients with symptoms concerning for CM at presentation (eg. headache, fever, or neck stiffness) were assumed to receive a lumbar puncture (LP) and treatment for baseline CM if diagnosed, consisting of Amphotericin B 0.7 mg/kg/day for 2 weeks, followed by Fluconazole 800 mg for 3 weeks and Fluconazole 400 for 9 weeks, with potential for future relapse [30]. All patients without initial CM disease could progress to develop CM, based on current literature estimates and adjusted based on model interventions such as receiving preemptive treatment. Given uncertainty in long-term progression rates, we focused on short/medium term progression over 5 years [31]. Patients that progressed to develop CM could either be detected and treated, or lost to follow-up. Untreated CM among PLWH was assumed to have 100% mortality [8]. Within each arm of the model, PLWH that were successfully treated for CM disease could still go on to have disease relapse (Fig. 1).

In order to evaluate the impact and cost-effectiveness of CRAG screening, rates of diagnosis and/or development and treatment of CM differed between the model arms based on usage of CRAG screening. In the 'no screening' arm, no CRAG screening was performed and no prophylactic antifungal therapy was administered.

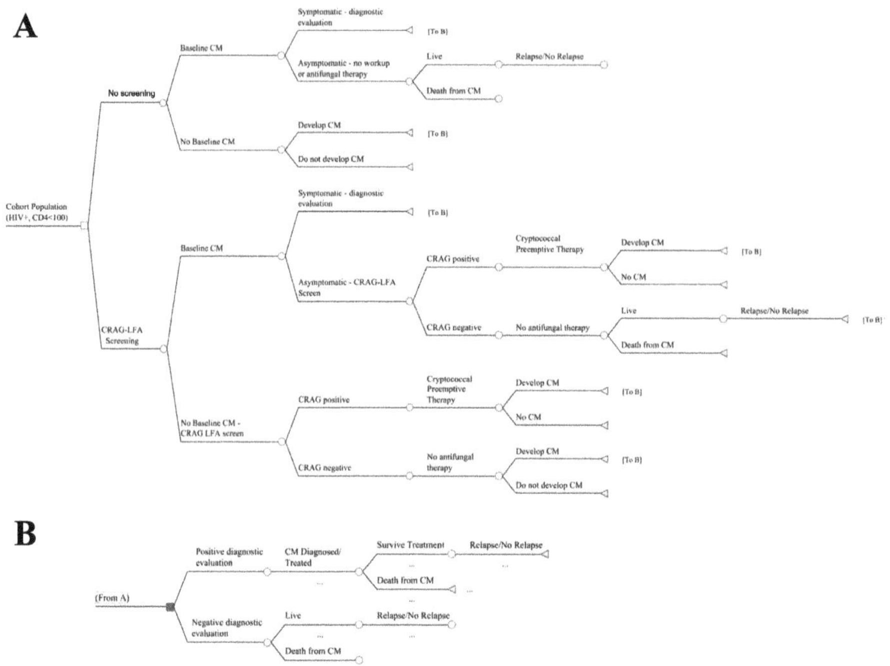

Fig. 1 Model Schematic. Abbreviations: CRAG-LFA—cryptococcal antigen lateral flow assay, CM—cryptococcal meningitis, ART—antiretroviral therapy. Decision-analytic model schematic. We modeled progression or relapse of CM over a 5 year time period for a cohort of PLWH with CD4 < 100. In both model arms, symptomatic patients at baseline receive evaluation for CM assumed to include a lumbar puncture (LP), and treatment if diagnosed with CM. We assumed ART initiation in all arms. The model compares two interventions for prevention of cryptococcal morbidity for those without a baseline diagnosis of CM: 1) No screening, in which patients receive no CM screening or prophylaxis 2) CRAG-LFA, in which all patients receive serum CRAG-LFA screening. Individuals with positive CRAG were assumed to receive the cryptococcal preemptive treatment for cryptococcal antigenemia with fluconazole 800 mg for 2 weeks, followed by fluconazole 400 mg for 8 weeks. CRAG-negative individuals receive no further antifungal therapy. **a** outlines the two main model arms. **b** demonstrates the diagnostic evaluation and treatment for suspected CM cases

Asymptomatic patients were assumed to receive no further immediate cryptococcal related care, while symptomatic patients received evaluation as described above; patients without baseline CM were considered at risk for development of CM with rates dependent on prevalence of (undetected) cryptococcal antigenemia.

In the CRAG screening intervention arm, patients received a serum CRAG test using the LFA to identify cryptococcal antigenemia. In the base case, symptomatic CRAG-positive patients received further evaluation as described above, while asymptomatic CRAG-positive patients received no further evaluation. All asymptomatic CRAG-positive patients received preemptive treatment for cryptococcal antigenemia (fluconazole 800 mg for 2 weeks followed by 400 mg for 8 weeks) along with ART initiation per current Ugandan guidelines [24, 30]. We incorporated the protective effect of preemptive treatment as a reduction in the risk of developing CM, and as partial treatment for those with subclinical baseline CM [25, 26, 29–33]. CRAG negative patients began ART without further testing or treatment, and were at risk for development of CM based on literature estimates (Table 1).

To aid in programmatic implementation, we conducted secondary analysis to explore alternative interventions for individuals with baseline CRAG positivity in the CRAG-screening intervention arm, including an intensified case-finding algorithm consisting of an LP for evaluation of CM in all CRAG positive patients regardless of symptoms (in base case analysis, only symptomatic patients receive LP and asymptomatic patients receive preemptive therapy). In this algorithm, CRAG positive patients diagnosed with CM disease after LP receive full CM treatment, while CRAG positive patients without a diagnosis of CM after LP are treated with preemptive therapy. We additionally explored provisions for full CM treatment to all CRAG positive patients, without requiring LP or additional diagnostic workup. The effect of each of these clinical algorithms on ICER values for CRAG-LFA screening was determined. Policy makers must also consider the costs and impact of scaling up new screening strategies. As such, in additional secondary analysis, we also modeled the net costs, effects, and cost-effectiveness of population level scale-up of CRAG screening, by varying the percentage of individuals (accessing HIV care in a given year) receiving CRAG screening, and compared these to the current practice arm. The absolute number of Ugandans enrolling in HIV care per year with CD4 < 100 was estimated to be 61,400 and was varied widely in sensitivity analysis [34].

Table 1 Key Parameter Estimates

Parameter name	Value	Range	Source
Epidemiology			
Number of patients enrolling in HIV care in Uganda per year	245,600	150,000–350,000	[34]
Total number of patients enrolling in HIV care per year with CD4 < 100 (% of total)	61,400 (25%)	13,000 (5%) -105,000 (30%)	[34]
Average age of cohort	37	32–44	[41]
Life Expectancy in years[a] (on ART)	19.1	17–23	[41]
CRAG-positive prevalence (at baseline)	8.80%	1–20%	[20, 29, 31, 32]
Percentage of CRAG+ patients with baseline CM disease	25%	0–50%	[33, 45]
Proportion developing CM among CRAG positive patients without treatment[b]	34%	10–75%	[21, 23, 31, 29]
Relative reduction in CM development among CRAG positive patients on CPET[b,c]	65%	10–90%	[51, 26, 29, 31]
Proportion developing CM among CRAG negative patients[b]	0.8%	0–2%	[10, 21, 29]
Treatment			
Survival of diagnosed CM with full CM treatment	70%	50–90%	[30]
Survival of CM without treatment	0%		
Relapse rate for treated CM[d]	12.50%	9–16%	[26, 43]
Disability Weights			
CM disease	0.615	0.46–0.77	[52, 53]
HIV (on ART)	0.053	0.039–0.066	[52, 53]
CM treatment	0.05	0.0375–0.0625	[52, 53] (Assumption)
Costs			
CRAG-LFA	$2.52	$1.50–$10.00	[38]
Lumbar Puncture	$8.08	$6.03–$10.42	[35, 38]
CM Diagnosis (lab and staff costs)	$7.07	$2.42–$12.79	[35–38]
Preemptive treatment: Fluconazole 800 mg daily for 2 weeks, then 400 mg daily for 8 weeks	$22.22	$17.00–$33.00	[24, 35]
CM Treatment: Amphotericin B 0.7 mg/kg/day for 2 weeks, then fluconazole 800 mg for 3 weeks and fluconazole 400 for 9 weeks	$343.28	$200–$600	[33–35]

Abbreviations: *CRAG-LFA* cryptococcal antigen lateral flow assay, *CPET* WHO Cryptococcal Pre-emptive therapy, *CM* cryptococcal meningitis, *ART* antiretroviral therapy

[a]Life expectancy was estimated to be reduced by 25% in CRAG positive individuals, independent of development of CM, to account for higher observed mortality in this population in recent cohort studies [20]

[b]CRAG-LFA testing was a component of only the CRAG-LFA screening intervention; However, risk of progression to CM for all model arms was stratified based on epidemiologic data on prevalence of baseline CRAG positivity

[c]Absolute and relative risk reduction were calculated based on available studies of fluconazole therapy in CRAG positive patients [26, 29, 31]. An estimated 15% of patients in all model arms were considered lost to follow up over the time horizon of the model, with higher rates of CM development and relapse. Sensitivity analysis was conducted around these parameters

[d]Assuming a 75% case detection rate for symptomatic CM disease

Epidemiologic, diagnostic, and treatment parameters

Key model parameters, values, and ranges are shown in Table 1. Variables including prevalence of cryptococcal antigenemia, percentage uptake, and percent of HIV patients with CD4 count <100 cells/μL were varied widely in sensitivity analysis to incorporate findings from multiple countries. For variables with limited data, uncertainty ranges were determined by varying base case values by ±75%. Probabilistic sensitivity analysis using Monte-Carlo simulation was conducted to simultaneously vary all parameters across their ranges to generate 95% uncertainty ranges (UR) for outcome estimates of costs, DALYs and cost-effectiveness.

Costs

Costs were derived from literature estimates as well as invoices from the Infectious Disease Institute in Kampala, Uganda and are presented in 2016 US dollars.

Costs of the CRAG LFA, lumbar puncture, and CM diagnosis were based on estimates accounting for personnel, materials, and outpatient visit costs, and are summarized in Table 1. Medication costs were based on prices available in Uganda from the Joint Medical Service [35–39]. Full CM treatment cost included the price of medication (Amphotericin B and Fluconazole), hospitalization, and therapeutic laboratory monitoring. Lifetime costs of ART and HIV care were not included in the base case analysis. However, to determine the impact of ART costs on the cost-effectiveness of CRAG screening, secondary analyses were performed to calculate the ICER inclusive of lifetime ART cost. Costs for future years were discounted at 3% [40–42].

Outcomes

The primary outcomes of the model were DALYs calculated based on disability attributable to CM disease with associated treatments, and years of life lost from CM-associated mortality (Table 1). We assumed near full life expectancy for individuals without CM disease with ART, based on site-specific data in Uganda for HIV-infected persons [41].

Cost-effectiveness was represented by the incremental cost-effectiveness ratio (ICER) comparing model arms, and assessed relative to WHO's suggested country-specific willingness-to-pay (WTP) threshold, defined in our analysis as per-capita Ugandan gross domestic product (GDP $572) per DALY averted [43, 44].

Results

Costs

Projected costs are summarized in Table 2. The incremental health system cost of the CRAG screening intervention in the base case scenario (i.e.100% implementation of CRAG screening for 1 year; total costs inclusive of a 5 year time period of downstream costs) was projected to be $1.52 (95%UR: $-5.46 to $9.42) more than 'no screening' per patient,. The diagnostic costs of the CRAG-LFA testing algorithm ($2.71 per person, inclusive of all diagnostic workup costs) were largely offset by averted costs associated with reduced development and treatment of CM when compared to costs of no screening (treatment costs for CRAG-LFA arm: $7.90 per person, compared to $8.85 for no screening).

Effectiveness

CRAG screening, implemented for all eligible individuals, resulted in improved health benefits compared to no screening (25 DALYs averted per hundred individuals), as summarized in Table 2. In the CRAG screening intervention arm, use of preemptive therapy among CRAG positive patients was projected to reduce CM development and thus early CM mortality. We estimated that implementation of CRAG screening resulted in a relative risk reduction in cryptococcal-associated mortality of 44% compared to CP (Absolute CM mortality projections: No screening 45 deaths per 1000 PLWH, CRAG screening 25 deaths per 1000 PLWH).

Cost-effectiveness

In the base case analysis, 100% implementation of CRAG screening (with preemptive therapy for CRAG-positive patients) was highly cost-effective compared to No screening ($6.14 per DALY averted, 95% UR: -$20.32 to $36.47) at current WTP thresholds for Uganda (Table 2). In secondary analysis, when including cost of lifetime ART, CRAG screening cost approximately $557 per DALY averted, still below the WTP threshold for cost-effectiveness in Uganda.

Secondary analysis

In the base case we assumed all asymptomatic CRAG-positive patients received preemptive treatment in the CRAG screening arm, without further evaluation for subclinical baseline CM. We explored alternative implementation algorithms for intensified diagnosis and treatment for CRAG-positive patients. If all CRAG-positive patients received a LP for intensified diagnosis of CM (with full CM treatment if diagnosed), the ICER for CRAG screening rose to $32 per DALY averted

Table 2 Costs, Effects, and ICER values of implementing universal CRAG screening

Intervention	Total Cost (95% UR)[a,c]	Incremental Cost[c]	DALYs	Incremental Effectiveness (DALYs averted)	ICER (cost per DALY averted)[c]
No screening	9.24 (7.31to 18.40)	REFERENCE	8.55 (6.70 to 10.90)	REFERENCE	REFERENCE
CRAG screening[b]	10.76 (8.39 to 12.29)	1.52 (−5.46 to 9.42)	8.30 (6.41to 10.79)	25 DALYs averted per 100 participants (13 to 47)	6.14 (−20.32 to 36.47)

Abbreviations: *CP* current practice, *CRAG-LFA* cryptococcal antigen lateral flow assay, *DALY* disability adjusted life-year, *ICER* incremental cost-effectiveness ratio

[a]Total costs represent total health systems costs, inclusive of diagnostic testing and treatment costs related to diagnosed cryptococcal antigenemia and/or cryptococcal meningitis over a 5 year time period, but excludes lifetime ART costs. DALYs were evaluated over a lifelong time horizon. Future years are discounted by 3% and ART costs are not included in base case analysis

[b]The CRAG-LFA intervention consists of screening all cohort patients for cryptococcal antigenemia with CRAG-LFA, followed by cryptococcal pre-emptive therapy (CPET) for those who screen positive

[c]In secondary analysis, the total costs inclusive of lifetime ART costs were $5772 and $5991 (incremental of139.48) for CP and CRAG-LFA screening arms, respectively. The ICER inclusive of lifetime ART costs was 558 per DALY averted

compared to No screening. Alternatively, if all CRAG positive patients were treated for CM (i.e. Amphotericin followed by fluconazole) irrespective of any additional evaluation, the ICER rises to $75 per DALY averted compared to No screening.

In further secondary analysis, we calculated the costs and effects of CRAG screening at four levels of programmatic scale-up (25, 50, 75, and 100% of eligible individuals, Table 3). We found that the incremental costs and DALYs averted were affected proportionally by percentage uptake of CRAG screening, and consequently the ICER for each level of implementation remained unchanged at $6.14 per DALY averted. However, the absolute costs and impact of varied by different levels of population level coverage of CRAG screening. The total (discounted) health system cost for an annual estimate of persons with HIV and CD4 < 100 cells/uL enrolling into care (inclusive of screening, further diagnostic evaluation when indicated, and treatment costs) of CRAG screening in Uganda was estimated at $651,454 at 100% uptake ($473,394, $303,930, $146,132 for 75%, 50%, 25% uptake respectively). Total mortality among this cohort from CM disease improved at each level of programmatic implementation (CM deaths averted compared to 'no screening': 307 at 25%, 614 at 50%, 921 at 75%, 1228 at 100% uptake). These estimates varied based on the estimated number of people enrolling in HIV care in Uganda as well as the estimated percentage with CD4 < 100 (Table 3).

Sensitivity analysis

We explored the impact of parameter uncertainty on our base case cost-effectiveness estimates (at 100% implementation) in one-way and multi-way sensitivity analyses (see Fig. 2 for selected one-way analyses). We did not identify any scenarios in which CRAG screening would not be considered highly cost-effective (i.e. where ICER dropped below the WTP threshold).

The variables that most impacted the ICER for CRAG screening included prevalence of cryptococcal antigenemia, relative reduction in CM progression among those who received preemptive therapy, and cost of CRAG-LFA testing. However, CRAG screening remained highly cost-effective at current WTP thresholds even at a CRAG prevalence of 0.5%, CRAG LFA cost of $9.80, and only 10% efficacy of preemptive treatment. Our model projected that if the proportion of CRAG positive cohort patients developing CM over a 5-year time period (despite ART usage) rose above 44%, CRAG screening became cost-saving compared to No screening. CRAG screening also became cost-saving if preemptive therapy reduced CM development by 90% compared to no therapy.

In probabilistic sensitivity analysis, CRAG screening was considered cost-effective compared to 'no screening' 100% of the time at a WTP threshold of GDP per capita. CRAG screening was considered cost-saving (both less expensive and more effective than No screening) in approximately 32% of simulations.

Discussion

Diagnosis and management of CM remains a significant clinical and infrastructural problem in Sub-Saharan Africa. Our study suggests that for HIV-infected patients with CD4 counts <100 cells/μL, incorporation of routine CRAG screening using the LFA would be highly cost-effective compared to no screening. Our model projects that CRAG screening with preemptive therapy for CRAG-positive individuals could reduce relative risk of CM mortality among PLWH with CD4 < 100 by over 40% while increasing costs by less than $2.00 per patient compared to no screening, suggesting that CRAG screening represents excellent value for money for HIV programs in these regions.

Our analysis also provides a unique assessment of alternative implementation algorithms for CRAG screening that have not been previously modeled, including intensified diagnostic evaluation with LP and providing full empiric treatment for CM among all CRAG-positive individuals. At $32 per DALY averted, incorporation of LP for all CRAG-positive patients remained well below WTP thresholds for Uganda and improved outcomes for patients with sub-clinical CM disease. While treatment of all CRAG-positive patients with full CM treatment also improved outcomes, it more than doubled the ICER compared to intensified diagnosis ($75 per DALY averted) with only a marginal mortality benefit. Our results suggest that, where feasible, intensified diagnostic evaluation of CRAG-positive patients with LP can improve detection of subclinical CM disease while remaining cost-effective [45].

Sensitivity analysis identified important parameters underlying the cost-effectiveness of CRAG screening. The prevalence of CRAG positivity among the cohort population had a significant influence on the ICER – as disease prevalence drops, CRAG screening identifies fewer high-risk patients and leads to fewer absolute benefits. Despite this, CRAG screening remained cost effective at the WTP threshold for Uganda even if prevalence declined to 1%; this result suggests that CRAG screening need not be limited to high-prevalence areas. Estimates of CRAG prevalence from various cohorts in Thailand and Sub-Saharan Africa including Ghana, Kenya, Ethiopia, Nigeria, and South Africa have reported a range of cryptococcal antigenemia from 2.2 to 21%, indicating that our results could be generalizable across much of Sub-Saharan Africa [7, 46]. The US and UK have previously estimated CRAG prevalences of 2.9 and 5% among cohorts of PLWH with CD4 < 100, suggesting that routine CRAG screening may be cost-effective in these populations as well, though further evaluation is warranted given the significant differences in practice and costs [47, 48].

Table 3 Absolute Costs and Effects for Various Levels of CRAG Screening

Implementation of CRAG screening (%)					Universal Screening
	0%	25%	50%	75%	100%
Number of Patients eligible for CRAG screening (CD4 < 100) enrolling in care per year	61,400 (13,000–105,000)	61,400 (13,000–105,000)	61,400 (13,000–105,000)	61,400 (13,000–105,000)	61,400 (13,000–105,000)
Number of patients receiving CRAG screening	0	15,350 (3250–26,250)	30,700 (6500–52,500)	46,050 (9750–78,750)	61,400 (13,000–105,000)
Total cost per patient[a,b]	$9.24 (7.31–18.40)	$9.52 (0.87–26.87)	$9.90 (1.28–27.29)	$10.28 (1.54–27.40)	$10.76 (1.85–28.26)
Incremental Cost per patient, compared to No screening[a,b]	REFERENCE	$0.37 (−6.44–8.47)	$0.75 (−6.03–8.89)	$1.13 (−5.77–9.09)	$1.52 (−5.46–9.42)
Total Program Cost	$559,968 (95,000–1,900,000)	$584,528 (123,000–1,930,000)	$607,860 (154,000–1,960,000)	$631,192 (178,000–1,990,000)	$651,454 (198,000–2,100,000)
Total Incremental Program Costs compared to No screening[a,b]	REFERENCE	$24,560 (12,000–36,000)	$47,892 (30,000–64,000)	$71,224 (54,000–96,000)	$91,486 (76,000–104,000)
DALYs accumulated per patient	8.55 (6.70–10.90)	8.48 (1.59–10.87)	8.42 (6.53–10.84)	8.36 (6.47–10.82)	8.3 (6.41–10.79)
Total DALYs averted compared to No screening	REFERENCE	4298	7982	11,666	15,350
Deaths from CM (proportion of cohort)	2763 (0.045)	2456 (0.04)	2149 (0.035)	1842 (0.03)	1535 (0.025)
CM deaths averted compared to No screening	REFERENCE	307	614	921	1228

Abbreviations: *CRAG-LFA* cryptococcal antigen lateral flow assay, *DALY* disability adjusted life-year, *ICER* incremental cost-effectiveness ratio

[a]Total costs represent total health systems costs, inclusive of diagnostic testing and treatment costs related to diagnosed cryptococcal antigenemia and/or cryptococcal meningitis over a 5 year time period, but excludes lifetime ART costs. Future years are discounted by 3% and ART costs are not included in base case analysis. Costs stratified by source: No screening – Diagnostic costs $0.27 per person, $16,500 total, Treatment costs $8.85 per person, $543,000 total. Universal CRAG screening – Diagnostic costs $2.71 per person, $166,000 total, Treatment costs $7.90 per person, $485,000 total

[b]Total cost per patient including lifetime ART: $5772 at 0%, $5807 at 25%, $5842 at 50%, $5876 at 75%, $5911 at 100%. Projected total program cost including lifetime ART: $354,400,800 at 0%, $89,133,613 at 25%, $179,318,700 at 50%, $270,601,313 at 75%, $362,935,400 at 100%

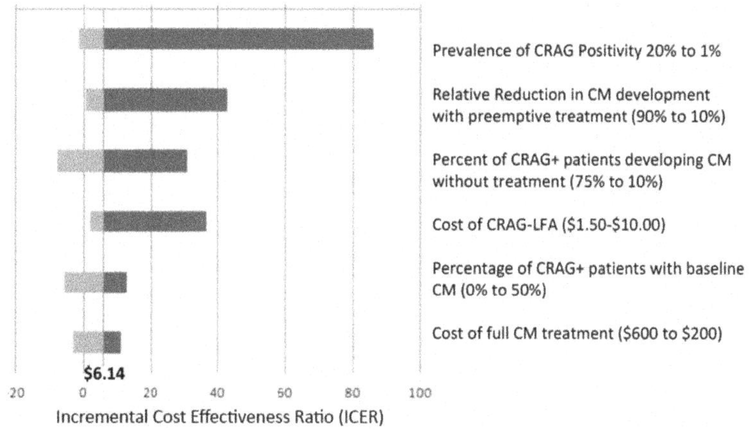

Fig. 2 Tornado Diagram demonstrating Impact of Model Variables on ICER. Abbreviations: CRAG-LFA –cryptococcal antigen lateral flow assay, CM – cryptococcal meningitis, CRAG – cryptococcal antigen. Tornado diagram demonstrating the effect of varying six pertinent variables on the ICER value for CRAG screening compared to CP. The vertical line at $6.14 represents the ICER for the base case analysis

There are several limitations to our study. Like all cost-effectiveness analyses, we are limited by the availability of data to inform estimates for key model parameters. When data were limited, we incorporated large ranges and conducted sensitivity analyses to assess their impact on cost-effectiveness. Overall, our model projections are consistent with empirically collected data from studies evaluating CRAG screening (31–57 deaths per 1000 PLWH) [2, 3, 8]. While base case analysis did not include ART costs, we performed secondary analysis to incorporate these costs into each intervention and calculate the ICER inclusive of ART cost. Our model assumes optimal implementation and uptake of CRAG screening; however this may not be possible in resource-limited settings. Additional research is needed to examine infrastructural and programmatic barriers associated with implementing a CRAG-LFA screening program.

Our study has significant strengths and differs from previous analyses in several important ways. First our model focuses on population-level effects of scaling-up CRAG screening in a low-income country in Sub-Sarahan Africa, a region with high cryptococcal burden and approximately 500,000 of the 625,000 yearly CM deaths [1]. Furthermore, we modeled the incorporation of preemptive therapy for clinical management of cryptococcal antigenemia and explored cost-effectiveness at varying degrees of preemptive treatment efficacy. We also incorporated relapse and loss-to-follow-up into our projections and modeled the intervention at various degrees of scale-up to estimate realistic implementation efforts. Our findings build on data from higher income settings and demonstrate the cost-effectiveness and projected implementation effects of CRAG-LFA screening for a high prevalence, low-income region.

Despite WHO recommendations for universal CRAG screening among eligible patients, implementation is of paramount importance and remains a challenge in overburdened, under-resourced clinics. Despite known survival benefit with CRAG screening, successful national implementation will require education of healthcare workers, training of laboratory workers, purchasing of CRAG LFA kits, and sufficient supply of fluconazole and ART. In our experience stock-outs of fluconazole are a common limiting factor. CRAG screening programs with high rates of loss to follow up, have proven unsuccessful [45]. Without an advocate in each clinic for those particularly vulnerable patients with a CD4 < 100 cells/uL, it remains challenging to successfully implement CRAG screening programs outside of research studies. Finally, CRAG screening programs need to be closely linked to ART initiation and retention in care. ART remains the most important intervention to decrease mortality in highly immunosuppressed HIV patients.

Notably, we project that a CRAG screening program, including preemptive treatment, costs approximately $10.76 per person per year in Uganda. In comparison, the mean annual price for first line ART is $100 per year in sub-Saharan Africa, and delivery of ART including lab monitoring and personnel costs is estimated between $150 and $500 US dollars per person-year, suggesting that CRAG screening is relatively inexpensive and could serve as a key peri-ART intervention for immunosuppressed patients [49, 50].

Conclusion

Taken together, our analysis suggests that CRAG screening would be a highly cost-effective policy intervention in Uganda, with potential application to much of sub-Saharan Africa. It also underscores the need for additional research such as case detection, rates of CM relapse and loss to follow-up in these regions. Further work should also focus on potential barriers to implementation and developing an optimized clinical algorithm for managing these patients. As access to ART continues to improve in these regions over time, median CD4 will rise and prevalence of CM will likely decrease – developing cost-effectiveness projections to model this progression will be useful in guiding allocation of care. As we move towards universal ART access, implementing CRAG screening has the potential to reduce the high burden of cryptococcal disease in Sub-Saharan Africa.

Abbreviations

PLWH: People living with HIV; ART: Antiretroviral therapy; CM: Cryptococcal meningitis; CRAG: Cryptococcal antigen; DALY: Disability-adjusted life year; ICER: Incremental cost-effectiveness ratio; LFA: Lateral-flow assay; LP: Lumbar puncture; WTP: Willingness-to-pay

Acknowledgements

Not applicable.

Funding

This project was funded with Federal funds from the National Institute of Allergy and Infectious Diseases, National Institutes of Health, under grant # K23AI089259, and the Infectious Disease Society of America. RR is supported by the National Institute of Allergy and Infectious Diseases (U01AI089244) and by the National Center for Advancing Translational Sciences of the National Institutes of Health (UL1TR000114). YM receives salary support from the Fogarty International Center, National Institutes of Health HIV co-infections in Uganda:TB, Cryptococcus, and viral hepatitis (D43TW009771).

Authors' contributions

AR conducted the primary analysis and authored the manuscript draft. MS supervised model construction and guided data analysis. YM defined the scope of the project and contextual relevance to practice in Uganda. RR provided key model data and contributed to the manuscript discussion. All authors reviewed and approved the manuscript.

Competing interests

All authors declare that they have no competing interests.

Consent for publication

Not applicable.

Author details

[1]Johns Hopkins University School of Medicine, 725 N. Wolfe St. PCTB building-224, Baltimore, MD 21205, USA. [2]Infectious Diseases Institute, Makerere University College of Health Sciences, Kampala, Uganda. [3]Division of Infectious Diseases and International Medicine, Department of Medicine, University of Minnesota, Minneapolis, MN, USA.

References

1. Park BJ, Wannemuehler KA, Marston BJ, Govender N, Pappas PG, Chiller TM. Estimation of the current global burden of cryptococcal meningitis among persons living with HIV/AIDS. AIDS. 2009;23(4):525–30.
2. French N, Gray K, Watera C, et al. Cryptococcal infection in a cohort of HIV-1-infected Ugandan adults. AIDS. 2002;16(7):1031–8.
3. Okongo M, Morgan D, Mayanja B, Ross A, Whitworth J. Causes of death in a rural, population-based human immunodeficiency virus type 1 (HIV-1) natural history cohort in Uganda. Int J Epidemiol. 1998;27(4):698–702.
4. Corbett EL, Churchyard GJ, Charalambos S, et al. Morbidity and mortality in South African gold miners: impact of untreated disease due to human immunodeficiency virus. Clin Infect Dis. 2002;34(9):1251–8.
5. WHO U. Towards Universal Access: Scaling up priority HIV/AIDS interventions in the health sector. Progress Report. World Health Organization. 2011; 53. Available at: http://www.who.int/hiv/topics/treatment/data/en/index2.html. Accessed 14 Jan 2015.
6. Jarvis JN, Harrison TS. HIV-associated cryptococcal meningitis. AIDS. 2007; 21(16):2119–29. doi:10.1097/QAD.0b013e3282a4a64d.
7. Meyer AC, Jacobson M. Asymptomatic cryptococcemia in resource-limited settings. Curr HIV/AIDS Rep. 2013;10(3):254–63.
8. Kambugu A, Meya DB, Rhein J, et al. Outcomes of cryptococcal meningitis in Uganda before and after the availability of highly active antiretroviral therapy. Clin Infect Dis. 2008;46(11):1694–701.
9. Chang LW, Phipps WT, Kennedy GE, Rutherford GW. Antifungal interventions for the primary prevention of cryptococcal disease in adults with HIV. Cochrane Database Syst Rev. 2005;2005(3):CD004773.
10. Parkes-Ratanshi R, Wakeham K, Levin J, et al. Primary prophylaxis of cryptococcal disease with fluconazole in HIV-positive Ugandan adults: a double-blind, randomised, placebo-controlled trial. Lancet Infect Dis. 2011;11(12):933–41.
11. Lindsley MD, Mekha N, Baggett HC, et al. Evaluation of a newly developed lateral flow immunoassay for the diagnosis of cryptococcosis. Clin Infect Dis. 2011;53(4):321–5.
12. Binnicker MJ, Jespersen DJ, Bestrom JE, Rollins LO. Comparison of four assays for the detection of cryptococcal antigen. Clin Vaccine Immunol. 2012;19(12):1988–90.
13. Hansen J, Slechta ES, Gates-Hollingsworth MA, et al. Large-scale evaluation of the immuno-mycologics lateral flow and enzyme-linked immunoassays for detection of cryptococcal antigen in serum and cerebrospinal fluid. Clin Vaccine Immunol. 2013;20(1):52–5.
14. McMullan BJ, Halliday C, Sorrell TC, et al. Clinical utility of the cryptococcal antigen lateral flow assay in a diagnostic mycology laboratory. PLoS One. 2012;7(11):e49541.
15. Boulware DR, Rolfes MA, Rajasingham R, et al. Multisite validation of cryptococcal antigen lateral flow assay and quantification by laser thermal contrast. Emerg Infect Dis. 2014;20(1):45–53.
16. Jarvis JN, Percival A, Bauman S, et al. Evaluation of a novel point-of-care cryptococcal antigen test on serum, plasma, and urine from patients with HIV-associated cryptococcal meningitis. Clin Infect Dis. 2011;53(10):1019–23.
17. Escandon P, Lizarazo J, Agudelo CI, Chiller T, Castaneda E. Evaluation of a rapid lateral flow immunoassay for the detection of cryptococcal antigen for the early diagnosis of cryptococcosis in HIV patients in Colombia. Med Mycol. 2013;51(7):765–8.
18. Kozel TR, Bauman SK. CrAg lateral flow assay for cryptococcosis. Expert Opin Med Diagn. 2012;6(3):245–51.
19. McKenney J, Smith RM, Chiller TM, et al. Prevalence and correlates of cryptococcal antigen positivity among AIDS patients–United States, 1986-2012. MMWR Morb Mortal Wkly Rep. 2014;63(27):585–7.
20. Liechty CA, Solberg P, Were W, et al. Asymptomatic serum cryptococcal antigenemia and early mortality during antiretroviral therapy in rural Uganda. Trop Med Int Health. 2007;12(8):929–35.
21. Jarvis JN, Lawn SD, Vogt M, Bangani N, Wood R, Harrison TS. Screening for cryptococcal antigenemia in patients accessing an antiretroviral treatment program in South Africa. Clin Infect Dis. 2009;48(7):856–62.
22. Ganiem AR, Indrati AR, Wisaksana R, et al. Asymptomatic cryptococcal antigenemia is associated with mortality among HIV-positive patients in Indonesia. J Int AIDS Soc. 2014;17:18821.
23. Feldmesser M, Harris C, Reichberg S, Khan S, Casadevall A. Serum cryptococcal antigen in patients with AIDS. Clin Infect Dis. 1996;23(4):827–30.
24. WHO. Rapid Advice: Diagnosis, Prevention and Management of Cryptococcal Disease in HIV-infected Adults, Adolescents and Children. 2011.
25. Mfinanga S, Chanda D, Kivuyo SL, et al. Cryptococcal meningitis screening and community-based early adherence support in people with advanced HIV infection starting antiretroviral therapy in Tanzania and Zambia: an open-label, randomised controlled trial. Lancet. 2015;385:2173–82.

26. Pac L, Horwitz M, Namutembi A. Integrated Pre-Antiretroviral Therapy Screening and Treatment for Tuberculosis and Cryptococcal Antigenemia. JAIDS. 2015. (in press).
27. Jarvis JN, Harrison TS, Lawn SD, Meintjes G, Wood R, Cleary S. Cost effectiveness of cryptococcal antigen screening as a strategy to prevent HIV-associated cryptococcal meningitis in South Africa. PLoS One. 2013;8(7):e69288.
28. Vallabhaneni S, et al. Implementation and Operational Research: Evaluation of a Public-Sector, Provider-Initiated Cryptococcal Antigen Screening and Treatment Program, Western Cape, South Africa. JAIDS. 2016;72(2):e37–42.
29. Pac L, Horwitz MM, Namutebi AM, Auerbach BJ, Semeere A, Namulema T, et al. Implementation and operational research: integrated pre-antiretroviral therapy screening and treatment for tuberculosis and cryptococcal antigenemia. J Acquir Immune Defic Syndr. 2015;68(5):e69–76.
30. Boulware DR, Meya DB, Muzoora C, et al. Timing of antiretroviral therapy after diagnosis of cryptococcal meningitis. N Engl J Med. 2014;370(26):2487–98.
31. Butler EK, Boulware DR, Bohjanen PR, Meya DB. Long term 5-year survival of persons with cryptococcal meningitis or asymptomatic subclinical antigenemia in Uganda. PLoS One. 2012;7(12):e51291.
32. Pongsai P, Atamasirikul K, Sungkanuparph S. The role of serum cryptococcal antigen screening for the early diagnosis of cryptococcosis in HIV-infected patients with different ranges of CD4 cell counts. J Infect. 2010;60(6):474–7.
33. Meyer AC, Kendi CK, Penner JA, et al. The impact of routine cryptococcal antigen screening on survival among HIV-infected individuals with advanced immunosuppression in Kenya. Trop Med Int Health. 2013;18(4):495–503.
34. UNAIDS. "The HIV/AIDS Uganda Country Progress Report 2014" http://www.unaids.org/sites/default/files/country/documents/UGA_narrative_report_2015.pdf. Accessed 14 May 2016
35. Joint Medical Store. Catalogue and Price Indicator. http://www.jms.co.ug/sites/default/files/resources/Catalogue%20Feb%202015_light%20version_0.pdf. Accessed 4 Mar 2016.
36. Ninci A, Ocakacon R. How Much Do Lab Tests Cost? Analysis of Lacor Hospital Laboratory Services. Health Policy Dev. 2004;2(2):44–150.
37. Rajasingham R, Meya DB, Boulware DR. Integrating cryptococcal antigen screening and pre-emptive treatment into routine HIV care. J Acquir Immune Defic Syndr. 2012;59(5):e85–91.
38. Rajasingham R, Rolfes MA, Birkenkamp KE, Meya DB, Boulware DR. Cryptococcal meningitis treatment strategies in resource-limited settings: a cost-effectiveness analysis. PLoS Med. 2012;9(9):e1001316.
39. Moreland S, Namisango E, Paxton A, Powell R. Measure Evaluation - The costs of HIV treatment, care, and support services in Uganda: a technical report. 2013.
40. Weinstein MC, Siegel JE, Gold MR, Kamlet MS, Russell LB. Recommendations of the Panel on Cost-effectiveness in Health and Medicine. JAMA. 1996; 276(15):1253–8.
41. Mills EJ, Bakanda C, Birungi J, et al. Life expectancy of persons receiving combination antiretroviral therapy in low-income countries: a cohort analysis from Uganda. Ann Intern Med. 2011;155(4):209–16.
42. Hirth RA, Chernew ME, Miller E, Fendrick AM, Weissert WG. Willingness to pay for a quality-adjusted life year: in search of a standard. Med Decis Making. 2000;20(3):332–42.
43. WHO. Cost-Effectiveness Thresholds. Available at: http://www.who.int/choice/costs/CER_levels/en/ . Accessed 4 Nov 2014.
44. World_Bank. GDP per capita by country.Available at: http://data.worldbank.org/indicator/NY.GDP.PCAP.CD?order=wbapi_data_value_2013+wbapi_data_value+wbapi_data_value-last&sort=asc. Accessed 4 Nov 2014.
45. Fiani D, Vedastus A, Neborak J et al. Maximizing detection and improving outcomes of cryptococcosis in rural Tanzania. 2016. Available at: http://www.croiconference.org/sites/default/files/posters-2016/760_0.pdf Accessed 14 Jun 2016
46. Govender N, Roy M, Mendes J, Zulu T, Chiller T, Karstaedt A. Evaluation of Screening and Treatment of Cryptococcal Antigenaemia among HIV-infected Persons in Soweto, South Africa. HIV Med. 2015;16:468–76.
47. Patel S, Shin GY, Wijewardana I, et al. The prevalence of cryptococcal antigenemia in newly diagnosed HIV patients in a Southwest London cohort. J Infect. 2013;66(1):75–9.
48. McKenney J, Bauman S, Neary B, et al. Prevalence, Correlates, and Outcomes o Cryptococcal Antigen Positivity Among Patients With AIDS, United States, 1986–2012. Clin Infect Dis. 2015;60(6):959–65.
49. Bendavid E, Leroux E, Bhattacharya J, Smith N, Miller G. The relation of price of antiretroviral drugs and foreign assistance with coverage of HIV treatment in Africa: retrospective study. BMJ. 2010;341:c6218.
50. Jain V, Chang W, Byonanebye DM, et al. Estimated Costs for Delivery of HIV Antiretroviral Therapy to Individuals with CD4+ T-Cell Counts >350 cells/uL in Rural Uganda. PLoS One. 2015;10(12):e0143433. doi:10.1371/journal.pone.0143433. Lima VD, ed
51. Meya DB, Manabe YC, Castelnuovo B, et al. Cost-effectiveness of serum cryptococcal antigen screening to prevent deaths among HIV-infected persons with a CD4+ cell count < or = 100 cells/microL who start HIV therapy in resource-limited settings. Clin Infect Dis. 2010;51(4):448–55.
52. WHO. Age-Specific Disability Weights for untreated and treated forms of sequelae included in the Global Burden of Disease Study. http://www.who.int/healthinfo/bodreferencedisabilityweights.xls. Accessed Jun 10, 2014.
53. Salomon JA, Vos T, Hogan DR, et al. Common values in assessing health outcomes from disease and injury: disability weights measurement study for the Global Burden of Disease Study 2010. Lancet. 2012;380(9859):2129–43.

High dose fluconazole in salvage therapy for HIV-uninfected cryptococcal meningitis

Hua-Zhen Zhao[1†], Rui-Ying Wang[1†], Xuan Wang[1], Ying-Kui Jiang[1], Ling-Hong Zhou[1], Jia-Hui Cheng[1], Li-Ping Huang[1], Thomas Stephen Harrison[2*†] and Li-Ping Zhu[1*†]

Abstract

Background: The 2010 Infectious Diseases Society of America (IDSA) guidelines for management of cryptococcal diseases recommend high dose fluconazole (≥ 800 mg/day), either alone or with other antifungal drugs, as alternative anticryptococcal choices. But evidence for its use in the treatment of HIV-uninfected cryptococcal meningitis (CM) remains sparse.

Methods: A retrospective analysis of HIV-uninfected CM patients who received fluconazole 800 mg/day for salvage therapy from January 2011 to December 2016 at Huashan Hospital, Shanghai, China was performed. Efficacy and safety were assessed, and mortality and prognostic factors evaluated.

Results: A total of 44 patients were studied including 19 refractory to amphotericin B induction therapy, 8 refractory to fluconazole consolidation therapy (400 mg/d), and 17 intolerant of antifungal drugs. For salvage, 11 patients received triple therapy of high dose fluconazole, amphotericin B and flucytosine, 20 received dual therapy of high dose fluconazole and flucytosine, 13 received monotherapy of high dose fluconazole. Median duration of high dose fluconazole in salvage regimens was 136.5 days (range, 1–667 days). Clinical response rates were 72.1% (31/43) and 83.7% (36/43) when assessed at 2 weeks and the end of salvage therapy, respectively. Adverse events possibly related to high dose fluconazole occurred in 54.5% (24/44) of the patients, and all were mild or moderate. From the initiation of salvage therapy, 1-year all-cause mortality was 13.6% (6 of 44 patients) among the study population with no significant difference in refractory or intolerant patients.

Conclusions: Adherence to guideline recommendations of high dose fluconazole, alone or in combination with other antifungals, was safe and often effective for salvage therapy of HIV-uninfected CM patients.

Keywords: High dose fluconazole, HIV-uninfected, Cryptococcal meningitis, Efficacy, Safety

Background

Cryptococcal meningitis (CM) is the most common opportunistic fungal infection of the central nervous system (CNS). The vast majority of cases are caused by *Cryptococcus neoformans*, while *Cryptococcus gattii* is more geographically restricted [1]. According to an updated estimate, over 220,000 cases of CM occur each year in HIV-infected patients, resulting in 181,000 deaths in 2014 [2]. Owing to the advent of highly active antiretroviral therapies, the incidence of HIV-infected CM has decreased and the long-term survival rate has increased in developed countries in recent years [3]. However, a growing number of CM cases occur in HIV-uninfected hosts with solid organ transplants, innate immunodeficiency and immune disorders, exogenous immunosuppressant administration, and even apparently normal immune status [4]. Mortality rate in these patients was as high as 25–40%, which was no lower than that in HIV-infected CM patients [5–8]. As a very heterogeneous group, HIV-uninfected CM patients pose great therapeutic challenges to clinicians.

Fluconazole is a triazole with excellent in vitro and in vivo activity against *Cryptococcus*. It has been widely used in CM as consolidation and maintenance therapy,

* Correspondence: tharriso@sgul.ac.uk; zhulp@fudan.edu.cn
†Hua-Zhen Zhao, Rui-Ying Wang, Thomas Stephen Harrison and Li-Ping Zhu contributed equally to this work.
[2]Institute of Infection and Immunity, St George's, University of London, London SW17, 0RE, UK
[1]Department of Infectious Diseases, Huashan Hospital, Fudan University, 12 Central Urumqi Road, Shanghai, China

usually at a dosage equal to or lower than 400 mg/day. In resource-limited areas, fluconazole alone has been used for induction therapy, and proved to be a poorly effective drug with 10-week mortality consistently > 50% even at high dosage [9–12]. But the efficacy was acceptable or favorable when high dose fluconazole was used in combination with other antifungal drugs or as enhanced consolidation therapy [13–18]. In the 2010 Infectious Diseases Society of America (IDSA) guidelines, higher dose fluconazole alone or in combination with other antifungals was recommended for both consolidation and salvage therapy in HIV-uninfected CM patients, compared with 400 mg/day in the 2000 version of these guidelines [19, 20]. However, evidence of high dose fluconazole for treatment of CM was mainly based on studies of HIV-infected populations, and remained sparse in HIV-uninfected patients. Therefore, we conducted a retrospective study among HIV-uninfected CM patients who received fluconazole 800 mg/day for salvage therapy, and evaluated the efficacy and safety of high dose fluconazole regimens.

Methods

Study design

This is a retrospective cohort study conducted among HIV-uninfected CM patients from January 2011 to December 2016 at Huashan Hospital, Fudan University (a tertiary health care center in Shanghai, China, with approximately 1200 hospital beds and 60,000 admissions per year). Patients who had been refractory to or intolerant of prior antifungal drugs and who then switched to salvage therapy with fluconazole 800 mg/day were included. This study was reviewed and approved by the local medical ethics committee.

Definitions

A proven diagnosis of CM was made if the patient met any of the following criteria: (1) positive culture of *Cryptococcus* from cerebrospinal fluid (CSF), (2) positive CSF ink smear, (3) cryptococcal capsular polysaccharide antigen detected in CSF on cryptococcal antigen (CrAg) lateral flow assay (IMMY, Inc., Norman, Oklahoma, USA) in CSF or (4) compatible histopathological findings, which are 5–10 μm encapsulated yeasts in brain tissue. Refractory CM was considered if any 2 of the following conditions were present after an adequate period of antifungal therapy (≥14 days): (1) persistently positive cultures of *Cryptococcus* in CSF, (2) deterioration of clinical signs and symptoms of disease, (3) new sites of disease or worsening of pre-existing lesions radiologically, and (4) decreasing level of glucose and increasing level of protein in CSF [21, 22]. Patients were considered as intolerance to antifungal drugs if they suffered severe or life-threatening toxicity from amphotericin B (AmB) based initial therapy [22].

Efficacy and safety assessment

Patients treated with high dose fluconazole for ≥1 week were included for efficacy evaluation. Response to salvage therapy was assessed at 2 weeks after initiation of salvage therapy, at the end of salvage therapy, and at the end of antifungal therapy. Efficacy of antifungal treatment was categorized as success (complete or partial response) or failure (stable response, disease progression, or death during the study period regardless of any cause) on the basis of clinical, radiological, and microbiological data according to previous criteria [21]. Adverse events (AEs) occurring during salvage therapy were recorded. The relationships of AEs and high dose fluconazole were evaluated with Naranjo probability scale [23]. High dose fluconazole related AEs were defined as one with a possible, probable or certain relationship.

Statistical analysis

Continuous variables were compared with t test or the non-parametric Mann-Whitney test. Proportions were compared with the $\chi 2$ test or Fisher's exact test, as appropriate. Log-rank test was used in univariate analysis for prognostic factors of 1-year survival, and Cox proportional hazards model for identification of independent prognostic predictors. A *P*-value of < 0 .05 was considered statistically significant.

Results

Demographics and manifestations

In total, 44 patients with proven CM were included in our study. Thirty-two also had pulmonary involvement and 6 cryptococcemia. The median age was 44 years, and 63.6% were male. Predisposing factors co-existed in 16 patients (36%). Detailed information is summarized in Table 1. Headache (100%) was the most common symptom, and 72.7% of them presented with fever, vomiting and meningeal irritation. Thirty-four patients presented with further neurological symptoms and signs, including altered mental status, epileptic seizures, cranial nerve deficits, limb weakness, uracratia and dysuria (Table 1).

Image findings

Cranial magnetic resonance imaging (MRI) was performed in all patients, with 41/44 (93.2%) yielding abnormal results. Local parenchymal lesions (86.4%) were most frequently observed, and common sites included frontal lobe (68.2%), parietal lobe (59.1%), periventricular region (29.5%) and basal ganglion (22.7%). Other abnormalities included meningeal enhancement

Table 1 Baseline characteristics, signs and symptoms of 44 cryptococcal meningitis patients treated with high dose fluconazole for salvage therapy

Variables	No. (%) of patients
Sex, male	28 (63.6)
Age, years	44 (range, 16–73)
Predisposing factors	
Evans syndrome	4 (9.1)
MDS	1 (2.3)
ITP	1 (2.3)
Lymphoma	1 (2.3)
Solid tumor[a]	2 (4.5)
SLE	5 (11.4)
Cirrhosis	2 (4.5)
Liver transplantation	1 (2.3)
Splenectomy	1 (2.3)
Type 2 diabetes mellitus	2 (4.5)
Steroids or immunosuppressants	10 (22.7)
Headache	44 (100)
Fever	32 (72.7)
Vomiting	32 (72.7)
Meningeal irritation	32 (72.7)
Seizure	16 (36.4)
Altered mental status[b]	12 (27.3)
Cranial nerve defect	
Impaired vision	16 (36.4)
Diplopia	8 (18.2)
Visual field defect	8 (18.2)
Ophthalmodynia	3 (6.8)
Hearing impairment	18 (40.9)
Facial paralysis	3 (6.8)
Limb weakness	14 (31.8)
uracratia	3 (6.8)
Dysuria	3 (6.8)

MDS myelodysplastic syndrome; *SLE* systemic lupus erythematosus; *ITP* idiopathic thrombocytopenia
[a]Including 1 gastric cancer and 1 cholangiocellular carcinoma
[b]Patients with scores less than 15 by Glasgow Coma Scale

(25 patients; 56.8%) and ventricular enlargement (12 patients; 27.3%). Most patients had 2 or more sites of involvement. Abnormalities on chest computer tomography (CT) scans were found in 32 of 44 patients (72.3%). The common findings were nodules and masses (47.7%), patches and strips (43.9%), pleural thickening (22.7%), pleural effusion (20.5%), lymph node enlargement (6.8%), air bronchogram sign (4.5%) and ground glass attenuation (2.3%). Some patients had mixed types of lesion on chest CT.

CSF findings

Before initiating salvage therapy, CSF examinations were performed in 43 patients including 42 samples from lumbar punctures, 1 from continuous lumbar cerebrospinal fluid drainage. CSF cultures were positive for *Cryptococcus* in 4 patients, and ink smears were positive in 18 patients. CSF CrAg tests were positive in all 43 patients, and 47.7% of them (21/43) had CrAg titer of at least 1:640. Median white blood cell count (WBC) of CSF was 29 /mm^3 (range, 0–550 /mm^3). Median levels of CSF protein and glucose were 824 mg/dL and 34 mg/dL, respectively. Of the 42 patients who had lumbar punctures, 21 had CSF opening pressure above 25 cm H_2O.

Antifungal therapy

As listed in Fig. 1, 19 patients (43.2%) were refractory to initial antifungal therapy, 8 (18.2%) were refractory to consolidation therapy, and 17 (38.6%) were intolerant of prior antifungals. AmB-based regimens were initially administered in all 44 patients, and daily dosage of AmB ranged from 20 to 40 mg (0.4–0.7 mg/kg/day). Median cumulative dose and duration of AmB were 1205 mg (range, 205–5775 mg) and 48.5 days (range, 9–212 days).

Of the 19 patients refractory to initial therapy, 11 received high dose fluconazole in combination with AmB and flucytosine for salvage, 6 received high dose fluconazole and flucytosine, and the remaining 2 received high dose fluconazole alone. For patients who were refractory to consolidation therapy, fluconazole dosage was increased from 400 mg/day to 800 mg/day and flucytosine co-administered in all but one patient. Of the 17 antifungal-intolerant patients, 10 received high dose fluconazole alone, and 7 others were treated with high dose fluconazole and flucytosine. Overall, triple therapy of high dose fluconazole, AmB and flucytosine was administered in 11 patients, 20 received dual therapy of high dose fluconazole and flucytosine, 13 received monotherapy of high dose fluconazole. Median duration of high dose fluconazole in salvage therapy for the 44 patients was 136.5 days (range, 1–667 days). Among the 31 patients (70.5%) receiving flucytosine, 27 were treated with flucytosine throughout the course, and the remaining 4 discontinued the drug for suspected side effects (3 with anemia, 1 with elevated transaminase). Median duration of flucytosine in salvage therapy for the 31 patients was 142 days (range, 22–561 days).

Efficacy and outcome

Except 1 patient who received high dose fluconazole less than 7 days and died of multiple organ failure (MOF), the other 43 patients were all included into efficacy evaluation. Two weeks after salvage therapy, partial response in 31 patients (72.1%), stable response in 11 patients (25.6%),

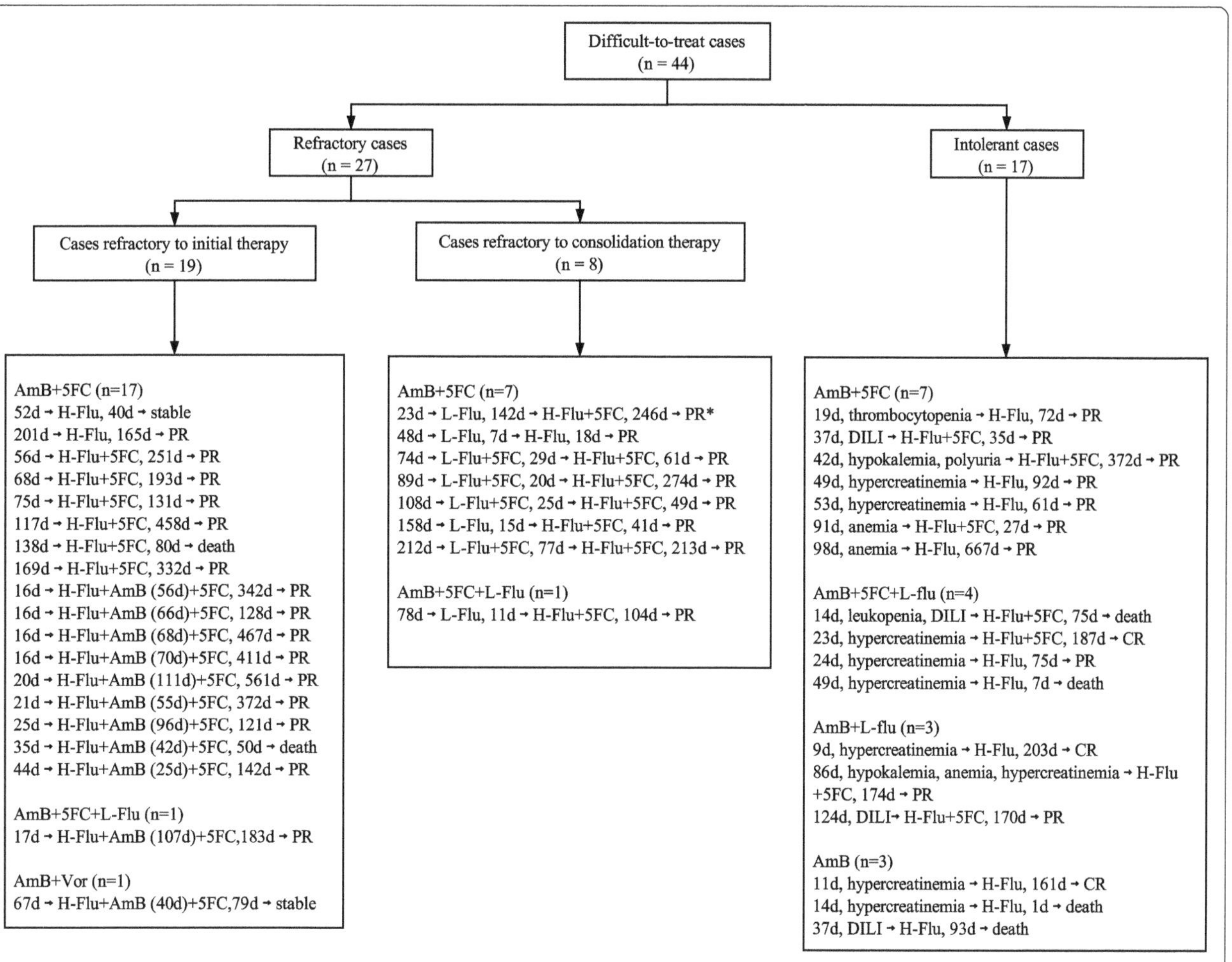

Fig. 1 Profiles of initial therapy and salvage therapy in 44 difficult-to-treat cryptococcal meningitis patients. *AmB* amphotericin B; *5FC* flucytosine; *Vor* voriconazole; *L-Flu* low dose fluconazole (≤ 400 mg/day); *H-Flu* high dose fluconazole (800 mg/day); CR complete response; *PR* partial response; *DILI* drug induced liver injury. Addition or removal of 5FC during initial and salvage therapy were not listed. An example for reading the figure: * means that the patient received AmB and flucytosine for a duration of 23 days as induction therapy, followed by consolidation therapy with low dose fluconazole for 142 days, and then switched to salvage therapy with high dose fluconazole for 246 days, and finally achieved partial response at the end of salvage therapy

and death caused by brain hernia in 1 patient (2.3%) were observed. At the end of salvage therapy, 3 patients (7.0%) achieved complete response, 33 (76.7%) achieved partial response, 2 (4.7%) achieved stable response, and 5 (11.6%) died. The overall efficacy rate was 83.7%. Of the 2 stable patients, 1 discontinued fluconazole, reinstituted with AmB and flucytosine and achieved partial response; the other was lost for follow-up 40 days after initiation of salvage therapy. Of the 4 patients who died after 2 weeks of salvage therapy, 1 was considered to have died of CM, 2 died from secondary infection and MOF, and 1 died from aggravation of lymphoma. Thirty-seven of 43 patients (86.0%) achieved clinical success and stopped antifungal drugs, 5 (11.6%) died and 1 (2.3%) was lost for follow-up. As shown in Table 2, we compared the response rates between patients treated with high dose fluconazole with or without flucytosie and those with combinations of AmB and high dose fluconazole with or without flucytosine.

Table 2 Clinical success rate in 43 cryptococcal meningitis patients treated with high dose fluconazole for salvage therapy

Time point	Total ($N = 43$)	H-Flu ±5FC ($N = 32$)	H-Flu + AmB ± 5FC ($N = 11$)	*P*-value
2-week of Salvage Therapy	31 (72.1)	20 (62.5)	11 (100)	0.019
End of Salvage Therapy	36 (83.7)	27 (84.4)	9 (81.8)	> 0.999
End of Antifungal Therapy	37 (86.0)	27 (84.4)	10 (90.9)	> 0.999

H-Flu high dose fluconazole (800 mg/day); *AmB* Amphotericin B; *5FC* flucytosine

Although a significant higher 2-week response rate was observed in the triple combination group (62.5% vs. 100%, $P = 0.019$), there was no apparent differences in efficacy at the end of salvage therapy (84.4% vs. 81.8%, $P > 0.999$) and the end of antifungal therapy (84.4% vs. 90.9%, $P > 0.999$). At 1-year follow-up after stopping antifungal drugs, all of the 37 successfully treated patients survived, and no relapses were observed.

Safety

All 44 patients were included in the safety assessment. Possible high-dose fluconazole related AEs were found in 54.5% (24/44) of them. No grade 3 or 4 AEs were observed. As shown in Table 3, the most frequent AE was elevated transaminase level in 11 patients. Transient grade 2 neutropenia and grade 1 thrombocytopenia occurred in 1 patient treated with fluconazole monotherapy. One patient presented with grade 2 anemia in the first week of salvage therapy, but his hemoglobin level recovered without discontinuance of fluconazole or flucytosine. Hypokalemia occurred in 3 patients, all of whom returned to normal condition after potassium supplementation (AmB were not co-administrated). There were no increased creatinine levels related to high dose fluconazole in our cases.

In terms of clinical manifestations, gastrointestinal side effects were common complaints. Skin lesions were documented in 2 patients. Photosensitive dermatitis occurred in 1 patient soon after initiation of fluconazole, and improved without fluconazole discontinuance. Rash developed in another patient several weeks after the salvage therapy and lasted until CM recovered and antifungal treatment finished. We also observed 1 patient with elevated D-dimer and deep venous thrombosis which was relieved after treatment with oral warfarin. None of these patients discontinued high dose fluconazole due to intolerance.

Table 3 High dose fluconazole related adverse events in 44 cryptococcal meningitis patients

Adverse events[a]	No. (%) of patients ($N = 44$)
Liver dysfunction	
GGT	10 (22.7)
ALT	5 (11.4)
AST	4 (9.1)
ALP	1 (2.3)
Hematocytopenia	
Anemia	1 (2.3)
Neutropenia	1 (2.3)
Thrombocytopenia	1 (2.3)
Hypokalemia	3 (6.8)
Nausea and vomitting	5 (11.4)
Constipation	3 (6.8)
Dry mouth	2 (4.5)
Dry eyes	1 (2.3)
Skin lesion	2 (4.5)
Numbness of upper limb	1 (2.3)
Thrombosis of lower limb	1 (2.3)

GGT gama-glutamyltransferase; *ALT* alanine aminotransferase; *AST* aspartate aminotransferase; *ALP* alkaline phosphatase
[a]All laboratory abnormalities were grade 1 or grade 2 only

Mortality and prognostic factors

From the beginning of salvage therapy, 1-year mortality related to all cause was 13.6% (6 of 44 patients) with no significant difference among 3 treatment groups (Fig. 2, $P = 0.258$). We assessed factors with a potential impact on all-cause mortality by means of univariate and multivariate analyses. In the univariate model, factors significantly associated with 1-year mortality were age ≥ 60 years ($P = 0.001$); serum albumin level < 35 g/L ($P = 0.001$); estimated glomerular filtration rate (eGFR) < 60 mL/min/1.73m^2 ($P = 0.015$); and CSF WBC count < 10 /mm^3 ($P = 0.002$). CSF CrAg titer ≥1280 was more frequently presented in mortality group but it did not reach a statistic significance ($P = 0.058$). By multivariate analysis, as shown in Table 4, factors significantly correlated with decreased survival in the overall population were serum albumin level < 35 g/L ($P = 0.014$) and CSF CrAg titer ≥1280 ($P = 0.048$).

Discussion

In 1996, Pappas et al. reported 12 HIV-uninfected CM patients who received high dose fluconazole, 800 mg/day, in

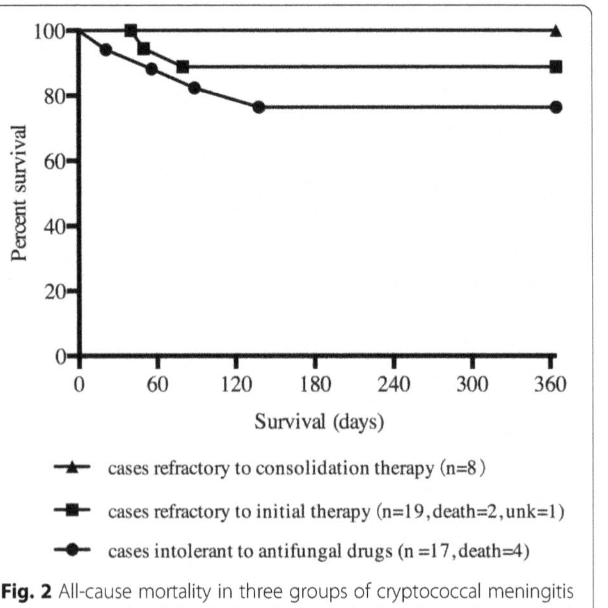

Fig. 2 All-cause mortality in three groups of cryptococcal meningitis patients treated with high dose fluconazole for salvage therapy. *Unk* status unknown

Table 4 Univariate and multivariate analysis of factors associated with 1-year mortality among 44 cryptococcal meningitis patients

Factor	Univariate Analysis			Multivariate Analysis	
	Total No. of patients	No. (%) of patients who died	*P*-value[b]	*P*-value	RR (95% CI)
Age ≥ 60 years	12	4 (33.3)	0.022		
Initial AmB course < 6 weeks	10	3 (30.0)	0.095		
Salvage therapy without 5FC	13	3 (23.1)	0.196		
Serum albumin level < 35 g/L	13	5 (38.5)	0.001	0.014	16.23 (1.78–148.19)
eGFR < 60 mL/min/1.73m^2	8	3 (37.5)	0.015		
CSF WBC count < 10 /mm^3[a]	14	4 (28.6)	0.012		
CSF glucose level < 36 mg/dL[a]	22	1 (4.5)	0.127		
CSF CrAg titer ≥ 1280[a]	17	4 (23.5)	0.058	0.048	9.30 (1.02–84.73)

AmB Amphotericin B; *5FC* flucytosine; *eGFR* estimated glomerular filtration rate; *CrAg* cryptococcal capsular antigen; *CSF* cerebrospinal fluid; *WBC* white blood cell
[a]Data of CSF WBC count, CSF glucose level and CSF cryptococcal antigen titter was unavailable in 1 dead patient
[b]Factor entered the initial univariate analysis included male, age ≥ 60 years, time before diagnosis ≥60 days, predisposing factors, pulmonary involvement, seizure, altered mental status, parenchyma lesions of brain MRI, initial AmB course < 6 weeks, salvage therapy without 5FC, serum albumin level < 35 g/L, eGFR < 60 mL/min/1.73m^2, CSF WBC count < 10 /mm^3, CSF protein level > 500 mg/dL, CSF glucose level < 36 mg/dL, CSF CrAg titer ≥1280. Only predictors with a *P*-value less than 0.2 were listed in the table

their induction therapy or as consolidation therapy [24]. However, since then, no published study has specifically addressed the use of high dose fluconazole in the management of HIV-uninfected cryptococcal infections. The results of our study showed that high dose fluconazole (800 mg/day) either alone or in combination with other antifungal drugs had favorable effects and was well tolerated among HIV-uninfected CM patients.

AmB-based regimens are recommended to optimize fungal clearance and survival for both HIV-infected and HIV-uninfected CM patients [19]. Despite given appropriate treatment, 25–35% patients experience refractory cryptococcal infections or drug intolerance [5, 6, 18, 25, 26]. In previous trials with AmB lipid complex, posaconazole and voriconazole used as salvage therapies, the overall efficacy rates were not impressive, with success rates no more than 50% [22, 27, 28]. Recombinant IFN-γ treatment as salvage therapy was tested only in case reports, and this form of adjunct could be detrimental in non-HIV infections, depending on host immune responses [29–31]. In our study, after salvage therapy with fluconazole 800 mg/day for a median of 137 days, 72% achieved effective response in 2 weeks, and 84% achieved effective response at the end of salvage therapy. Consistent with our findings, the good efficacy of high dose fluconazole as salvage therapy was also reported in HIV-infected CM patients, with 6 out of 8 patients (75%) achieving microbiological improvement after a mean course of 4.5 months, showed as either sterile CSF culture or decreased CSF CrAg titers [32]. Compared with patients treated with high dose fluconazole with or without flucytosine, there was significantly improved efficacy at 2 weeks in patients treated with AmB and high dose fluconazole with or without flucytosine. However, no apparent differences were showed in the long term outcomes between the two groups at the end of salvage therapy and the end of antifungal therapy.

In our study, no significant difference in 1-year mortality rates was found among patients with refractory infections and those intolerant of prior antifungal drugs. Factors linked with poor prognosis in our patients were older age, renal dysfunction, lower CSF white cell count, and high CSF CrAg titers, as consistent with previous reports in HIV-uninfected population [5, 6, 25, 33]. Though previous reports found altered mental status to be an additional factor, it was more common in patients died of active disease and not significant in our present study. Compared with an overall mortality rate of 25–40% reported in the previous studies of HIV-uninfected CM population [5–7], a relatively lower mortality rate of 13.6% after 1 year of salvage therapy was observed in our study.

In previous studies of treatment for cryptococcal or other fungal infections, fluconazole was well tolerated at dosages from 800 to 2000 mg/day [9–13, 34–37]. Consistent with previous studies, nausea and vomiting were common in patients treated with fluconazole, especially early in the course of treatment. Liver enzyme abnormalities were usually asymptomatic and self-limiting. In our study, 10 of the 17 antifungal-intolerant patients had AmB-related renal insufficiency and switched to salvage regimens. Of note, further deterioration of renal function related to high dose fluconazole was not observed, suggesting that high dose fluconazole with or without flucytosine were well tolerated for patients with AmB induced renal impairment.

There were some limitations to this work. As we included a limited number of cases in the present study and did not include a group of patients who received low dose fluconazole as a control, the results should be interpreted with caution. Only a few patients were culture positive when changed to salvage therapy. For these patients, the reasons for "failure" may be due to the poor efficacy of previous therapy, dysfunctional immune responses, or associated underlying conditions, and some may have done well if the previous antifungal therapy had been continued. Hence, multicenter randomized controlled trials are needed for making a further objective evaluation.

Conclusions

Evidence for the use of high dose fluconazole in HIV-uninfected CM patients remains sparse. Our study specifically addressed the efficacy and safety of high dose fluconazole in this population and suggested that fluconazole 800 mg/day alone, or in combination with other antifungal drugs was a safe and promising choice for HIV-uninfected CM patients. Either refractory cases or those intolerant to prior antifungal drugs can achieve favorable outcomes after receiving high dose fluconazole as salvage therapy.

Abbreviations

AEs: Adverse events; AmB: Amphotericin B; CM: Cryptococcal meningitis; CNS: Central nervous system; CrAg: Cryptococcal antigen; CSF: Cerebrospinal fluid; CT: Computerized tomography; HIV: Human immunodeficiency virus; IDSA: Infectious Diseases Society of America; MOF: Multiple organ failure; MRI: Cranial magnetic resonance imaging; WBC: White blood cell

Acknowledgements

The authors thank all the patients and healthcare workers for their contribution and participation in this study.

Funding

Not applicable.

Authors' contributions

LPZ and TSH designed this study. YKJ, LHZ, JHC and LPH collected the data from medical records. HZZ, RYW and XW analyzed and interpreted the data. HZZ and RYW were equal contributors in writing the manuscript. All authors read and approved the final manuscript.

Consent for publication

Not applicable.

Competing interests

TSH reports an investigator award and honoraria from Gilead Sciences, advisory board fees from Viamet, gift of tests for research from Immuno-Mycologics, and honoraria from Pfizer. All authors declare no competing interests.

References

1. Cogliati M. Global molecular epidemiology of *Cryptococcus neoformans* and *Cryptococcus gattii*: an atlas of the molecular types. Scientifica (Cairo). 2013; 2013:675213.
2. Rajasingham R, Smith RM, Park BJ, et al. Global burden of disease of HIV-associated cryptococcal meningitis: an updated analysis. Lancet Infect Dis. 2017;17:873–81.
3. Pyrgos V, Seitz AE, Steiner CA, Prevots DR, Williamson PR. Epidemiology of cryptococcal meningitis in the US: 1997-2009. PLoS One. 2013;8:e56269.
4. Pappas PG. Cryptococcal infections in non-HIV-infected patients. Trans Am Clin Climatol Assoc. 2013;124:61–79.
5. Pappas PG, Perfect JR, Cloud GA, et al. Cryptococcosis in human immunodeficiency virus-negative patients in the era of effective azole therapy. Clin Infect Dis. 2001;33:690–9.
6. Zhu LP, Wu JQ, Xu B, Ou XT, Zhang QQ, Weng XH. Cryptococcal meningitis in non-HIV-infected patients in a Chinese tertiary care hospital, 1997-2007. Med Mycol. 2010;48:570–9.
7. Nguyen MH, Husain S, Clancy CJ, et al. Outcomes of central nervous system cryptococcosis vary with host immune function: results from a multi-center, prospective study. J Inf Secur. 2010;61:419–26.
8. Liao CH, Chi CY, Wang YJ, et al. Different presentations and outcomes between HIV-infected and HIV-uninfected patients with Cryptococcal meningitis. J Microbiol Immunol Infect. 2012;45:296–304.
9. Longley N, Muzoora C, Taseera K, et al. Dose response effect of high-dose fluconazole for HIV-associated cryptococcal meningitis in southwestern Uganda. Clin Infect Dis. 2008;47:1556–61.
10. Nussbaum JC, Jackson A, Namarika D, et al. Combination flucytosine and high-dose fluconazole compared with fluconazole monotherapy for the treatment of cryptococcal meningitis: a randomized trial in Malawi. Clin Infect Dis. 2010;50:338–44.
11. Rothe C, Sloan DJ, Goodson P, et al. A prospective longitudinal study of the clinical outcomes from cryptococcal meningitis following treatment induction with 800 mg oral fluconazole in Blantyre, Malawi. PLoS One. 2013;8:e67311.
12. Gaskell KM, Rothe C, Gnanadurai R, et al. A prospective study of mortality from cryptococcal meningitis following treatment induction with 1200 mg oral fluconazole in Blantyre, Malawi. PLoS One. 2014;9:e110285.
13. Milefchik E, Leal MA, Haubrich R, Bozzette SA, Tilles JG, Leedom JM, et al. Fluconazole alone or combined with flucytosine for the treatment of AIDS-associated cryptococcal meningitis. Med Mycol. 2008;46:393–5.
14. Loyse A, Wilson D, Meintjes G, et al. Comparison of the early fungicidal activity of high-dose fluconazole, voriconazole, and flucytosine as second-line drugs given in combination with amphotericin B for the treatment of HIV-associated cryptococcal meningitis. Clin Infect Dis. 2012;54:121–8.
15. Pappas PG, Chetchotisakd P, Larsen RA, et al. A phase II randomized trial of amphotericin B alone or combined with fluconazole in the treatment of HIV-associated cryptococcal meningitis. Clin Infect Dis. 2009;48:1775–83.
16. Rolfes MA, Rhein J, Schutz C, et al. Cerebrospinal fluid culture positivity and clinical outcomes after amphotericin-based induction therapy for cryptococcal meningitis. Open Forum Infect Dis. 2015;2:ofv157.
17. Mootsikapun P, Chetchotisakd P, Anunnatsiri S, Choksawadphinyo K. The efficacy of fluconazole 600 mg/day versus itraconazole 600 mg/day as consolidation therapy of cryptococcal meningitis in AIDS patients. J Med Assoc Thail. 2003;86:293–8.
18. Day JN, Chau TT, Wolbers M, et al. Combination antifungal therapy for cryptococcal meningitis. N Engl J Med. 2013;368:1291–302.
19. Perfect JR, Dismukes WE, Dromer F, et al. Clinical practice guidelines for the management of cryptococcal disease: 2010 update by the infectious diseases society of america. Clin Infect Dis. 2010;50:291–322.
20. Saag MS, Graybill RJ, Larsen RA, et al. Practice guidelines for the management of cryptococcal disease. Infectious Diseases Society of America Clin Infect Dis. 2000;30:710–8.
21. Segal BH, Herbrecht R, Stevens DA, et al. Defining responses to therapy and study outcomes in clinical trials of invasive fungal diseases: mycoses study group and European Organization for Research and Treatment of Cancer consensus criteria. Clin Infect Dis. 2008;47:674–83.
22. Pitisuttithum P, Negroni R, Graybill JR, et al. Activity of posaconazole in the treatment of central nervous system fungal infections. J Antimicrob Chemother. 2005;56:745–55.
23. Rehan HS, Chopra D, Kakkar AK. Physician's guide to pharmacovigilance: terminology and causality assessment. Eur J Intern Med. 2009;20:3–8.
24. Pappas P, Hamill R, Kauffman C, Bradsher R, McKinsey D, We GC. Treatment of cryptococcal meningitis in non-HIV infected patients – a randomized comparative trial. Clin Infect Dis. 1996;23:873.
25. Dismukes WE, Cloud G, Gallis HA, et al. Treatment of cryptococcal meningitis with combination amphotericin B and flucytosine for four as compared with six weeks. N Engl J Med. 1987;317:334–41.
26. Bennett JE, Dismukes WE, Duma RJ, et al. A comparison of amphotericin B alone and combined with flucytosine in the treatment of cryptoccal meningitis. N Engl J Med. 1979;301:126–31.

27. Walsh TJ, Hiemenz JW, Seibel NL, et al. Amphotericin B lipid complex for invasive fungal infections: analysis of safety and efficacy in 556 cases. Clin Infect Dis. 1998;26:1383–96.
28. Perfect JR, Marr KA, Walsh TJ, et al. Voriconazole treatment for less-common, emerging, or refractory fungal infections. Clin Infect Dis. 2003;36:1122–31.
29. Netea MG, Brouwer AE, Hoogendoorn EH, et al. Two patients with cryptococcal meningitis and idiopathic CD4 lymphopenia: defective cytokine production and reversal by recombinant interferon-gamma therapy. Clin Infect Dis. 2004;39:e83–7.
30. Nierenberg NE, Thompson GR, Lewis JS, Hogan BK, Patterson TF. Voriconazole use and pharmacokinetics in combination with interferon-gamma for refractory cryptococcal meningitis in a patient receiving low-dose ritonavir. Med Mycol. 2010;48:532–6.
31. Gamaletsou MN, Sipsas NV, Kontoyiannis DP, et al. Successful salvage therapy of refractory HIV-related cryptococcal meningitis with the combination of liposomal amphotericin B, voriconazole, and recombinant interferon-gamma. Diagn Microbiol Infect Dis. 2012;74:409–11.
32. Berry AJ, Rinaldi MG, Graybill JR. Use of high-dose fluconazole as salvage therapy for cryptococcal meningitis in patients with AIDS. Antimicrob Agents Chemother. 1992;36:690–2.
33. Diamond RD, Bennett JE. Prognostic factors in cryptococcal meningitis. A study in 111 cases. Ann Intern Med. 1974;80:176–81.
34. Haubrich RH, Haghighat D, Bozzette SA, Tilles J, McCutchan JA. High-dose fluconazole for treatment of cryptococcal disease in patients with human immunodeficiency virus infection. The California Collaborative Treatment Group. J Infect Dis. 1994;170:238–42.
35. Anaissie EJ, Kontoyiannis DP, Huls C, et al. Safety, plasma concentrations, and efficacy of high-dose fluconazole in invasive mold infections. J Infect Dis. 1995;172:599–602.
36. Stevens DA, Diaz M, Negroni R, et al. Safety evaluation of chronic fluconazole therapy. Fluconazole pan-American study group. Chemotherapy. 1997;43:371–7.
37. Menichetti F, Fiorio M, Tosti A, et al. High-dose fluconazole therapy for cryptococcal meningitis in patients with AIDS. Clin Infect Dis. 1996;22:838–40.

18

Total delay in treatment among tuberculous meningitis patients in China

Yu He[1,5*], Chao Han[2], Kai-Feng Chang[3], Mao-Shui Wang[4] and Tian-Ren Huang[5*]

Abstract

Background: Currently, there is limited data on the risk factors associated with treatment delay in tuberculous meningitis (TBM). This study aimed to assess the duration of delay in the treatment TBM and to investigate its determinants.

Methods: During the period from September 2009 to February 2016, a retrospective cohort study of consecutive TBM patients admitted to our hospital was conducted to determine the risk factors associated with treatment delay in TBM. Treatment delay duration was defined as the time interval from onset of symptoms (by patient recall) to initiation of treatment and was stratified into two categories: ≤ 20 days, >20 days (median delay day is 20 days). Data collected included demography, comorbidity, cerebrospinal fluid (CSF) examinations and others. Univariable and multivariable logistic regression analysis was used to evaluate the determinants of treatment delay.

Results: A total of 161 TBM patients were included in our study, all were confirmed by CSF mycobacterial culture. The median treatment delay for all patients included in the study was 20 days [interquartile range, 14–60 days]. Multivariate analysis revealed that age (≤21 years old, OR = 0.202, 95% CI: 0.079, 0.521), fever (OR = 0.414, 95% CI: 0. 180, 0.952), and headache (OR = 0.204, 95% CI: 0.095, 0.442) had significantly lower risk for treatment delay, while multiple healthcare contact (>3 times) (OR = 3.938, 95% CI: 1.326, 11.691) as well as CSF chloride (>111 mmol/L) (OR = 2.479, 95% CI: 1.143, 5.377) had significantly higher risk of the delay.

Conclusions: Our findings indicate that multiple healthcare contact and high CSF chloride predict the risk of long delay, while young age, fever and headache are associated with short delay. Maintained focus on awareness of TBM in the population and in healthcare systems, and continuous implementation of diagnostic methods for TBM to detect the disease early, may reduce the mortality and morbidity.

Keywords: Tuberculous meningitis, Factor, Treatment delay

Background

Tuberculosis (TB) remains a severe global public health threat. In 2014, 9.6 million people are estimated to have fallen ill with TB, and 1.5 million people died from TB [1]. TB usually affects the lungs, but it also can affect any other organ of the body, e.g. lymph nodes, pleura, or meninges. Tuberculous meningitis (TBM) occurs in approximately 1% of all patients with active TB, but is disproportionately important because it kills or severely disables about half of the people affected [2].

TBM is the most severe form of TB and a medical emergency. A number of factors have been reported to be associated with poor outcome. Some of these factors are diagnosis delay; severity of TBM at the time of admission; the presence of headache, fever and hydrocephalus; high cerebrospinal fluid (CSF) protein and lactate concentration [3, 4]. Rapid diagnosis and early treatment before the occurrence of progression of stage are crucial for the outcome of TBM. A study conducted in Taiwan, showed that 47.6% of patients experienced delay in initiating appropriate treatment [3]. Until now,

* Correspondence: heyu31@163.com; tianrenhuang@sina.com
[1]Department of Clinical Laboratory, First Affiliated Hospital of Guangxi Medical University, Nanning, China
[5]Department of Epidemiology, Affiliated Tumor Hospital of Guangxi Medical University, 71#, Hedi Road, Nanning 530021, China
Full list of author information is available at the end of the article

several studies have proved that treatment delay is strongly associated with poor outcomes in adults or children [2, 5–9].

Factors affecting treatment delay are of key importance in TB management as delay may increase mortality [10]. Understanding the factors related to delay in treatment of disease is essential to reduce morbidity and mortality of TBM, and decreases the risk of mortality. However, there is limited data on the risk factors associated with treatment delay. This study aimed to assess the duration of delay in the treatment of TBM and to investigate its determinants. The findings of our study may be useful for management of TBM in the field of improving diagnosis, increasing physician awareness, control planning and policies in China.

Methods

Study design and population

This study was approved by the Human Research Ethics Committees of Shandong Provincial Chest Hospital (SPCH) and First Affiliated Hospital of Guangxi Medical University. This retrospective study was carried out in Jinan city, China during the period from September 2009 to February 2016.

We conducted a retrospective cohort study of consecutive TBM patients admitted to SPCH to determine the risk factors associated with treatment delay. TBM was defined as positive CSF mycobacterial culture. Delay was measured in days. Treatment delay duration was defined as the time interval from onset of symptoms (by patient recall) to initiation of treatment and was stratified into two categories: ≤ 20 days (short delay), >20 days (long delay).

Data collection

Data were collected by a questionnaire filled out by accessing medical records. Data collected included (1) demography (gender, age, symptoms (fever, headache, cough, vomiting, coma), previous anti-tuberculosis therapy, smoking habit, contact history of TB, hydrocephalus, and time during hospitaliziation); (2) comorbidity (pulmonary TB, extrapulmonary TB, diabetes mellitus, rheumatic diseases, miliary TB, recurrent TB); (3) CSF examinations (white blood cell (WBC), mononuclear cells, polynuclear cells, glucose, lactate, tryptophan, aspartate transaminase, lactate dehydrogenase, total protein, α-hydrooxybutyrate dehyrogenase, chloride, adenosine deaminase); (4) others (serum glucose).

Data analysis

Patient characteristics were summarised using means and standard deviations for continuous variables and counts/percentages for categorical variables. Univariate analysis was carried out using the $\chi 2$ test or Fisher exact test for categorical data and the Mann-Whitney *U* test for continuous variables. Beyond descriptive statistics, associations between the dependent variables (treatment delay) and the independent variables were analyzed by calculating the Odds Ratios (OR) and 95% confidence interval (CI). Multivariate logistic regression analysis was used to evaluate risk factors for the delay, using selection of factors associated with delay in univariate analysis ($P < 0.1$) or those known to have clinical significance. The Hosmer-Lemeshow goodness-of-fit test was performed to assess the overall fit of the model. A two-sided *P*-value <0.05 was considered significant for all analyses. Data analysis was carried out using SPSS 18.0 (IBM Corp., Armonk, United States).

Results

Baseline patient characteristics

Table 1 shows the characteristics of the participants of this study. A total of 161 TBM patients were included in our study, all were confirmed by CSF mycobacterial culture. Males comprised 54.7% of the participants. Smokers constituted 16.8% of participants. Nineteen patients had anti-TB therapy before admission to our hospital, and 18 patients had contact of TB history. Among them, 109 (67.7%) participants had pulmonary tuberculosis, 48 (29.8%) had extrapulmonary tuberculosis (excluding TBM), 8 had rheumatic diseases, 11 had diabetes mellitus, 51 had millary TB, 12 had recurrent TB. Fever was the most frequently reported symptom (72.0%) followed by headache (55.9%), vomiting (19.3%), cough (18.6%) and hydrocephalus (11.2%). Twenty five patients (15.5%) were diagnosed after one health care contact, 63 (39.1%) after two visits, 48 (29.8%) after three visits, 17 (10.6%) after four visits, and 8 (5.0%) after five or more visits. Results of CSF examinations are also summarized in Table 1.

Treatment delay

The median treatment delay for all patients included in the study was 20 days (interquartile range, 14–60 days). For 77 (47.8%) patients, the treatment delay was >20 days. Table 1 shows the univariate analysis on risk factors, comparing patients with total delay of >20 days with patients with total delay of ≤20 days. The delay was associated with age, previous anti-TB therapy, multiple healthcare contact, symptoms (fever, headache, vomiting and cough), and CSF examinations (mononuclear and polynuclear cell concentration, and chloride) (all $P < 0.05$) (Table 1).

Further multivariate analysis revealed that age (≤21 years old, OR = 0.202, 95% CI: 0.079, 0.521), fever (OR = 0.414, 95% CI: 0.180, 0.952), and headache (OR = 0.204, 95% CI: 0.095, 0.442) had significantly lower risk for treatment delay, while multiple healthcare contact (>3 times) (OR = 3.938, 95% CI: 1.326, 11.691) as well as CSF chloride

Table 1 Univariate analysis of risk factors associated with treatment delay in TBM patients

	Short delay	Long delay	Total	*P* value
N	84	77	161	
Age (years)	28.3 ± 16.9	34.1 ± 17.2	31.1 ± 17.2	0.037
Sex (male)	48	40	88	0.509
Time during hospitalization (days)	56.6 ± 44.6	64.6 ± 47.1	60.4 ± 45.9	0.273
Fees ($)	78,721 ± 71,922	98,186 ± 108,770	88,030 ± 91,645	0.192
Previous anti-TB therapy	5	14	19	0.022
Smoking habit (pack-years)	2.82 ± 9.10	3.36 ± 11.9	3.08 ± 10.50	0.746
Contact history of TB	10	8	18	0.761
No. of Healthcare visits	2.3 ± 0.9	2.8 ± 1.3	2.5 ± 1.1	0.010
Comorbidity				
Pulmonary TB	54	55	109	0.334
Extrapulmonary TB	23	25	48	0.481
Rheumatic diseases	3	5	8	0.401
Diabetes mellinus	3	8	11	0.434
Milliary TB	22	29	51	0.120
Recurrent TB	3	9	12	0.064
Symptoms				
Fever	68	48	116	0.010
Headache	63	27	90	0.000
Vomitting	23	8	31	0.008
Cough	10	20	30	0.025
Hydrocephalus	13	5	18	0.147
Abnormalty in brain CT	37	27	64	0.941
CSF examination				
WBC (10^9/L)	207 ± 210	187 ± 183	198 ± 198	0.524
Mononuclear cells (%)	64 ± 28	54 ± 28	59 ± 29	0.041
Polynuclear cells (%)	36 ± 29	46 ± 28	41 ± 28	0.037
Glucose (mmol/L)	1.96 ± 1.21	2.26 ± 1.81	2.11 ± 1.53	0.223
Tryptophan (+)	59	49	108	0.708
Lactate (mmol/L)	6.75 ± 2.37	6.40 ± 2.43	6.58 ± 2.39	0.410
AST (U/L)	18.7 ± 16.5	17.8 ± 10.5	18.3 ± 13.9	0.671
LDH (U/L)	136 ± 209	120 ± 138	129 ± 178	0.569
CSF-PR (mg/L)	1323 ± 649	1456 ± 758	1387 ± 704	0.230
α-HBDH (U/L)	131 ± 402	70 ± 73	102 ± 296	0.257
Chloride (mmol/L)	108 ± 8	111 ± 8	109 ± 8	0.038
ADA (U/L)	8.1 ± 8.1	8.5 ± 6.4	8.3 ± 7.3	0.738
CSF/Serum glucose	0.32 ± 0.18	0.32 ± 0.18	0.32 ± 0.18	0.932
Serum glucose (mmol/L)	6.30 ± 1.54	7.07 ± 3.27	6.66 ± 2.53	0.084

(>111 mmol/L) (OR = 2.479, 95% CI: 1.143, 5.377) had significantly higher risk of the delay (Table 2).

Discussion

Although TBM is a medical emergency, our study shows that a significant delay in treatment among TBM patients. Here, we found a median treatment delay time of 20 days in TBM patients. Early detection of cases and treating TBM patients are one of the strategies to reduce the disease's morbidity and mortality throughout the world. The treatment delay in TBM can be divided into the length of patient delay and the diagnosis delay [11]. Identifying the

Table 2 Multivariate analysis of risk factors associated with treatment delay in TBM patients

	P value	OR	95% CI
Age (≤21 years old)	0.001	0.202	0.079, 0.521
Fever	0.038	0.414	0.180, 0.952
Headache	0.000	0.204	0.095, 0.442
No. of Healthcare visits (>3 times)	0.014	3.938	1.326, 11.691
Chloride (>111 mmol/L)	0.022	2.479	1.143, 5.377

sources of delay is a critical issue for TBM therapy. In our study, the main factors associated with treatment delay in multivariate analysis were age (≤21 years old, OR = 0.202), fever (OR = 0.414), headache (OR = 0.204), multiple healthcare contact (OR = 3.938), and CSF chloride (>111 mmol/L, OR = 2.479). These may be likely explained by three main factors: perceived severity of illness and symptom recognition, lack of specific and rapid diagnostic methods in TBM and quality of health service provision.

Firstly, in the study, we found a clear association between treatment delay and clinical symptoms at inclusion, which has not been described before. Our results showed that symptoms, including fever and headache, were protective factors for shortening treatment delay. The two, headache and fever, can be a sign of infection that is localized to central nervous system, which consists of brain and spinal cord, such as meningitis, encephalitis, and a brain abscess. The combination may raise awareness of TBM among them. Younger age was also a protective factor for shortening the delay. This may be explained by the two reasons: 1) student is free of economic pressures, he can spend more time seeking health care; 2) in China, the One-child Policy forced parents to cherish their only child, and it saves much time in seeking health care for their children.

Secondly, diagnosing TBM remains a challenge. The early diagnosis of TBM is fundamental to avoiding treatment delay. However, it is always difficult to confirm the clinical suspicion of TBM. TBM presents in a non-specific manner and it is rare to confirm the diagnosis microbiologically even in high resource settings. Currently, there is no single test with optimal sensitivity in patients with suspected TBM. Routine assays, i.e., acid-fast bacillus staining and mycobacterial culture, are insensitive and slow. It was reported that only 10 to 20% of TBM patients were detected by CSF AFB staining [12], while other tests like Xpert MTB/RIF have several limitations including high cost, requirement for a stable electricity supply and short shelf life of consumables [13]. CSF adenosine deaminase has been evaluated and may be used as a supportive test in diagnosis, but is not recommended as a routine diagnostic test for TBM [2, 14, 15].

In our study, CSF chloride (>111 mmol/L) had significantly higher risk of the delay. This may be associated with the two reasons: 1) In practice, once the diagnosis of bacterial meningitis has been excluded, uncommonly low CSF chloride values (<110 mmol/L) may be associated with TBM but not with viral meningitis [16]. Therefore, TBM may be rapid and timely diagnosed relying on the rule by practitioners; 2) decreased CSF chloride was associated with increased intracranial pressure. This may be helpful to shorten the time between symptom onset and first visit to any health care provider.

Thirdly, the mean number of visits to health care facilities before the diagnosis was 2.5. This finding could be related to diagnostic challenge in TBM and lack of awareness of TB among health care workers. Under these circumstances, it is easy to neglect many important issues in TBM diagnosis and management, resulting from a lack of experience and expertise which had previously been found to be associated with diagnosis delays [17].

Moreover, in China, poverty has been reported as central factor causing delay in health care seeking [18–20]. Among the TB patients identified in the 4th National TB Survey, 37% ascribed their delays in clinical consultation to financial problems [21]. A majority of health providers believe there would be improved TB treatment compliance and overall control of TB infections if there was a decreased financial burden for patients and families [11]. Besides extent of the free TB diagnosis and treatment, educational attainment and knowledge of TB possibly enhances detection of TBM and shorten diagnosis delays [11].

This study has potential limitations. First, there is no agreed definition of what constitutes an "acceptable" delay. It probably depends on the local health services and the local epidemiological situation, with a shorter delay to be expected when incidence is high [22]. In our study, we used a cut-off interval of 20 days for subsequent analysis which was similar to that found by other authors in TB [7, 23–25]. Second, considering that it was difficult to access to the results of previous CSF examinations and remarkable difference existed in the principles of CSF assays between hospitals, these results of CSF examinations performed at our hospital were used, which may have overestimated the clinical severity. Third, TB is a chronic disease with an insidious start, making it difficult for patients to remember exactly when the symptoms started. Thus, recall bias may occur. Fourth, the results of our study need to be carefully interpreted because this data was based on a single hospital experience, which was not enough to represent the characteristics of TBM in the entire Chinese population. In addition, although several risk factors were discovered, additional studies are required to validate our findings.

Conclusions

Our findings represent a population-based analysis over a long time period and are based on a large dataset. The results clearly show that total delay in treatment of TBM is still high in the study area. Our findings indicate that multiple healthcare contact and high CSF chloride predict the risk of long delay, while younger age, fever and headache are associated with short delay. Maintained focus on awareness of TBM in the population and in healthcare systems and continuous implementation of diagnostic methods for TBM to detect the disease early, may reduce the mortality and morbidity.

Abbreviations

CI: Confidence interval; CSF: Cerebrospinal fluid; OR: Odds ratios; TB: Tuberculosis; TBM: Tuberculous meningitis; WBC: White blood cell

Acknowledgments

We thank the medical doctors and nurses of the Shandong Provincial Chest Hospital for their assistance in participant inclusion and data collection, especially the members of our department.

Funding

Not applicable.

Authors' contributions

HTR and HY conceived and designed the study. WMS supervised data collection. HC and CKF collected data. HY have been involved in the analysis and interpretation of data. HY and WMS wrote the manuscript. All authors read and approved the final manuscript.

Competing interests

The authors declare that they have no competing interest.

Consent for publication

Not applicable.

Author details

[1]Department of Clinical Laboratory, First Affiliated Hospital of Guangxi Medical University, Nanning, China. [2]Department of Geriatrics, Shandong Mental Health Center, Jinan, China. [3]Department of Infection Prevention, Pingyi Center for Disease Control and Prevention, Pingyi, China. [4]Department of Lab Medicine, Shandong Provincial Chest Hospital, Jinan, China. [5]Department of Epidemiology, Affiliated Tumor Hospital of Guangxi Medical University, 71#, Hedi Road, Nanning 530021, China.

References

1. World Health Organization Global tuberculosis report. http://www.who.int/tb/publications/global_report/en/. Accessed: 3 Oct 2015.
2. Thwaites G, Fisher M, Hemingway C, Scott G, Solomon T, Innes J. British Infection Society guidelines for the diagnosis and treatment of tuberculosis of the central nervous system in adults and children. J Inf Secur. 2009;59(3):167–87.
3. Sheu JJ, Yuan RY, Yang CC. Predictors for outcome and treatment delay in patients with tuberculous meningitis. Am J Med Sci. 2009;338(2):134–9.
4. Lu CH, Chang WN, Chang HW. The prognostic factors of adult tuberculous meningitis. Infection. 2001;29(6):299–304.
5. Karstaedt AS, Valtchanova S, Barriere R, Crewe-Brown HH. Tuberculous meningitis in south African urban adults. QJM. 1998;91(11):743–7.
6. Hosoglu S, Ayaz C, Geyik MF, Kokoglu OF, Ceviz A. Tuberculous meningitis in adults: an eleven-year review. Int J Tuberc Lung Dis. 1998;2(7):553–7.
7. Bang ND, Caws M, Truc TT, Duong TN, Dung NH, Ha DT, Thwaites GE, Heemskerk D, Tarning J, Merson L, et al. Clinical presentations, diagnosis, mortality and prognostic markers of tuberculous meningitis in Vietnamese children: a prospective descriptive study. BMC Infect Dis. 2016;16(1):573.
8. Gunes A, Uluca U, Aktar F, Konca C, Sen V, Ece A, Hosoglu S, Tas MA, Gurkan F. Clinical, radiological and laboratory findings in 185 children with tuberculous meningitis at a single centre and relationship with the stage of the disease. Ital J Pediatr. 2015;41:75.
9. Verdon R, Chevret S, Laissy JP, Wolff M. Tuberculous meningitis in adults: review of 48 cases. Clin Infect Dis. 1996;22(6):982–8.
10. Lienhardt C, Rowley J, Manneh K, Lahai G, Needham D, Milligan P, McAdam KP. Factors affecting time delay to treatment in a tuberculosis control programme in a sub-Saharan African country: the experience of the Gambia. Int J Tuberc Lung Dis. 2001;5(3):233–9.
11. Long Q, Li Y, Wang Y, Yue Y, Tang C, Tang S, Squire SB, Tolhurst R. Barriers to accessing TB diagnosis for rural-to-urban migrants with chronic cough in Chongqing, China: a mixed methods study. BMC Health Serv Res. 2008;8:202.
12. Shao Y, Xia P, Zhu T, Zhou J, Yuan Y, Zhang H, Chen J, Hu X. Sensitivity and specificity of immunocytochemical staining of mycobacterial antigens in the cytoplasm of cerebrospinal fluid macrophages for diagnosing tuberculous meningitis. J Clin Microbiol. 2011;49(9):3388–91.
13. Trebucq A, Enarson DA, Chiang CY, Van Deun A, Harries AD, Boillot F, Detjen A, Fujiwara PI, Graham SM, Monedero I, et al. Xpert(R) MTB/RIF for national tuberculosis programmes in low-income countries: when, where and how? Int J Tuberc Lung Dis. 2011;15(12):1567–72.
14. Tuon FF, Higashino HR, Lopes MI, Litvoc MN, Atomiya AN, Antonangelo L, Leite OM. Adenosine deaminase and tuberculous meningitis–a systematic review with meta-analysis. Scand J Infect Dis. 2010;42(3):198–207.
15. Xu HB, Jiang RH, Li L, Sha W, Xiao HP. Diagnostic value of adenosine deaminase in cerebrospinal fluid for tuberculous meningitis: a meta-analysis. Int J Tuberc Lung Dis. 2010;14(11):1382–7.
16. Ramkissoon A, Coovadia HM. Chloride levels in meningitis. S Afr Med J. 1988;73(9):522–3.
17. Chen TC, Lu PL, Lin WR, Lin CY, Lin SH, Lin CJ, Lo WC, Chen YH. Diagnosis and treatment of pulmonary tuberculosis in hospitalized patients are affected by physician specialty and experience. Am J Med Sci. 2010;340(5):367–72.
18. Gao J, Qian J, Tang S, Eriksson BO, Blas E. Health equity in transition from planned to market economy in China. Health Policy Plan. 2002;17(Suppl):20–9.
19. Yip WC, Wang H, Liu Y. Determinants of patient choice of medical provider: a case study in rural China. Health Policy Plan. 1998;13(3):311–22.
20. Li Y, Ehiri J, Tang S, Li D, Bian Y, Lin H, Marshall C, Cao J. Factors associated with patient, and diagnostic delays in Chinese TB patients: a systematic review and meta-analysis. BMC Med. 2013;11:156.
21. Dye C, Watt CJ, Bleed D. Low access to a highly effective therapy: a challenge for international tuberculosis control. Bull World Health Organ. 2002;80(6):437–44.
22. Ward J, Siskind V, Konstantinos A. Patient and health care system delays in Queensland tuberculosis patients, 1985-1998. Int J Tuberc Lung Dis. 2001; 5(11):1021–7.
23. Almeida CP, Skupien EC, Silva DR. Health care seeking behavior and patient delay in tuberculosis diagnosis. Cad Saude Publica. 2015;31(2):321–30.
24. Lin HP, Deng CY, Chou P. Diagnosis and treatment delay among pulmonary tuberculosis patients identified using the Taiwan reporting enquiry system, 2002-2006. BMC Public Health. 2009;9:55.
25. Gebeyehu E, Azage M, Abeje G. Factors associated with patient's delay in tuberculosis treatment in Bahir Dar City administration, Northwest Ethiopia. Biomed Res Int. 2014;2014:701429.

Sporadic isolated congenital asplenia with fulminant pneumococcal meningitis

Shigeo Iijima

Abstract

Background: Isolated congenital asplenia (ICA) is a rare and life-threatening condition that predisposes patients to severe bacterial infections. Most of the reported cases are familial and the mode of inheritance is usually autosomal dominant. Here, we report a case of sporadic isolated asplenia and review the literature while focusing on sporadic cases.

Case presentation: We report the case of an 11-month-old female infant who developed fulminant pneumococcal meningitis. The pneumococcal vaccine-unimmunized patient was hospitalized with fever, irritability, and purpura, and was diagnosed as having meningitis, septic shock, and disseminated intravascular coagulation. *Streptococcus pneumoniae* was isolated from both cerebrospinal fluid and blood. She was successfully treated with prompt antibiotic therapy. During hospitalization, abdominal ultrasonography and computed tomography findings, scintigraphy results, and Howell-Jolly body-containing red blood cells indicated the presence of asplenia without any visceroarterial anomalies. Moreover, the findings of peripheral blood smears and spleen ultrasonographic examinations of her parents were normal.

Conclusions: Majority of sporadic ICA cases were detected only after the onset of overwhelming infection and had a high mortality. In cases of severe invasive pneumococcal disease, a systematic search for Howell-Jolly bodies on blood smears and the presence of asplenia on abdominal imaging are essential for detecting ICA even in the absence of any family history. After the diagnosis of ICA, patient and parent education, vaccinations, antibiotic prophylaxis, and prompt empiric treatment of febrile episode should be provided.

Keywords: Sporadic asplenia, Isolated congenital asplenia, Pneumococcal meningitis, Howell-jolly body

Background

The spleen is critical in the predominantly innate immune response to infections from encapsulated bacterial pathogens such as *Streptococcus pneumoniae* [1]. Congenital asplenia often occurs as part of a recognized malformation syndrome, with anomalies of the heart, great vessels, and viscera [2]. The best known among these syndromes is the congenital asplenia/polysplenia syndrome associated with visceroarterial heterotaxy; its incidence is estimated at approximately 1/10,000 to 1/40,000 live births [3]. In contrast, isolated congenital asplenia (ICA) occurs less frequently. A recent French nationwide study indicated that the prevalence of ICA is 0.51 per million births [3]. Patients with congenital asplenia have increased susceptibility to invasive infections along with a high mortality rate despite aggressive therapy. Although the initial symptoms may be mild and nonspecific, it can progress rapidly to Waterhouse-Friderichsen syndrome with full-blown septic shock and disseminated intravascular coagulation (DIC). Compared to congenital asplenic syndrome, the diagnosis of ICA is more difficult due to the lack of other anomalies. In particular, in sporadic ICA, the condition may remain undetected until the postmortem autopsy.

Here, we present the case of a girl with sporadic ICA who developed overwhelming meningitis due to *S. pneumoniae* and compared the clinical manifestations between sporadic and familial ICA cases by reviewing the literature.

Correspondence: sige_pd@yahoo.co.jp
Department of Pediatrics, Hamamatsu University School of Medicine, Hamamatsu, Japan

Case presentation

A previously healthy 11-month-old female infant (the first child of non-consanguineous Japanese parents) was referred to our hospital with clinical signs of septic shock and purpura, which were preceded by fever for 2 days and signs of upper respiratory tract infection (URI) for 1 week. She had previously received oral antibiotic treatment for the URI. The patient had not received pneumococcal or *Haemophilus influenzae* type b (Hib) vaccination because these vaccines were not included in the routine immunization program at that time in Japan. On admission, she had a body temperature of 39.4 °C, heart rate of 180 bpm, blood pressure of 83/46 mmHg, and cold extremities with a capillary refill of >5 s. She was irritable without any focal neurological deficits. She was found to have purpura fulminans with ecchymoses of the face and trunk and purpura of her limbs and ears. Her neck was stiff. Laboratory examination indicated a white blood cell count of 35.1×10^9/L, with 67% neutrophils and 25% lymphocytes; platelet count of 8.1×10^9/L; hemoglobin level of 10.9 g/dL; and C-reactive protein level of 18.5 mg/dL. Prolonged prothrombin time and activated partial thromboplastin time and elevated levels of plasma fibrinogen degradation products (235 μg/mL: normal <5 μg/mL) indicated the presence of DIC. A lumbar puncture indicated the presence of pleocytosis in the cerebrospinal fluid (CSF), including 11,527 cells/μL (95% polymorphonuclear cells), 11 mg/dL glucose (blood glucose level; 87 mg/dL), and 425 mg/dL protein. The gram stains of CSF revealed the presence of gram-positive diplococci. We diagnosed the patient with bacterial meningitis followed by DIC and treated her with intravenous antibiotics (ampicillin and cefotaxime) empirically and addressed the DIC using anticoagulants. On the day after admission, blood and CSF cultures indicated positive results for *S. pneumoniae* (serotype not available). The minimum inhibitory concentration for penicillin was <0.06 μg/mL. The patient received antibiotic therapy for 14 days with a good clinical response and was discharged without any sequelae.

Over the clinical course, abdominal ultrasonography (US) was performed to detect adrenal hemorrhage as we suspected Waterhouse-Friderichsen syndrome; however, US did not indicate the presence of a spleen (Fig. 1a). In addition, no spleen was visible on abdominal computed tomography (Fig. 1b). Careful blood smear assessment indicated the presence of Howell-Jolly bodies (HJB) (Fig. 1c). Based on the suspicion of asplenia, scintigraphy with Tc-99 m phytate colloid was performed and no functioning splenic tissue was detected (Fig. 1d). The patient had no history of splenectomy. No other malformations such as heart defects, anomalous systemic or pulmonary venous connections, and abdominal heterotaxia were detected, leading to the diagnosis of ICA. Moreover, peripheral blood smears and spleen US examinations of the parents indicated normal results. After that, antibiotic prophylaxis with amoxicillin was initiated as

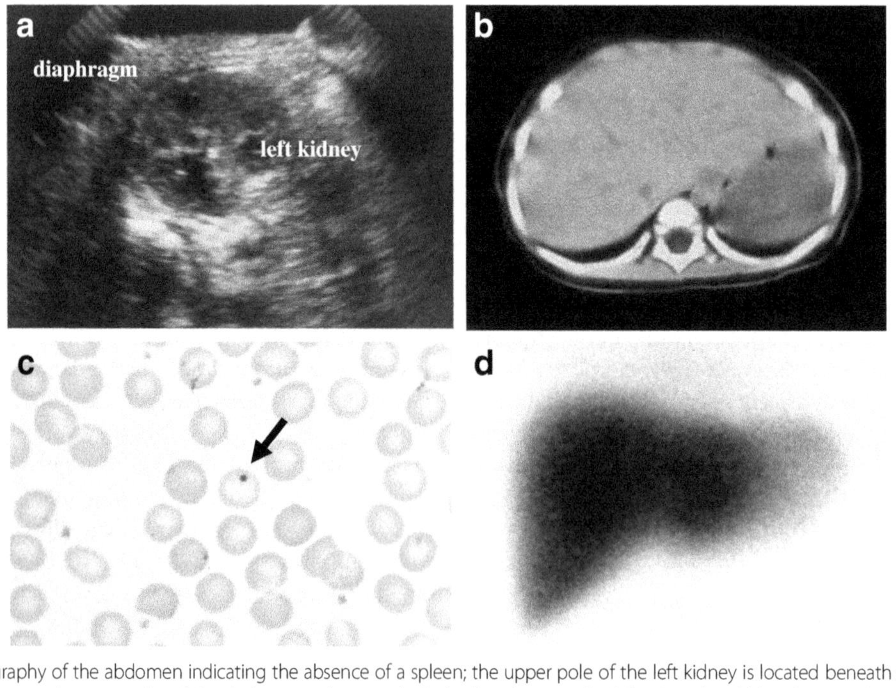

Fig. 1 **a** Ultrasonography of the abdomen indicating the absence of a spleen; the upper pole of the left kidney is located beneath the diaphragm. **b** Nonenhanced computed tomography of the abdomen indicating the lack of a spleen on the left. **c** Peripheral blood smear showing the presence of Howell-Jolly body (arrow). **d** Scintigraphy with Tc-99 m phytate colloid showing no functional spleen tissue

well as vaccinations using 7-valent pneumococcal conjugate vaccine (PCV7) and Hib vaccine, followed by 23-valent pneumococcal polysaccharide vaccine (PPSV23) when she was 2 years old. The parents were counseled about the need for prompt medical attention after the onset of fever. Subsequently, the patient has not experienced any invasive infections for >5 years.

Discussion

The congenital absence of the spleen has been recognized as a condition for more than 270 years. The first two cases, reported in 1740, were observed independently by Pohl and Jauch; in each of these young adult male cases, absence of the spleen was noted on autopsy [4]. Putschar and Manion described 11 cases (including the two mentioned above) of spleen agenesis without any other malformations in 1956 [4]; to our knowledge, that is the first series on ICA and 70 such patients have been reported to date [5].

In congenital asplenic syndrome, different modes of inheritance have been reported; mostly autosomal recessive, exceptionally autosomal dominant or X-linked. Two human genes are reportedly involved in this syndrome, connexin 43 and *ZIC3*, which are involved in an X-linked form [6]. On the other hand, most of the reported ICA cases are familial and the mode of inheritance is usually autosomal dominant, although recessive inheritance patterns have also been observed [3, 6]. Given the isolated abnormality of spleen development, mutations in the *Hox 11* have been reported in mice with ICA [7]. Moreover, a recent study in humans with autosomal dominant ICA demonstrated that germline mutations in *RPSA* lead to a spleen-specific developmental defect [8]. However, the genetic etiology of ICA remains unknown. With respect to sporadic ICA cases, Gilbert et al. described 13 of 31 cases of ICA between 1956 and 2000 [6], and Mahlaoui et al. documented 29 of 65 cases between 1956 and 2009 [3]; these researchers speculated that sporadic cases might be related to either the low penetrance of ICA or de novo mutations. In the present report, we reviewed 73 cases with ICA in the literature between 1956 and 2016 using the Medline database and identified 32 sporadic cases [3, 5, 9–27]. Their clinical details are summarized in Table 1. The first sign of ICA was severe invasive bacterial infection in 25 of 32 cases (78%), and 12 patients died. Of the 25 patients, only four had multiple episodes of invasive infections, including two episodes in three cases (two deaths) and three episodes in one case (no death). In a total of 29 episodes of overwhelming sepsis, the causative pathogen was *S. pneumoniae* in 18 episodes (62%), *H. influenzae* in six episodes (21%), and *Escherichia coli* in two episodes (7%). Of the 12 patients who died, at least nine (75%) died within the first 48 h of hospital admission and seven (58%) died within the first 24 h. The mortality rate for overwhelming postsplenectomy infection (OPSI) has been estimated as approximately 50–70% despite aggressive therapy [28], and >50% died within the first 48 h of hospital admission [29]. Similar to OPSI, overwhelming infection in ICA is a virulent entity that leads to death within 48 years in most cases. Hence, the diagnostic workup should never delay the initiation of empiric antibiotic therapy [30]. A delay of only a few hours may lead to death. Moreover, overwhelming infection in asplenia may also occur at any time after birth and should also be considered in adults, as demonstrated in our case series. As individuals who have undergone splenectomy can be identified as having infection by themselves or by clinicians, some OPSI cases may still be preventable. When asplenia develops as part of heterotaxy syndrome, it is often identified due to the presence of other congenital anomalies, and appropriate management may be instituted to prevent severe infection. However, in the case of ICA, there are no other physical clues for diagnosis and overwhelming infection may be the first sign of the disease [9–11]. In the 73 cases available for review, we compared the clinical characteristics between sporadic and familial ICA using the Mann-Whitney U-test (the Statistical Package for Social Sciences version 23, Tokyo, Japan) (Table 2). The analysis showed that event-free cases were significantly more common in familial ICA ($p = 0.001$). In a familial case, the identification of other family members with the condition may provide an important clue for the diagnosis. However, in sporadic cases, the condition may remain undetected even at the presentation with pneumococcal disease. In the present case, the diagnosis of asplenia in the context of sepsis was confirmed through US of the abdomen and identification of HJB on blood smears. In the case series, HJBs were identified in at least 18 patients (60%). Abdominal US and HJB assessment are important tests to perform in the first-degree relatives of affected individuals for the diagnosis of asplenia.

As for post-diagnosis management, immunization against encapsulated bacteria is an indispensable strategy to ensure the survival of asplenic patients. Moreover, PCVs enhance immunity in asplenic patients because PCVs can induce antibody responses in the absence of a spleen [31, 32]. Therefore, in ICA cases, the use of active immunizations including pneumococcal (not only PPSV but also PCV), Hib, and meningococcal vaccines could prevent overwhelming sepsis and save lives [33, 34]. In Japan, Hib conjugate vaccine has been available on a voluntary basis since 2008, and PCV has been available since 2010; however, the vaccination rate was estimated to be <10% in those years [35]. Subsequently, these two vaccines have been included in the routine

Table 1 Reported cases of sporadic congenital isolated asplenia

Case no.	Age at diagnosis	Sex	Clinical events	Pathogens	Howell-Jolly bodies	Outcome	Reference
1	2 months	Female	Meningitis	*H. influenzae*	Yes	Survived	[13]
2	4 months	Unknown	Sepsis	*E. coli*	NA	Died	[11]
3	6 months	Unknown	Sepsis	*S. Pneumoniae*	NA	Survived	[11]
4	6 months	Female	Sepsis, purpura fulminans	Unknown	Yes	Survived	[3]
5	7 months	Male	Sepsis, bilateral adrenal hemorrhage	*H. influenzae*	NA	Died in 12 h	[15]
6	7 months	Female	Asymptomatic	No infection	Yes	Alive	[3]
7	10 months	Unknown	Sepsis	*H. influenzae*	NA	Survived	[11]
8	10 months	Male	Sepsis, purpura fulminans	*S. pneumoniae*	Yes	Died in 20 h	[3]
9	11 months	Female	Meningitis, purpura fulminans	*S. pneumoniae*	Yes	Survived	Present case
10	12 months	Female	Sepsis, purpura fulminans	*S. pneumoniae*	Yes	Survived	[3]
11	12 months	Male	Meningitis (twice), osteomyelitis	*S. pneumoniae*	Yes	Survived	[14]
12	20 months	Female	Sepsis	Unknown	Yes	Survived	[3]
13	21 months	Unknown	Sepsis	*S. pneumoniae*	NA	Survived	[11]
15	1 years	Unknown	Sepsis	*S. pneumoniae*	NA	Survived	[27]
16	2 years	Male	Sepsis, bilateral adrenal hemorrhage	*H. influenzae*	NA	Died in 32 h	[15]
17	2 years	Female	Meningitis (3 times)	*E. coli, S. pneumoniae H. influenzae*	Yes	Survived	[5]
18	3 years	Unknown	Sepsis	*H. influenzae*	NA	Died in 24 h	[11]
19	4 years	Female	Sepsis, bilateral adrenal hemorrhage	*S. pneumoniae*	NA	Died in 12 h	[18]
20	5 years	Male	Sepsis, meningitis	*S. pneumoniae*	NA	Died	[23]
21	10 years	Female	Sepsis, arthritis (twice)	*S. pneumoniae*	NA	Died in 24 h	[21]
22	15 years	Male	Meningitis (twice), bilateral adrenal hemorrhage	*S. pneumoniae*	Yes	Died in 3 h	[12]
23	28 years	Male	Sepsis	Group B *streptococcus*	Yes	Survived	[24]
24	20 years	Male	Tonsillitis	Unknown	Yes	Alive	[22]
25	36 years	Male	Meningitis, bilateral adrenal hemorrhage	*S. pneumoniae*	NA	Died in 29 h	[10]
26	37 years	Female	Thrombocytosis	No infection	Yes	Alive	[16]
27	44 years	Female	Thrombocytosis	No infection	Yes	Alive	[25]
28	56 years	Female	Thrombocytosis	No infection	Yes	Alive	[20]
29	56 years	Male	Thrombocytosis	No infection	Yes	Alive	[20]
30	60 years	Female	Meningitis	*S. pneumoniae*	Yes	Survived	[19]
31	67 years	Female	Sepsis	*S. pneumoniae*	NA	Died in 24 h	[26]
32	72 years	Male	Thrombocytosis	No infection	Yes	Alive	[28]

NA Not available

immunization program since 2013. In fact, the present patient did not receive the PCV or Hib vaccine before the septicemic onset because these vaccinations were voluntary at the time. Moreover, meningococcal vaccine has not been approved yet in Japan. In contrast, in Western countries, greater efforts, including the publication of national guidelines, have been made to improve the management of asplenic patients [33, 34]. As for the latest recommendations, asplenic patients should receive vaccines including 13-valent PCV (PCV13) and Hib vaccine for children aged <2 years as recommended routinely for immunocompetent persons based on the Centers for Disease Control and Prevention annual schedule, followed by PPSV23 at 2 years of age or older, with a recommendation for a second dose of PPSV23 5 years later. Moreover, some European public health agencies recommend PPSV23 reimmunization of asplenic individuals every 5 years [36]. Meningococcal vaccine

Table 2 Comparison of clinical characteristics between sporadic and familial cases of isolated congenital asplenia

	Sporadic $n = 32$	Familial $n = 41$	P value
Age at diagnosis, years	2.1 (0.8–34.2)	1.0 (0.6–3.0)	0.04
Male sex	11[a] (44)	25(61)	0.18
Clinical events			
Sepsis and/ or meningitis	25(78)	24 (58)	0.08
Others	6 (19)	2 (5)	0.06
Asymptomatic	1 (3)	15 (37)	0.001
Pathogens			
S. pneumoniae	16[b] (62)	14[c] (56)	0.69
H. influenzae	5[b] (19)	3[c] (12)	0.48
Others	3[b] (12)	0[c] (0)	0.08
Howell- Jolly bodies	18 (56)	17 (41)	0.21
Outcome			
Death	12 (38)	16 (39)	0.68

Values are presented as median (interquartile range) or number (percentage). $P < 0.05$ is considered to be significant. [a]data from 25 patients were available. [b]data from 26 patients were available. [c]data from 25 patients were available

should also be administered to asplenic patients aged ≥2 months. In addition, yearly influenza vaccination is recommended for all asplenic patients aged >6 months because the influenza virus is an important risk factor for secondary pneumococcal and *H. influenzae* infections [34]. However, vaccination does not fully eliminate the risk of invasive infection [32]. The second major strategy is antibiotic prophylaxis and treatment. Daily antibiotic prophylaxis against pneumococcal infections is recommended due to evidence of good efficacy in patients with sickle cell anemia (functional asplenia) [37, 38]. However, the appropriate duration of prophylaxis in asplenic patients is unknown. The use of life-long penicillin prophylaxis has potential disadvantages as it can be associated with the development of bacterial resistance, may have side effects including allergy, and may be associated with poor adherence [39]. The American Academy of Pediatrics recommends prophylaxis until the child is 5 years of age [38]. In contrast, British guidelines recommend life-long penicillin prophylaxis in high-risk patients defined as those <16 or >50 years of age, those with an inadequate serological response to pneumococcal vaccination, and those who have had a previous episode of invasive pneumococcal disease [34]. Education for asplenic patients and their parents is also important to enable them to understand that all febrile illnesses are potentially serious in asplenic patients and that patients developing such signs must be given systemic antibiotics and admitted to hospital. If an asplenic patient travels to or resides in an area where medical care is not accessible, an appropriate antibiotic agent should be readily available and the child's caregiver should be instructed in its appropriate use [38]. Patients and parents should also be advised about animal handling as overwhelming sepsis (due to *Capnocytophaga canimorsus*) may result from dog, cat, or other animal bites [40]. Furthermore, these patients require specific advice regarding travel as they are at increased risk of severe malaria (mosquito bites) and babesiosis (tick bites) in endemic areas [34, 38].

Conclusions

In the case of severe invasive pneumococcal disease, a systematic search for HJB on blood smears and imaging examination of the abdomen for the presence of asplenia are vital for detecting ICA, even in the absence of a family history. If asplenia is detected, life-saving vaccination with a series of PCV13 and Hib vaccines, followed by PPSV23, in addition to penicillin prophylaxis, preemptive investigation, and empiric treatment early in the course of illnesses should be provided.

Considering the limitations of the literature review, this article may have incomplete data about the full syndrome of asplenia. The inclusion of unwritten, unpublished, or repetitive cases, or cases published in grey literature might have influenced the findings.

Abbreviations

CSF: Cerebrospinal fluid; DIC: Disseminated intravascular coagulation; Hib: *Haemophilus influenzae* type b; HJB: Howell-Jolly bodies; ICA: Isolated congenital asplenia; OPSI: Overwhelming postsplenectomy infection; PCV7: 7-valent pneumococcal conjugate vaccine; PPSV23: 23-valent pneumococcal polysaccharide vaccine; URI: Upper respiratory tract infection; US: Ultrasonography

Acknowledgements

Not applicable.

Funding

No funding sources.

Authors' contributions

SI conceived the study and was responsible for data collection. SI performed data analysis, interpreted the data, and prepared the first draft of the manuscript.

Consent for publication

A written informed consent was obtained from the patient's parents for publication of this case report and any accompanying images.

Competing interests

The authors declare that they have no competing interests.

References

1. Bisno AL, Freeman JC. The syndrome of asplenia, pneumococcal sepsis, and disseminated intravascular coagulation. Ann Int Med. 1970;72:389–93.
2. Ivemark BI. Implications of agenesis of the spleen on the pathogenesis of controtruncus anomalies in childhood; an analysis of the heart malformations in the splenic agenesis syndrome, with fourteen new cases. Acta Paediatr. 1955;44(Supple 104):7–110.
3. Mahlaoui N, Minard-Colin V, Picard C, Bolze A, Ku CL, Tournilhac O, et al. Isolated congenital asplenia: a French nationwide retrospective survey of 20 cases. J Pediatr. 2011;158:142–8.
4. Putschar WGJ, Manion WC. Congenital absence of the spleen and associated anomalies. Am J Clin Pathol. 1956;26:429–70.
5. Uchida Y, Matsubara K, Wada T, Oishi K, Morio T, Takada H, et al. Recurrent bacterial meningitis by three different pathogens in an isolated asplenic child. J Infect Chemother. 2012;18:576–80.
6. Gilbert B, Menetrey C, Belin V, Brosset P, de Lumley L, Fisher A. Familial isolated congenital asplenia: a rare, frequently hereditary dominant condition, often detected too late as a cause of overwhelming pneumococcal sepsis. Report of a new case and review of 31 others. Eur J Pediatr. 2002;161:368–72.
7. Roberts CW, Shutter JR, Korsmeyer SJ. Hox11 controls the genesis of the spleen. Nature. 1994;368:747–9.
8. Bolze A, Mahlaoui N, Byun M, Turner B, Trede N, Ellis SE, et al. Ribosomal protein SA haploinsufficiency in humans with isolated congenital asplenia. Science. 2013;340:976–8.
9. Myerson RM, Koelle WA. Congenital absence of the spleen in an adult: report of a case associated with recurrent Waterhouse-Friderichsen syndrome. N Engl J Med. 1956;254:1131–2.
10. Waldman JD, Rosenthal A, Smith AL, Shurin S, Nadas AS. Sepsis and congenital asplenia. J Pediatr. 2002;90:555–9.
11. Gopal V, Bisno AL. Fulminant pneumococcal infections in "normal" asplenic hosts. Arch Intern Med. 1977;137:1526–30.
12. Honingman R, Lanzkowsky P. Isolated congenital asplenia: an occult case of overwhelming sepsis. Am J Dis Child. 1979;133:552–3.
13. Gill DG, Kara M. Septicaemia and adrenal hemorrhage in congenital asplenia. Arch Dis Child. 1991;66:1366.
14. Dyke MP, Martin RP, Berry PJ. Septicaemia and adrenal haemorrhage in congenital asplenia. Arch Dis Child. 1991;66:636–7.
15. Rose C, Quesnel B, Facon T, Fenaux P, Jouet JP, Bauters F. Congenital asplenia, a differential diagnosis of essential thrombocythemia. Presse Med. 1993;22:1748.
16. Ferlicot S, Emile JF, Le Bris JL, Cheron G, Brousse N. Congenital asplenia. A childhood immune deficit often detected too late. Ann Pathol. 1997;17:44–6.
17. Kanthan R, Moyana T, Nyssen J. Asplenia as a cause of sudden unexpected death in childhood. Am J Forensic Med Pathol. 1999;20:57–9.
18. Germing U, Perings C, Steiner S, Peters AJ, Heintzen MP, Aul C. Congenital asplenia detected in a 60-year-old patient with septicemia. Eur J Med Res. 1999;4:283–5.
19. Chanet V, Tournilhac O, Dieu-Bellamy V, Boiret N, Spitz P, Baud O, et al. Isolated spleen agenesis: a rare cause of thrombocytosis mimicking essential thrombocythemia. Haematologica. 2000;85:1211–3.
20. Halbertsma FJJ, Neeleman C, Weemaes CM, van Deuren M. The absent and vanishing spleen: congenital asplenia and hyposplenism-two case reports. Acta Paediatr. 2005;94:369–71.
21. Almoznino-Sarafian D, Dotan E, Sandbank J, Gorelik O, Chachashvily S, Shteinshnaider M, et al. Unusual manifestations of myelofibrosis in a patient with congenital asplenia. Acta Haematol. 2007;118:226–30.
22. Araújo AR, Maciel I, Lima L, Chacim I, Barbot J. Congenital asplenia and severe visceral toxocariasis. Pediatr Infect Dis J. 2008;27:478.
23. Thiruppathy K, Privitera A, Jain K, Gupta S. Congenital asplenia and group B streptococcus sepsis in the adult: case report and review of the literature. FEMS Immunol Med Microbiol. 2008;53:437–9.
24. Takahashi F, Uchida K, Nagaoka T, Honma N, Cui R, Yoshioka M, et al. Isolated congenital spleen agenesis: a rare cause of chronic thromboembolic pulmonary hypertension in an adult. Respirology. 2008;13:913–5.
25. Vincentelli C, Molina EG, Robinson MJ. Fatal pneumococcal Waterhouse-Friderichsen syndrome in a vaccinated adult with congenital asplenia. Am J Emerg Med. 2009;27:751.e3–5.
26. Shachor-Meyouhas Y, Sprecher H, Kassis I. Isolated congenital asplenia—a rare cause of severe pneumococcal sepsis. Harefuah. 2010;149:486–9.
27. Imashuku S, Kudo N, Kubo K, Takahashi N, Tohyama K. Persistent thrombocytosis in elderly patients with rare hyposplenias that mimic essential thrombocythemia. Int J Hematol. 2012;95:702–5.
28. Okabayashi T, Hanazaki K. Overwhelming postsplenectomy infection syndrome in adults-a clinically preventable disease. World J Gastroenterol. 2008;14:176–9.
29. Brigden ML, Pattullo AL. Prevention and management of overwhelming postsplenectomy infection-an update. Crit Care Med. 1999;27:836–42.
30. Lynch AM, Kapila R. Overwhelming postsplenectomy infection. Infect Dis Clin N Am. 1996;10:693–707.
31. Breukels MA, Zandvoort A, van Den Dobbelsteen GP, van Den Muijsenberg A, Lodewijk ME, Beurret M, et al. Pneumococcal conjugate vaccines overcome splenic dependency of antibody response to pneumococcal polysaccharides. Infect Immun. 2001;69:7583–7.
32. Forstner C, Plefka S, Tobudic S, Winkler HM, Burgmann K, Burgmann H. Effectiveness and immunogenicity of pneumococcal vaccination in splenectomized and functionally asplenic patients. Vaccine. 2012;30:5449–52.
33. Rubin LG, Levin MJ, Ljungman P, Davies EG, Avery R, Tomblyn M, Bousvaros A, Dhanireddy S, Sung L, Keyserling H, Kang I. Infectious Diseases Society of America. 2013 IDSA clinical practice guideline for vaccination of the immunocompromised host. Clin Infect Dis. 2014;58:309–18.
34. Davies JM, Lewis MP, Wimperis J, Rafi I, Ladhani S, Bolton-Maggs PH. British Committee for Standards in Haematology. Review of guidelines for the prevention and treatment of infection in patients with an absent or dysfunctional spleen: prepared on behalf of the British Committee for Standards in Haematology by a working party of the Haemato-oncology task force. Br J Haematol. 2011;155:308–17.
35. Ishiwada N, Hishiki H, Nagasawa K, Naito S, Sato Y, Chang B, et al. The incidence of pediatric invasive Haemophilus influenzae and pneumococcal disease in Chiba prefecture, Japan before and after the introduction of conjugate vaccines. Vaccine. 2014;32:5425–31.
36. Mourtzoukou EG, Pappas G, Peppas G, Falagas ME. Vaccination of asplenic or hyposplenic adults. Br J Surg. 2008;95:273–80.
37. Hirst C, Owusu-Ofori S. Prophylactic antibiotics for preventing pneumococcal infection in children with sickle cell disease. Cochrane Database Syst Rev. 2014;11:CD003427.
38. American Academy of Pediatrics. Children with asplenia or functional asplenia. In: Kimberlin DW, Brady MT, Jackson MA, Long SS, editors. Red book: 2012 report of the committee on infectious diseases. 29th ed. Elk Grove Village, IL: American Academy of Pediatrics; 2012. p. 88–90.
39. Keenan RD, Boswell T, Milligan DW. Do post-splenectomy patients take prophylactic penicillin? Br J Haematol. 1999;105:509–10.
40. Zajkowska J, Król M, Falkowski D, Syed N, Kamieńska A. Capnocytophaga canimorsus – an underestimated danger after dog or cat bite – review of literature. Przegl Epidemiol. 2016;70:289–95.

20

Ischemic stroke as a complication of cryptococcal meningitis and immune reconstitution inflammatory syndrome

Jayne P. Ellis[1,2*], Newton Kalata[1], Elizabeth C. Joekes[3], Samuel Kampondeni[4], Laura A. Benjamin[5], Thomas S. Harrison[6], David G. Lalloo[7] and Robert S. Heyderman[1,8*]

Abstract

Background: Cryptococcal meningitis remains the leading cause of adult meningitis in Sub-Saharan Africa. Immune Reconstitution Inflammatory Syndrome (IRIS) following anti-retroviral therapy (ART) initiation is an important complication. Here we report the first documented case of a IRIS reaction presenting as an ischemic stroke.

Case presentation: A 38 year old newly diagnosed HIV-infected, ART naive Malawian male presented to a tertiary referral hospital in Blantyre, Malawi with a 2 week history of headache. A diagnosis of cryptococcal meningitis was made and the patient was started on 1200 mg fluconazole once daily and flucytosine 25 mg/kg four times daily as part of the Advancing Cryptococcal Treatment for Africa (ACTA) clinical trial. There was an initial clinical and microbiological response to anti-fungal treatment and anti-retroviral therapy was started at week 4. The patient re-presented 16 days later with recurrence of headache, fever, and a sudden onset of left sided weakness in the context of rapid immune reconstitution; peripheral CD4 count had increased from a baseline of 29 cells/µl to 198 cells/µl. Recurrence of cryptococcal meningitis was excluded through CSF examination and fungal culture. Magnetic Resonance Imaging (MRI) of the brain demonstrated multi-focal DWI (diffusion weighted imaging) positive lesions consistent with an ischemic stroke. Given the temporal relationship to ART initiation, these MRI findings in the context of sterile CSF with raised CSF protein and a rapid immune reconstitution, following an earlier favorable response to treatment is most consistent with a paradoxical Immune Reconstitution Inflammatory Syndrome.

Conclusions: Stroke is an increasing cause of morbidity and mortality amongst HIV infected persons. Ischemic stroke is a recognized complication of cryptococcal meningitis in the acute phase and is thought to be mediated by an infectious vasculitis. This is the first time an ischemic stroke has been described as part of a paradoxical IRIS reaction. This report adds to the spectrum of clinical IRIS presentations recognized and highlights to clinicians the potential complications encountered at ART initiation in severely immunocompromised patients.

Keywords: HIV, Cryptococcal meningitis, Immune reconstitution inflammatory syndrome, Stroke

* Correspondence: j.ellis@doctors.org.uk; r.heyderman@ucl.ac.uk
[1]Malawi-Liverpool-Wellcome Trust Clinical Research Programme, College of Medicine, Chichiri, Blantyre, Malawi
Full list of author information is available at the end of the article

Background

Cryptococcal meningitis (CM) remains a common opportunistic infection in settings with high HIV prevalence and is the leading cause of adult meningitis in Sub-Saharan Africa [1]. Mortality remains high in Africa, ranging from 24% [2] to 100% [3] depending upon the anti-fungal regimen used. With roll out of anti-retroviral therapy (ART), Immune Reconstitution Inflammatory Syndrome (IRIS) has emerged as a prominent early complication in CM patients. Cryptococcal IRIS (C-IRIS) is believed to be caused by the recovery of cryptococcus-specific immune responses following ART initiation resulting in a pathological inflammatory response [4]. Two distinct forms of C-IRIS are recognised: paradoxical and unmasking IRIS. Paradoxical IRIS is characterized by a clinical deterioration and severe inflammation in a patient with previously diagnosed cryptococcal disease following ART initiation despite an earlier favorable response to anti-fungal therapy [4]. Paucity of viable organisms in the CSF despite severe inflammation is characteristic of paradoxical C-IRIS [5]. In contrast, unmasking IRIS is seen in patients with sub-clinical/undiagnosed cryptococcosis presenting with meningitis soon after ART initiation [4].

C-IRIS is therefore a highly heterogeneous condition which may result in a variety of clinical syndromes with both central nervous system (CNS) and non-CNS features. CNS C-IRIS presentations reported in the literature include: aseptic meningitis and intracranial cryptococcomas [6], spinal cord abscess [7], recalcitrant raised intracranial pressure [8], optic nerve oedema [9] and cranial nerve lesions [10]. Non-CNS manifestations of C-IRIS include chorioretinitis [11], lymphadenitis [12], soft tissue abscess, hypercalcaemia, cavitatory pulmonary disease [13] and lobar pneumonitis [11].

Here we present the history of a Malawian man who developed an ischemic stroke in the context of a paradoxical C-IRIS reaction. We aim to highlight the diagnostic challenges encountered when a patient with known CM presents with recurrence of symptoms and to add to the literature describing the spectrum of clinical IRIS presentations.

Case presentation

A 38 year old newly diagnosed HIV-infected, ART naive Malawian male presented to Queen Elizabeth Central Hospital, a large teaching hospital in Blantyre, Malawi. He reported a 2 week history of headache and vomiting. He had no past medical history of smoking, hypertension or diabetes. On examination, his blood pressure was 122/80 mmHg, pulse 124 beats/min and temperature 36.7 °C. He had a Glasgow Coma Score (GCS) of 15/15, there was evidence of meningism but no focal neurological deficit. A lumbar puncture (Additional file 1: Table S1) showed a WCC (white cell count) $6.0 \times 10^6/\mu L$, glucose < 2.22 mmol/L (normal range 2.22–4.44 mmol/L), protein 1.68 g/L (normal range 0.15–0.45 g/L) and a positive lateral flow assay for cryptococcal antigen (crAg; IMMY, Norman, OK) (Additional file 1: Table S1). Cerebrospinal fluid (CSF) opening pressure was 28 cm H_20 (normal range 5–20 cm H_20). Quantitative cryptococcal culture (QCC) demonstrated 740,000 colony forming units (cfu) /ml (normal < 0 cfu/ml). CD4 count at admission was 29 cells/μl, Hb 11.6 g/dL, WCC 7.5 $10^3/\mu L$, lymphocytes 0.9 $10^3/\mu L$. A diagnosis of CM was made and the patient started on 1200 mg fluconazole once daily and flucytosine 25 mg/kg four times daily as part of the Advancing Cryptococcal Treatment for Africa (ACTA) clinical trial (Open label, multicentre randomised trial; trial no. ISRCTN45035509). The patient received 14 days of treatment as an inpatient as per protocol. He required twice daily lumbar punctures until day 7 to manage his persistently raised intra-cranial pressure (ICP). His day 7 QCC was 22,300 cfu/ml and his QCC prior to discharge on day 14 was 30 cfu/ml.

The patient re-presented 5 days post discharge with recurrence of severe headaches, neck pain, drowsiness and vomiting. On examination, he had a GCS (Glasgow coma scale) of 15/15 and had no neurological deficit. CSF opening pressure was 28 cm H_20 and his CSF was crAg positive, WCC 0 $10^6/\mu L$, glucose 2.88 mmol/L and protein 1.22 g/L (Additional file 1: Table S1). The patient was commenced on amphotericin to treat suspected CM relapse whilst awaiting cryptococcal culture. The culture was subsequently negative and amphotericin was discontinued. He continued on 800 mg fluconazole once daily and was discharged 19 days later with no ongoing symptoms of meningitis. ART was started according to national guidelines (TDF/3TC/EFV) at day 39.

The patient re-presented to hospital at day 54 (16 days post ART commencement) with recurrence of headache and fever, and a sudden onset of left sided weakness. He reported adherence to his fluconazole and ART. On examination, temperature was 38.2 °C, blood pressure 135/92 mmHg, pulse 89 beats/min, respiratory rate 22 breaths/min. He had a new left sided hemiparesis involving both the upper limb and lower limb (power 4/5 using the Medical Research Council (MRC) scale), and there was no sensory deficit. The CSF opening pressure was 21 cm H20. The CSF crAg remained positive, CSF WCC 0 $10^6/\mu L$, CSF protein was high, 3.26 g/L. Culture remained negative (Additional file 1: Table S1).

His peripheral CD4 count had increased from a baseline of 29 cells/μl to 198 cells/μl. Magnetic Resonance Imaging (MRI) of the brain (performed on day 5 of symptom onset) demonstrated multi-focal DWI positive lesions in the right corona radiata (Fig. 1), right posterior limb of the internal capsule, right cerebral peduncle and

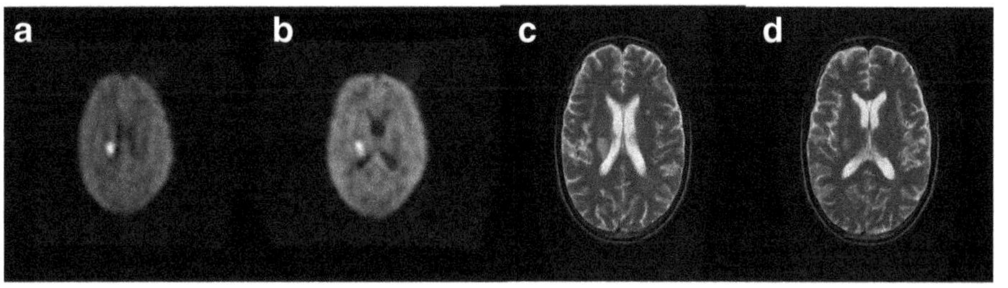

Fig. 1 **a-d** are MRI sequences taken on day 5 of an acute presentation of left arm and leg weakness; **a-b** are DWI axial B-900 sequences, showing restriction in the right corona radiata (**a**) and posterior limb of the internal capsule (**b**). **c** and **d** (T2 axial sequences) showed high signal in the corresponding areas to the DWI lesions; consistent with an acute ischemic stroke. High T2 signal was also seen in the left deep white matter (**c**); Not shown but there was increased T2 signal (with DWI restricted diffusion) in the right cerebral peduncle and the brainstem (without DWI changes); suggesting further ischaemia

1 month later, the right caudate nucleus; these changes were consistent with an acute ischemic stroke. There was high T2 signal without DWI restricted diffusion in the right brainstem and left deep white matter, suggesting previous ischemia. The MRI findings and raised CSF protein in the context of rapid immune reconstitution, following an earlier favorable clinical and microbiological response to anti-fungal treatment and a sterile CSF is consistent with paradoxical C-IRIS as opposed to acute CM infection. Because of the involvement of both anterior and posterior circulation, this met the criteria for probable cerebral vasculitis[12]. The 0.35 T GE MRI scanner used, does not support an ADC sequence. However, given the sudden onset of the symptoms, these focal DWI changes, in the corresponding anatomical location, occurring within a vascular territory, the etiology is unlikely to be anything other than vascular.

The development of an ischemic stroke was considered to be either a late manifestation of the CM infection or due to intensification of HIV- or CM- associated inflammation with immune reconstitution[8]. Fluconazole at a dose of 400 mg was continued with ART and the patient achieved good functional improvement. Corticosteroids were not given.

An MRI scan performed one month later demonstrated maturation of the ischemic stroke (Fig. 2), and a new DWI lesion in the right caudate, consistent with C-IRIS. The patient however reported complete resolution of the left sided weakness and remained well at day 185.

Discussion and conclusions

This case demonstrates the diagnostic challenges encountered when a patient with known CM presents with recurrence of symptoms following commencement of ART. Paradoxical C-IRIS complicates around 15% of cases of CM in ART naïve patients [14], usually during the first ten months of ART [4]. There is no definitive diagnostic test for IRIS but by adopting the clinical criteria checklist approach set out by the International Network for the Study of HIV-associated IRIS [4] (Additional file 1: Table S2), we were able to diagnose paradoxical C-IRIS in this low resource setting. This patient had several of the recognized risk factors for paradoxical IRIS including: low CD4 count at ART initiation, high fungal burden [15] and lack of initial CSF inflammation (WBC < 25 cells/μl and CSF protein < 50 mg/dL) [16]. These characteristics are not uncommon in patients with CM in Sub-Saharan Africa.

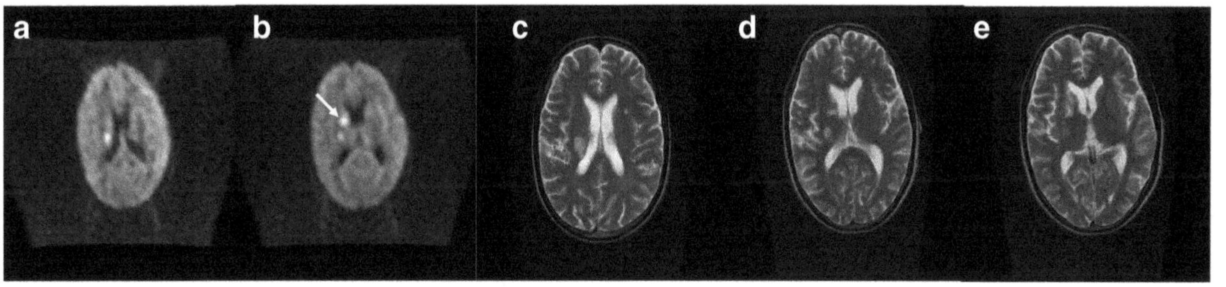

Fig. 2 **a-e** are MRI sequences taken 1 month later from symptom onset and on the background of a resolved left sided weakness. **a-b**; shows a new DWI lesion (**b** – arrow) suggesting evolving inflammation. However, the burden of the previous DWI changes reported in (1) is less. **c-d** (T2 axial) shows maturation of previously reported infarct

In line with current treatment guidelines, ART for this patient was not commenced until after week 4 of treatment, and was continued despite the diagnosis of paradoxical C-IRIS [17]. Although the reported mortality risk associated with C-IRIS is highly variable (0–83% [4]), ART and successful immune reconstitution is key to survival in HIV and so ART was not interrupted or discontinued due to IRIS. For non-life threatening IRIS manifestations, there are no specific definitive treatments recommended and symptoms should resolve spontaneously within weeks to months. For deteriorating patients with CNS inflammation leading to raised intra-cranial pressure, with no alternative diagnosis, corticosteroids should be considered (0.5 mg – 1.0 mg/kg per day of prednisolone) [17]. As our patient was clinically stable with improving neurology, steroids were not given.

Ischemic stroke is a recognized complication of CM in the acute phase and is thought to be mediated by an infectious vasculitis, primarily causing an endarteritis obliterans [18]. In this case however, the progressive parenchymal disease in the presence of sterile CSF and absence of traditional vascular risk factors, is most consistent with an immuno-pathological process. The increased risk of cerebrovascular disease in patients with HIV is well documented [19]. The pathophysiology is likely multifactorial with proposed mechanisms including increased prevalence of traditional vascular risk factors, infectious vasculitis, HIV-associated vasculopathy, and coagulopathy [20]. In a case-control study of 222 Malawian adults with MRI confirmed acute stroke, the highest risk of stroke in patients with untreated HIV infection was in the first 6 months after starting antiretroviral therapy (ART) (aOR 15.6 [4.21–46.6], $p < 0.001$) [19]. These results have led to the hypothesis that IRIS may be contributing to the disease.

In conclusion, this case report adds to the spectrum of clinical IRIS presentations encountered while managing CM. Whilst ART is essential in improving survival outcomes in these patients, clinicians should be aware of the complications of ART initiation including C-IRIS and stroke.

Abbreviations

ART: Anti-retroviral therapy; C-IRIS: Cryptococcal – immune reconstitution inflammatory syndrome; CM: Cryptococcal meningitis; CNS: Central nervous system; CSF: Cerebrospinal fluid; DWI: Diffusion weighted imaging; GCS: Glasgow coma scale; HIV: Human immunodeficiency virus; ICP: Intracranial pressure; MRC: Medical research council; MRI: Magnetic Resonance Imaging; QCC: Quantitative cryptococcal culture

Acknowledgements

We thank all the participants and their families, and gratefully acknowledge the support offered by the staff at all trial sites.

Funding

The ACTA trial was funded by the MRC (UK) (Grant ID: 100504), and ANRS (France) (Grant ID: ANRS12275). The MLW Clinical Research Programme was funded by a strategic award from the Wellcome Trust UK. The funding body was not involved in the design of the study and collection, analysis, and interpretation of data or in writing the manuscript.

Authors' contributions

JE, NK, RH, EJ and SK were all directly involved in the clinical management of this case. JE drafted the original manuscript under the guidance of RH, DL and TH. SK, EJ and LB offered expert radiological opinion on the case and on presentation of the results for publication. All authors read and approved the final manuscript.

Consent for publication

The study participant has signed a written consent form giving his consent for publication of this case in an academic journal.

Competing interests

The authors declare that they have no competing interests.

Author details

[1]Malawi-Liverpool-Wellcome Trust Clinical Research Programme, College of Medicine, Chichiri, Blantyre, Malawi. [2]Hospital for Tropical Diseases, University College London Hospitals NHS Foundation Trust, London, UK. [3]Department of Radiology, The Royal Liverpool University Hospitals NHS Trust, Liverpool, UK. [4]Blantyre Malaria Project, Blantyre, Malawi. [5]Brain Infections Group, Walton Centre NHS Foundation Trust, and Institute of Infection and Global Health, University of Liverpool, Liverpool, UK. [6]Institute for Infection and Immunity, St George's, University of London, London, UK. [7]Department of Clinical Sciences, Liverpool School of Tropical Medicine, Liverpool, UK. [8]Division of Infection and Immunity, University College London, London, UK.

References

1. Jarvis JN, Meintjes G, Williams A, Brown Y, Crede T, Harrison TS. Adult meningitis in a setting of high HIV and TB prevalence: findings from 4961 suspected cases. BMC Infect Dis. 2010;10(1):67. https://doi.org/10.1186/1471-2334-10-67.
2. Bicanic T, Wood R, Meintjes G, et al. High-dose amphotericin B with Flucytosine for the treatment of Cryptococcal meningitis in HIV-infected patients: a randomized trial. Clin Infect Dis. 2008;47(1):123–30. https://doi.org/10.1086/588792.
3. Mwaba P, Mwansa J, Chintu C, et al. Clinical presentation, natural history, and cumulative death rates of 230 adults with primary cryptococcal meningitis in Zambian AIDS patients treated under local conditions. Postgrad Med J. 2001;77(914):769–73.
4. Haddow LJ, Colebunders R, Meintjes GA, et al. Cryptococcal immune reconstitution inflammatory syndrome in HIV-1-infected individuals: proposed clinical case definitions. Lancet Infect Dis. 2010;10(11):791–802. https://doi.org/10.1016/S1473-3099(10)70170-5.
5. Walker NF, Scriven J, Meintjes G, Wilkinson RJ. Immune reconstitution inflammatory syndrome in HIV-infected patients. HIV AIDS (Auckl). 2015;7:49–64. https://doi.org/10.2147/HIV.S42328.
6. Pettersen KD, Pappas PG, Chin-Hong P, Baxi SM. A paradoxical decline: intracranial lesions in two HIV-positive patients recovering from cryptococcal meningitis. BMJ Case Rep. 2015;2015:bcr2015212108. https://doi.org/10.1136/bcr-2015-212108.
7. Rambeloarisoa J, Batisse D, Thiebaut J-B, et al. Intramedullary abscess resulting from disseminated cryptococcosis despite immune restoration in a patient with AIDS. J Inf Secur. 2002;44(3):185–8. https://doi.org/10.1053/jinf.2001.0955.
8. Cinti SK, Armstrong WS, Kauffman CA. Case report. Recurrence of increased intracranial pressure with antiretroviral therapy in an AIDS patient with cryptococcal meningitis. Mycoses. 2001;44(11–12):497–501.
9. Werner AC, Vuong LN, Hedges TR, Baumal CR. Immune reconstitution inflammatory syndrome causing progressive optic nerve edema in cryptococcal meningitis. Retin Cases Brief Rep. 2017. https://doi.org/10.1097/ICB.0000000000000582 [Epub ahead of print].
10. Khanna N, Nüesch R, Buitrago-Tellez C, Battegay M, Hirsch HH. Hearing loss after discontinuing secondary prophylaxis for cryptococcal meningitis: relapse or immune reconstitution? Infection. 2006;34(3):163–8. https://doi.org/10.1007/s15010-006-4042-y.

11. Kambugu A, Meya DB, Rhein J, et al. Outcomes of Cryptococcal meningitis in Uganda before and after the availability of highly active antiretroviral therapy. Clin Infect Dis. 2008;46(11):1694–701. https://doi.org/10.1086/587667.
12. Sethupathi M, Yoganathan K. Late onset of cryptococcal cervical lymphadenitis following immune reconstitution inflammatory syndrome in a patient with AIDS. BMJ Case Rep. 2015;2015(jan06 1):bcr2014206601-bcr2014206601). https://doi.org/10.1136/bcr-2014-206601.
13. Jenny-Avital ER, Abadi M. Immune reconstitution cryptococcosis after initiation of successful highly active antiretroviral therapy. Clin Infect Dis. 2002;35(12):e128–33. Epub 2002 Nov 20. https://doi.org/10.1086/344467.
14. Jarvis JN, Bicanic T, Loyse A, et al. Determinants of mortality in a combined cohort of 501 patients with HIV-associated cryptococcal meningitis: Implications for improving outcomes. Clin Infect Dis. 2014;58(5):736–45. https://doi.org/10.1093/cid/cit794 Epub 2013 Dec 6.
15. Longley N, Harrison TS, Jarvis JN. Cryptococcal immune reconstitution inflammatory syndrome. Curr Opin Infect Dis. 2013;26(1):26–34. https://doi.org/10.1097/QCO.0b013e32835c21d1.
16. Boulware DR, Bonham SC, Meya DB, et al. Paucity of initial cerebrospinal fluid inflammation in cryptococcal meningitis is associated with subsequent immune reconstitution inflammatory syndrome. J Infect Dis. 2010;202(6): 962–70. https://doi.org/10.1086/655785.
17. Saag MS, Graybill RJ, Larsen RA, et al. Practice guidelines for the management of cryptococcal disease. Infectious Diseases Society of America. Clin Infect Dis. 2000;30(4):710–8. https://doi.org/10.1086/313757.
18. Martin-Blondel G, Delobel P, Blancher A, et al. Pathogenesis of the immune reconstitution inflammatory syndrome affecting the central nervous system in patients infected with HIV. Brain. 2011;134(4):928–46. https://doi.org/10.1093/brain/awq365.
19. Benjamin LA, Corbett EL, Connor MD, et al. HIV, antiretroviral treatment, hypertension, and stroke in Malawian adults: a case-control study. Neurology. 2016;86(4):324–33. https://doi.org/10.1212/WNL.0000000000002278.
20. Benjamin LA, Bryer A, Lucas S, et al. Arterial ischemic stroke in HIV: defining and classifying etiology for research studies. Neurol Neuroimmunol Neuroinflamm. 2016;3(4):e254. https://doi.org/10.1212/NXI.0000000000000254.

21

Progressive cutaneous Cryptococcosis complicated with meningitis in a myasthenia gravis patient on long-term immunosuppressive therapy

Nguyen Thi Cam Huong[1,6*], Ahmed M. A. Altibi[2], Nguyen My Hoa[1,6], Le Anh Tuan[1,6], Samar Salman[3], Sara Morsy[4], Nguyen Thi Bich Lien[5], Nguyen Thanh Truong[6], Nguyen Thi Hoang Mai[8,6], Pham Thi Le Hoa[1,6], Nguyen Ba Thang[9] and Van The Trung[7*]

Abstract

Background: Cryptococcosis is an opportunistic infection caused by the encapsulated yeast *Cryptococcus neoformans* and most remarkably manifests in HIV-infected individuals, especially in the settings of very low CD4 count. Development of cryptococcosis in HIV-uninfected individuals is exceedingly rare and usually signifies a marked immunodeficiency. Cryptococcosis in association with myasthenia gravis or thymoma has been previously documented in only very few cases in the literature.

Case presentation: We reported a complicated case of severe cutaneous cryptococcosis in a 39-year-old Vietnamese male patient with myasthenia gravis on long-term immunosuppressive therapy. The patient presented with a five month history of recurrent and progressive skin lesions that later on progressed into cryptococcal meningitis.

Conclusion: Through this case, we aimed to emphasize the importance of including cutaneous cryptococcosis in the differential diagnosis of cutaneous lesions in patients on chronic immunosuppressive therapy. The cutaneous manifestations of cryptococcosis can be the first clue for a disseminated disease, which makes early recognition crucial and life-saving.

Keywords: Cryptococcus, Cutaneous Cryptococcosis, Cryptococcus meningitis, Myasthenia gravis

Background

Cryptococcosis is an infection caused by two species of the encapsulated yeast *Cryptococcus*: *Cryptococcus neoformans* (*C. neoformans*) and *Cryptococcus gatti (C. gatti). C. neoformans* is a rare opportunistic infection that is typically reported causing disease in immunocompromised patients, while *C. gatti* is an endemic infection in the tropical parts of the continent of Africa and Australia and is capable of causing disease in non-immunocompromised individuals.

Cryptococcosis, caused by *C. neoformans*, was known for a long time as an opportunistic infection that occurs exclusively in patients with HIV. Nowadays, many case-studies proved that this pathogen can cause disease in immunocompetent patients as well [1–3] and can also be fatal in patients without known immunosuppression history [3].

The pathogen can cause a wide range of diseases, ranging from isolated cutaneous cryptococcosis to fatal meningoencephalitis and disseminated disease affecting lungs, lymph nodes, skin, and brain [2]. It is transmitted to humans primarily by inhalation of the fungus present in the soil contaminated with avian excreta or decaying wood in the hollows of trees [4]. Other rare methods of

* Correspondence: camhuong37@yahoo.com; vanthetrungdhyd@yahoo.com
[1]Department of Infectious Diseases, University of Medicine and Pharmacy at Ho Chi Minh City , Ho Chi Minh city, Vietnam
[7]Department of Dermatology, University of Medicine and Pharmacy at Ho Chi Minh City, Ho Chi Minh City, Vietnam
Full list of author information is available at the end of the article

transmission have been reported, including organ transplantation and from contact with birds [5, 6].

Although it is well-known for causing meningoencephalitis, pulmonary and cutaneous cryptococcosis were reported in many cases. Cutaneous cryptococcosis is present in 5 % of patients with meningoencephalitis with increasing prevalence in patients with organ transplantation and disseminated disease [7]. However, this is not always the case, cutaneous cryptococcosis has been recently reported in patients with no signs of systemic infection and can present solely as localized cutaneous lesions with positive cultures for *Cryptococcus* species [7]. This predominantly cutaneous presentation is reported in both immunocompetent and immunocompromised patients [1].

Cryptococcosis is also reported in immunocompromised HIV-uninfected patients. This includes patients with organ transplantation, prolonged corticosteroids or immunosuppressive therapy. Cryptococcosis has also been rarely reported in myasthenia gravis (MG) patients.

MG is an autoimmune disease with auto-antibodies that attack specific receptors located on the surface of muscle cells preventing acetylcholine from binding to them, and thus, preventing the muscle from responding to the nerve signal. That is why although treatment with anticholinesterase agents produce some benefit, the prognosis remains poor. More recently, with the use of immunosuppressive therapy or surgical removal of thymus gland the general outlook for MG has improved dramatically [8]. Generalized immune suppression from the MG treatment compromises the immune system as a whole with increased susceptibility to infections, including opportunistic infections, and neoplasia [9–11]. Here, we reported a complicated case of a predominantly cutaneous cryptococcosis that progressed later to meningitis in a myasthenia gravis patient on chronic immunosuppressive therapy.

Case presentation

A 39-year-old Vietnamese male presented with a five month history (from June to November 2016) of recurrent and progressive skin lesion. Initially, the patient had painless papules distributed at multiple locations, including the chest, arms, hands, thighs, and feet. The papules then progressed into nodules, which later on expanded, ulcerated and became painful.

At the age of 27, the patient was diagnosed with myasthenia gravis (MG), was treated with prednisolone and pyridostigmine since August 2004 and had surgical removal of thymus gland on November 2004. The regimen for his MG from 2010 to 2016 was methyl prednisolone and periodically combined with IMDH inhibitors (mycophenolate or azathioprine) based on his weakness. The starting dose on September 2010 were azathioprine 100 mg/day and methyl prednisolone 48 mg/day. These doses were adjusted afterwards under the consultance of his doctor for 2 years and he did self adjusted later by his objective feeling of weakness. At the time of admission, he was under azathioprine 50 mg/day and methyl prednisolone 16 mg/day.

The patient was also diagnosed with type II diabetes one month after his first eruption (July 2016). Since then, his blood glucose level has been monitored and controlled by dietary modification, his periodically HbA1C were under 6%. From June to September 2016, the patient had completed twelve weeks of directly-acting antivirals (DAAs) for his chronic hepatitis C and he had gained virologic response (HCV RNA negative after 3 months of stop treatment).

Additionally, he had been diagnosed with TB pneumonia at the Pham Ngoc Thach Hospital which is one of the top ranked TB centers in Vietnam for his cough, hemoptysis, shortness of breath, prolonged fever with body temperature from 38 °C - 39 °C, abnormal chest X ray and the Acid-fast bacilli positivity of the sputum. He was started on anti-tuberculosis regimen (2RHZE/4RHE) since September 2016. The regimen consisted of rifampin, isoniazid, pyrazinamide and ethambutol for two months, then withdrawn pyrazinamide for the next four months. His symptoms and chest X ray improved after two weeks of RHZE treatment. He was still on the last week of the first 2RHZE at the time of admission.

The chronological order of the patient's medical history is shown in Fig. 1.

It is worth mentioning that the patient had been breeding birds and had close contact with them for the past three years. He had no history of skin trauma within 1 month before the outbreak of painless papules.

On admission, the patient's main complaints were mild fever, painful and persistent skin lesions with painful and swollen left knee that made him unable to stand or walk. For the past few days, he also had headache that was dull in nature, extended from anterior to posterior and was worse in the afternoon. He also had 5–6 bowel movements/day with loose stool. He did not have symptoms of cough and short breaths during this illness.

He looked thin, pale, anemic, and was only able to sit with support. His temperature was 38.5 °C. He had no neck stiffness, no hepatosplenomegaly or lymphadenopathy. His left leg had intense inflammation (red, swollen, hot, and tender) that resembled cellulitis.

He also had multiple ulcers on his body. The 10 × 15 cm ulcer on his left chest (Fig. 2) was deep with visible capillaries at the base, purulent and bleeding. A group of skin lesions 5 × 10 cm was seen on his right arm (Fig. 3). There were multiples papules, which some of them progressed into nodules and ulcers (Fig. 3). The largest and deepest ulcer (15 × 20 cm) was on his right

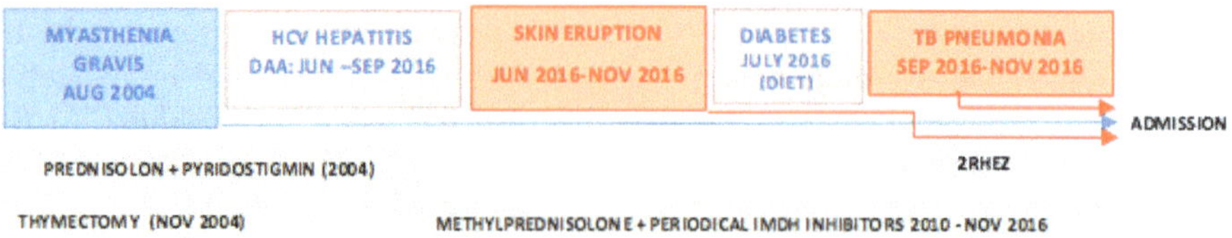

Fig. 1 Chronological order of the patient's medical history

thigh (Fig. 4). It was necrotic, purulent, bleeding, and had visible capillaries and small bullous with cloudy fluid in the margins. The presentation of the ulcerative skin lesions simulated Pyoderma gangrenosum.

On complete blood count, the patient was found to have low hemoglobin (7.6 g/dL) and low red blood cells (RBC) count (2.64 M/mL). The white blood cells (WBC) and platelets counts were within the normal ranges. The first blood culture was negative. HIV testing was negative while his CD4 count was remarkably low (236 cells/mL). The MRI of the head did not reveal any lesions in the brain and the chest X-Ray was normal.

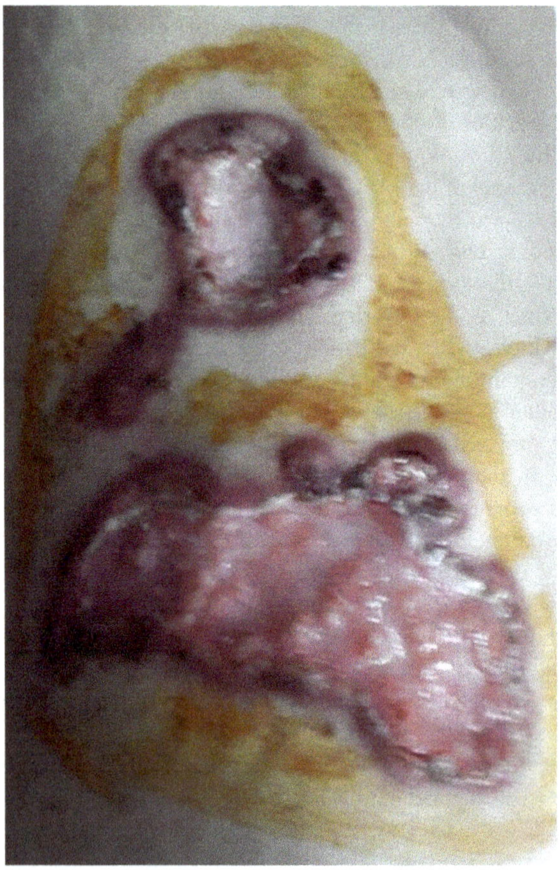

Fig. 2 Large, deep, ulcers on the left chest at 1st day of admission. *Cryptococcus neoformans* was detected upon culturing fluids expressed from these ulcers

The fluids from his bullous skin lesions were collected for microbiology stain and culture. These results came back negative for bacteria. Despite the negative culture, the patient was treated empirically with a combination of meropenem and vancomycin for fourteen days. During the time under antibiotics, the patient was still fever. The headache and skin lesions and were not improved.

The skin biopsy of the chest and leg ulcers was performed subsequently. The histopathological results detected the spores of cryptococcosis inside the macrophages (Figs. 5 and 6).

The patient underwent a lumbar puncture at admission. The cerebral spinal fluid opening pressure was 9 cm H_20 and all the opening pressures afterwards were normal. The analysis of the cerebral spinal fluid (CSF) detected elevated protein levels (1.61 g/L), mildly decreased glucose level (2.14 mmol/L, serum glucose: 4.84 mmol/L), lactate of 3.76 mmol/L and a white cell count of 112 cells/μL with neutrophilic predominance (78%). Lateral flow assay (LFA) test of the CSF was positive for cryptococcal antigen. The CSF cultures, however, were negative for both bacteria and fungi. Hence, the second culture of the smear of the skin ulcers was performed and was positive for *C. neoformans* and negative for bacteria.

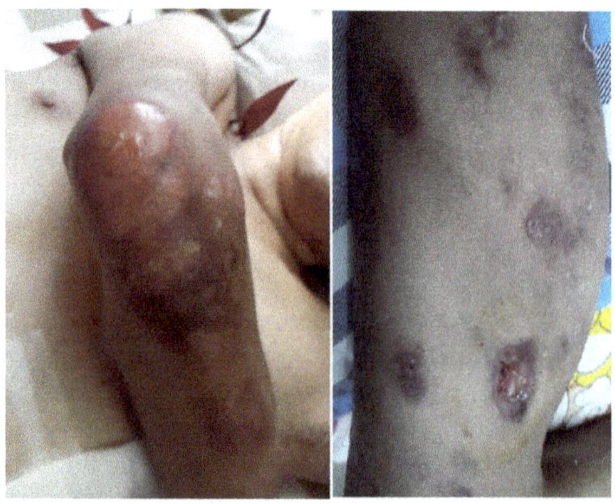

Fig. 3 The cutaneous lesions at 1st day of admission: right arm (left) and left leg (right)

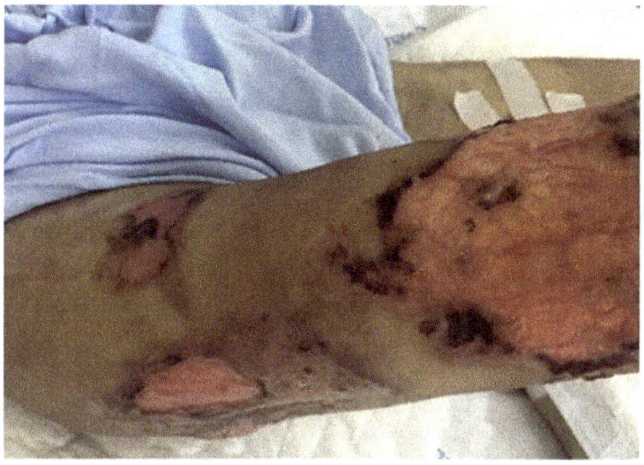

Fig. 4 Ulcers on the right thigh at day 11 after admission. The ulcers were deep and with pus and bled when it was cleaned by nurse

Subsequently, the patient was started on amphotericin B (1 mg/kg/day) and fluconazole (800 mg/day) firstly in parallel with methyl prednisolone, azathioprine, pyridostigmine and anti-tuberculosis regimen. As planned, amphotericin B and fluconazole would be continued for 28 day. Fluconazole, for consolidation, would be continued for 11 months later.

The fever subsided after 4 days of treatment with amphotericin B and fluconazole but the patient still complained a severe headache. The neurologist considered the immune suppression effect of azathioprine, the stable status of MG and the low CD4 cell count and decided stopping azathioprine and lowered the methyl prednisolone dose to 4 mg/day for better control of Cryptococcal infection. The patient's hypokalemia, attributed to amphotericin B, was also corrected via oral potassium replacement.

A dramatic clinical and microbiologic improvement was observed after 11 days of treatment: the anemic status improved with hemoglobin level increasing to 9.0 g/dL without RBC transfusion, the headache subsided, the meningeal signs disappeared and the patient became afebrile. The ulcers became smaller, with no exudates, granulated and improved quickly. The culture of skin ulcers on day 10 post-treatment was negative for both bacteria and fungi.

On day 14 of treatment, the WBC count of the CSF dropped to 19 cells/mL and the LFA test became negative; the glucose level was 3.53 mmol/L (serum glucose: 10.87 mmol/L) and the protein remained high (1.66 g/L).

On day 28 of treatment, the WBC count of the CSF was 12 cells/mL, the protein was 1.34 g/L, the glucose was 2.82 mmol/L (serum glucose: 6.02 mmol/L). The lactate level dropped to 2.48 mmol/L but the LFA test was positive again although the fungus culture was still negative in the CSF. The skin ulcer cultures were negative also for both bacteria and fungi.

After 28 days of treatment, amphotericin B was stopped and fluconazole (1000 mg) was consolidated until 12 months of treatment as recommended. We used a high dose of fluconazole because the patient was using rifamycin (anti-tuberculosis) which is known to reduce the level of fluconazole.

The patient was finally discharged on day 32. He had also been advised to avoid contact with birds. The cutaneous lesions on the day of discharge are shown on (Fig. 7).

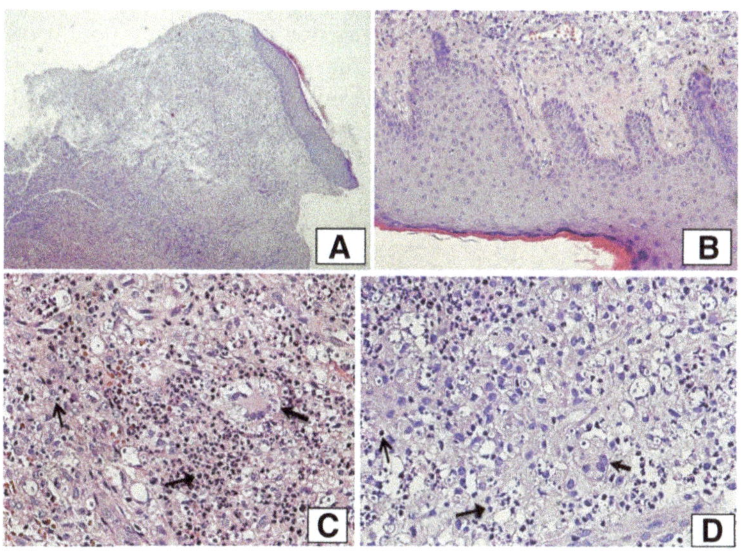

Fig. 5 a and **b.** Light microscopic view (HE ×200 and HE ×400) of ulcer tissue from chest and leg shows loss of the epidermis and some portions of the dermis and subcutaneous fat. Lymphocyte and macrophages infiltrates with neutrophiles. **c** and **d:** The dermal infiltrates consisted of lymphocytes (↑) and a few monocytes-macrophages (**←**); and numerous neutrophils (**→**) created sporadic focal abscesses

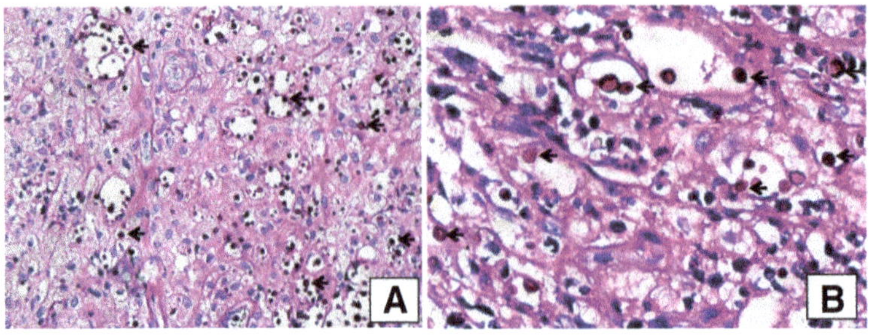

Fig. 6 a and **b.** PAS-stained (PAS ×400 & PAS ×1000) showing numerous Cryptococcal spores inside macrophages (←) that stain positive with PAS. *Ziehl-Neelson stain was negative for acid-fast bacilli*

The patient will be re-examined every two months during the time of fluconazole maintenance.

Discussion

Cryptococcosis in HIV-uninfected patients almost always develops in the setting of immunocompromised status, such as patient with organ transplant, with malignancies or on chronic immunosuppressive treatment (e.g., corticosteroids) [12]. The development of cutaneous cryptococcosis is exceedingly rare in HIV-uninfected population.

Here, our patient has multiple risk factors. He has been on prolonged immunosuppressive therapy and had a low $CD4^+$ cell count (236 cells/mL). Additionally, he had also been diagnosed with diabetes mellitus which is considered a clue for immune dysfunction [13]. Moreover, the patient also had tuberculosis, which most likely resulted from reactivation of a latent infection, another warning for weakening of the immune system. All of these coexisting factors in this patient revealed a high susceptibility to opportunistic agents such as *Cryptococcus neoformans.*

Our patient had a prolonged course of cutaneous lesions (more than 5 months) before the final diagnoses was figured out. This can be justified by the great variation in cutaneous cryptococcus presentations and the rarity of this kind of infection in HIV-uninfected patients.

Additionally, in our case the initial bacterial culture of the fluid from the skin lesions was negative. Nevertheless, by the time of histopathological detecting of spores from the ulcer, the repeated culture of the smear from skin lesion for both fungal and bacteria was also positive for *Cryptococcus.* This adds to the complexity of making the diagnosis and provides an additional evidence that histopathology has a core role in making a rapid diagnosis of the disease – as many times the culture fails to flourish the pathogen [14]. The culture of the bullous fluid or smears from the ulcers was more sensitive for bacterial pathogens, but less helpful for fungal pathogens, especially when suspected fungal pathogens were not specifically notified by the clinician.

From this case, we recommended physicians to perform a culture for yeast in all skin lesions in immunosuppressed patients or to perform a Lateral Flow Assay (LFA). The cryptococcal antigen LFA is a rapid, very sensitive, easy-to-perform assay with a demonstrated usefulness as a point-of-care assay for diagnosing cryptococcosis in resource-limited countries. The availability of this assay in remote locations could have a meaningful impact on early diagnosis of cryptococcosis [15].

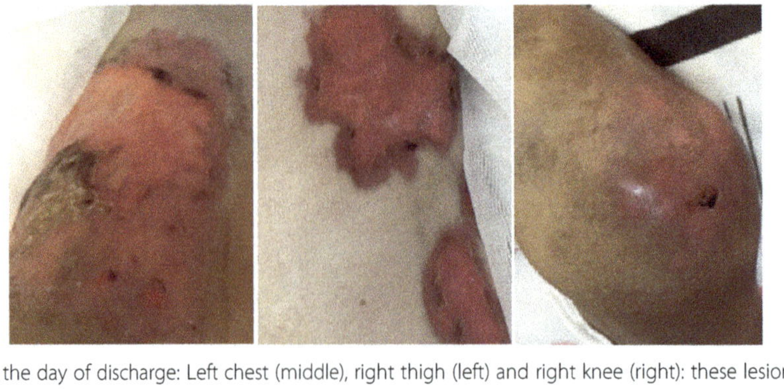

Fig. 7 Cutaneous lesions at the day of discharge: Left chest (middle), right thigh (left) and right knee (right): these lesions were reduced in size compared to initial lesions

Despite being reported many times in the literature, arguments continue on the existence of primary cutaneous cryptococcosis versus cutaneous cryptococcosis being only secondary to hematogenous dissemination [16].

The patient had no history of skin trauma but he had bred birds many months in the past. He could had skin cuts once or several times without his notification. We could not precisely conclude whether he was acquired the cryptococcus through skin lesion or through respiratory aspiration of Cryptococcal spores. However, in case of aspiration the chronological sequence should be: firstly presentation of lung infection with respiratory symptoms and signs, bacteremia later, and lastly meningitis or skin appearances. His true progression was reversed with the skin ulcer were found several months in advance, the meningeal affect (headache, fever) progressed much later after the presentation of skin lesions, and the lung was not been affected at the time of menigitis. Therefore, the patient should be a case of primary cutaneous Cryptococosis, circulatory disseminated and secondary menigitis.

It is worth mentioning that, similar to our case, systemic or disseminated infections can firstly present solely with skin lesions and later progress to involve other organs such as the meninges [17]. Hence, a high index of suspicion is required to reach to an early diagnosis.

The treatment recommendation for HIV-uninfected patients who are diagnosed with cryptococcal meningoencephalitis is to give induction therapy with amphotericin B for 2–4 weeks followed by consolidation with fluconazole (400–800 mg/day) for 12 months [12]. In our case, however, after induction with Amphotericin B, we adjusted the dose of fluconazole into 900–1000 mg/day as the patient was receiving rifampicin which is known to reduce the blood level of fluconazole [18].

In case of cryptococcosis persisted during treatment or recurred after sufficient therapy, then we should consider antifungal resistance, relapse or immune reconstitution inflammatory syndrome. Resistance, that comes if we never achieve CSF sterility, could occur with low dose of fluconazole, especially if it is used as a monotherapy. We could deal with relapse by re-induction therapy with amphotericin at high doses (1 mg/kg/day) for at least seven days and fluconazole dose could be increased up to 1200 mg/day [19]. On the other hand, sudden onset deterioration with worsening meningitis symptoms along with CSF sterility or stable titers of cryptococcal antigen support the diagnosis of immune reconstitution inflammatory syndrome [20].

This is not the first case in literature to report cryptococcosis in patients with MG [8–11, 21–23]. And although not surprising in a MG patient on chronic immunosuppression, this is only the eighth case reporting on such association. Infections in previously reported cases were in the forms of meningitis in three cases [8, 9, 11], prostatic abscess in one case [21], prosthetic joint infection in one case [22], cryptococcal cellulitis [10] in one case and disseminated cryptococcal infection in one case [23].

However, despite the fact that patients with diseases of the lymphatic systems are prone to fungal infections [11], this simultaneous occurrence of cryptococcosis and MG could be only a pure coincidence and directly attributed to the steroids-induced immunosuppression status.

Conclusion

This case is an opportunity to emphasize on the importance of including cutaneous cryptococcosis in the differential diagnosis of cutaneous lesions in patients on chronic immunosuppressive therapy, especially if the skin lesions are resistant to empiric antibiotic treatment. The cutaneous manifestations of cryptococcosis can be the first clue for a disseminated disease, which makes early recognition crucial and life-saving.

Abbreviations

C. gatti: *Cryptococcus gatti*; *C. neoformans*: *Cryptococcus neoformans*.; CSF: Cerebral spinal fluid.; DAAs: Directly-acting antivirals.; LFA: Lateral flow assay.; MG: Myasthenia gravis.; RBC: Red blood cells.; WBC: White blood cells.

Acknowledgment

Not applicable.

Funding

The authors declare that they have no funding source.

Authors' contribution

All authors have read and approved the final manuscript. All authors (NTCH, NMH, LAT, NTBL, NTT, NTHM, AMAA, SM, SS, NBT, VTT and PTLH) helped on the diagnosis, data collection and scientific writing.

Competing interests

The authors declare that they have no competing interests.

Author details

[1]Department of Infectious Diseases, University of Medicine and Pharmacy at Ho Chi Minh City , Ho Chi Minh city, Vietnam. [2]Faculty of Medicine, University of Jordan, Amman, Jordan. [3]Dermatology and Venereology Department, Tanta University Hospital, Tanta, Egypt. [4]Biochemistry Department, Faculty of Medicine, Tanta University, Tanta, Egypt. [5]Ho Chi Minh City Hospital of Dermatology-Venereology, Ho Chi Minh City, Vietnam. [6]The Hospital for Tropical Diseases, Ho Chi Minh City, Vietnam. [7]Department of Dermatology, University of Medicine and Pharmacy at Ho Chi Minh City, Ho Chi Minh City, Vietnam. [8]Oxford University Clinical Research Unit, Ho Chi Minh City, Vietnam. [9]Department of Neurology, University of Medicine and Pharmacy at Ho Chi Minh City, Ho Chi Minh City, Vietnam.

References

1. Christianson JC, Engber W, Andes D. Primary cutaneous cryptococcosis in immunocompetent and immunocompromised hosts. Med Mycol. 2003; 41(3):177–88.
2. Murakami Y, Oki M, Saka H, Kajikawa S, Murakami A, Ishida A. Disseminated cryptococcosis presenting as mediastinal and hilar lymphadenopathy in an immunocompetent patient. Respirology Case Reports. 2016;4(4):e00167.

3. Raberahona M, Rakotoarivelo RA, Randriamampionona N, Rakotomalala AF, Razafinambinintsoa T, Bénet T, Vanhems P, Randria MJDD, Cornet M, Rakoto-Andrianarivelo M: Rapid Fatal Outcome of Cryptococcal Meningoencephalitis in a Non-HIV Immunocompromised Patient with a Low Fluconazole Susceptibility Isolate: A Case Report from Madagascar Case Reports in Infectious Diseases 2016, 2016: ID 3492504, http://dx.doi.org/10.1155/2016/3492504.
4. Chowdhary A, Rhandhawa HS, Prakash A, Meis JF. Environmental prevalence of *Cryptococcus neoformans* and Cryptococcus gattii in India: an update. Crit Rev Microbiol. 2012;38(1):1–16.
5. Baddley JW. Schain dc Fau - Gupte AA, Gupte aa Fau - Lodhi SA, Lodhi Sa Fau - Kayler LK, Kayler Lk Fau - Frade JP, Frade Jp Fau - Lockhart SR, Lockhart Sr Fau - Chiller T, Chiller T Fau - Bynon JS, Jr., Bynon Js Jr Fau - bower WA, bower WA: transmission of *Cryptococcus neoformans* by organ transplantation. Clin Infect Dis. 2011;52:e94–8.
6. Lagrou K. Van Eldere J Fau - Keuleers S, Keuleers S Fau - Hagen F, Hagen F Fau - Merckx R, Merckx R Fau - Verhaegen J, Verhaegen J Fau - Peetermans WE, Peetermans we Fau - Boekhout T, Boekhout T: zoonotic transmission of *Cryptococcus neoformans* from a magpie to an immunocompetent patient. Journal of Internal of Medicine. 2005;257(4):385–8.
7. Neuville S, Dromer F, Morin O, Dupont B, Ronin O, Lortholary O. French Cryptococcosis study G: primary cutaneous Cryptococcosis: a distinct clinical entity. Clin Infect Dis. 2003;36(3):337–47.
8. Schmidt S, Padberg F. Late onset immunodeficiency in a patient with recurrent thymic carcinoma and myasthenia gravis. J Neurol Sci. 1998;157(2):201–5.
9. Lorenzoni PJ, Scola RH, Kay CS, Almeida SM, Muro MD, Burigo IP, Carraro H Jr, Werneck LC. Myasthenia gravis complicated with cryptococcal meningitis after thymectomy and long-term immunosuppressive therapy. Arq Neuropsiquiatr. 2011;69(2b):410–1.
10. Lafleur L, Beaty S, Colome-Grimmer MI, LaForte RA, Dotson AD. Cryptococcal cellulitis in a patient on prednisone monotherapy for myasthenia gravis. Cutis. 2004;74(3):165–70.
11. Rowland LP, Griffiths CO, Kabat EA. Myasthenia gravis, thymoma and cryptococcal meningitis. N Engl J Med. 1965;273(12):620–7.
12. Pappas PG. Cryptococcal infections in non-Hiv-infected patients. Trans Am Clin Climatol Assoc. 2013;124:61–79.
13. Geerlings SE, Hoepelman AI. Immune dysfunction in patients with diabetes mellitus (DM). FEMS Immunol Med Microbiol. 1999;26(3–4):259–65.
14. Gonzalez Santiago TM, Pritt B, Gibson LE, Comfere NI. Diagnosis of deep cutaneous fungal infections: correlation between skin tissue culture and histopathology. J Am Acad Dermatol. 2014;71(2):293–301.
15. Lindsley MD, Mekha N, Baggett HC, Surinthong Y, Autthateinchai R, Sawatwong P, Harris JR, Park BJ, Chiller T, Balajee SA, et al. Evaluation of a newly developed lateral flow immunoassay for the diagnosis of cryptococcosis. Clinical infectious diseases : an official publication of the Infectious Diseases Society of America. 2011;53(4):321–5.
16. Neuville S, Dromer F, Morin O, Dupont B, Ronin O, Lortholary O, Group FCS. Primary cutaneous cryptococcosis: a distinct clinical entity. Clin Infect Dis. 2003;36(3):337–47.
17. Nascimento E. Bonifacio da Silva ME, Martinez R, von Zeska Kress MR: primary cutaneous cryptococcosis in an immunocompetent patient due to Cryptococcus gattii molecular type VGI in Brazil: a case report and review of literature. Mycoses. 2014;57(7):442–7.
18. Ayudhya DPN, Thanompuangseree N, Tansuphaswadikul S. Effect of rifampicin on the pharmacokinetics of fluconazole in patients with AIDS. Clin Pharmacokinet. 2004;43(11):725–32.
19. Musubire AK, Boulware DR, Meya DB, Rhein J. Diagnosis and Management of Cryptococcal Relapse. *Journal of AIDS & clinical research*. Suppl. 2013;3(3):S3–003.
20. Boulware DR, Bonham SC, Meya DB, Wiesner DL, Park GS, Kambugu A, Janoff EN, Bohjanen PR. Paucity of initial cerebrospinal fluid inflammation in cryptococcal meningitis is associated with subsequent immune reconstitution inflammatory syndrome. The Journal of infectious diseases. 2010;202(6):962–70.
21. Yip SK, Cheng C, Wong MY, Tan BH, Sim CS, Lim SH. Cryptococcal prostatic abscess in an immunocompromised patient: a case report and review of the literature. Ann Acad Med Singap. 1998;27(6):873–6.
22. Shah NB, Shoham S, Nayak S. *Cryptococcus neoformans* Prosthetic joint infection: case report and review of the literature. Mycopathologia. 2015; 179(3–4):275–8.
23. Narayanan S, Banerjee C, Holt PA. Cryptococcal immune reconstitution syndrome during steroid withdrawal treated with hydroxychloroquine. Int J Infect Dis. 2011;15(1):e70–3.

22

New molecular tools for meningitis diagnostics in Ethiopia – a necessary step towards improving antimicrobial prescription

Guro K. Bårnes[1,2], Esayas Kebede Gudina[3], Melkamu Berhane[3], Alemseged Abdissa[3], Getnet Tesfaw[3], Gemeda Abebe[3,5], Siri Laura Feruglio[1], Dominique A. Caugant[1,2*] and Hannah Joan Jørgensen[1,4]

Abstract

Background: Meningitis remains a top cause of premature death and loss of disability-adjusted life years in low-income countries. In resource-limited settings, proper laboratory diagnostics are often scarce and knowledge about national and local epidemiology is limited. Misdiagnosis, incorrect treatment and overuse of antibiotics are potential consequences, especially for viral meningitis.

Methods: A prospective study was conducted over three months in a teaching hospital in Ethiopia with limited laboratory resources. Cerebrospinal fluid (CSF) samples from patients with suspected meningitis were analysed using a multiplex PCR-based system (FilmArray, BioFire), in addition to basic routine testing with microscopy and culture. Clinical data, as well as information on treatment and outcome were collected.

Results: Two hundred and eighteen patients were included; 117 (54%) neonates (0–29 days), 63 (29%) paediatrics (1 month-15 years) and 38 (17%) adults (≥16 years). Of 218 CSF samples, 21 (10%) were PCR positive; 4% in neonates, 14% in paediatrics and 18% in adults. Virus was detected in 57% of the PCR positive samples, bacteria in 33% and fungi in 10%. All CSF samples that were PCR positive for a bacterial agent had a white cell count ≥75 cells/mm^3 and/or turbid appearance. The majority (90%) of patients received more than one antibiotic for treatment of the meningitis episode. There was no difference in the mean number of different antibiotics received or in the cumulative number of days with antibiotic treatment between patients with a microorganism detected in CSF and those without.

Conclusions: A rapid molecular diagnostic system was successfully implemented in an Ethiopian setting without previous experience of molecular diagnostics. Viral meningitis was diagnosed for the first time in routine clinical practice in Ethiopia, and viral agents were the most commonly detected microorganisms in CSF. This study illustrates the potential of rapid diagnostic tests for reducing antibiotic usage in suspected meningitis cases. However, the cost of consumables for the molecular diagnostic system used in this study limits its use in low-income countries.

Keywords: Cerebrospinal fluid, FilmArray, Multiplex PCR, Viral meningitis, Bacterial meningitis

* Correspondence: dominique.caugant@fhi.no
[1]Division for Infection Control and Environmental Health, Norwegian Institute of Public Health, Oslo, Norway
[2]Faculty of Medicine, University of Oslo, Oslo, Norway
Full list of author information is available at the end of the article

Background

Meningitis remains a major cause of mortality and morbidity worldwide. In Ethiopia, it is an important cause of premature death and disability, being the 9th most common cause of years of life lost and loss of disability-adjusted life years [1]. In addition to the morbidity and mortality associated with meningitis, the disease also represents a huge burden on affected families and the health care system, especially in low-income countries. One case of meningococcal disease in sub-Saharan Africa has been estimated to cost the household 90 US dollar (USD), equal to 34% of the annual gross domestic product per capita, and an additional 154 USD if the disease leads to sequelae [2].

Early treatment is essential in the clinical management of meningitis. A delay in therapy negatively affects the prognosis for patients with both bacterial [3] and viral [4] meningitis/encephalitis. Empiric antimicrobial therapy is therefore initiated on suspicion, before laboratory results are available [5, 6]. Traditionally, laboratory diagnostics of meningitis have included examination of cerebrospinal fluid (CSF) for white blood cells (WBC), measurement of glucose and protein levels, and Gram staining. These are rapid, low-cost analyses but do not have satisfactory specificity alone [7, 8]. When septicemia is additionally suspected, peripheral blood WBC count is usually obtained, but this analysis also suffers from a lack of sensitivity and specificity [9, 10]. Positive bacterial cultures from CSF can provide a definite diagnosis, but may take several days and quality requirements are high. Therefore, rapid molecular diagnostics have become routine in meningitis diagnostics in high-income countries.

In many low-income countries, poor laboratory services impede the quality of health care. Ethiopia is experiencing high gross domestic product growth, but the per capita income remains one of the lowest in the world [11]. Healthcare in Ethiopia is under-resourced, and laboratory services are weak. Inadequate and delayed microbiological services foster distrust in the value of laboratory testing among clinicians, and reduce their inclination to submit clinical samples for analyses. Ultimately, this compromises patient care, prevention of infectious diseases and antibiotic stewardship.

More often than not, in Ethiopia and other low-resource settings patients receive an inadequate diagnostic workup [12] and decisions to treat meningitis are based on clinical findings alone. This approach lacks accuracy [13, 14] and ultimately results in unjustified prescriptions of antibiotics [12]. Incorrect use of antimicrobials is a recognized challenge in Ethiopia, with delayed initiation, unindicated use, duplication of broad spectrum antimicrobials and unnecessarily long duration of treatment being the major problems [15]. Fortunately, in the last few years greater attention has been paid to antimicrobial resistance also in Ethiopia, where it is becoming an increasing concern [16].

Recently, a rapid molecular diagnostic system (FilmArray, BioFire; http://www.biomerieux-usa.com/clinical/biofire-film-array) was developed for multiplex testing for the most common causes of infectious syndromes. The system is closed and integrates nucleic acid extraction and nested PCR for detection of the pathogens included in the panels. It is easy to use, has a low risk of sample contamination, requires little hands-on time and limited prior training in molecular diagnostics. For each sample, a kit that contains all necessary reagents is used, and sample preparation takes only a couple of minutes. These features are advantageous in settings with limited experience and limited facilities for molecular analyses. The main limitation for use in such settings is the high cost of test-kits.

The aim of this study was to investigate which infectious agents were responsible for meningitis in a region of Ethiopia where treatment decisions are usually made without microbiological results. We demonstrated that an easy-to-use and reliable molecular diagnostic instrument could set the ground for improving patient management and reducing usage of antimicrobials in a resource-limited setting.

Methods

Study design and population

This prospective study was performed between March 20th and June 20th 2017, at Jimma University Specialized Hospital (JUSH), one of the oldest public hospitals in Ethiopia, established in 1937. It is the only teaching and referral hospital in the southwestern part of the country and serves a catchment population of 15–20 million. The hospital has 600 beds and 1621 staff members, providing services for 218,095 outpatients, 16,778 inpatients, 14,207 emergencies and 5,973 deliveries yearly (data from September 2016 to September 2017). Other public health services in the catchment area include five primary hospitals, one army hospital, 118 health centres and 482 health posts.

All patients with a clinical suspicion of meningitis and from whom a CSF sample was available for analyses were eligible for inclusion. The study was run as an integrated part of routine practice and inclusion was done by the treating physicians. A written consent was given by the participants, or by parents or guardians in the case of children or unconscious patients. As samples were taken as part of routine diagnostic practice, participation in the study required no additional interventions.

Before the start of the study, a general introduction of the project aims and procedures, to the new instrument and interpretation of results was given to all medical doctors at the pediatric and internal medicine department. A four-hour training on how to perform analysis with the FilmArray was given to four dedicated JUSH staff members at the bacteriology department. Results of the PCR analysis are generated automatically by the FilmArray software and are reported as either negative, or positive with a defined species. Two senior medical doctors (study investigators) associated with the pediatric and medical wards, respectively, acted as supervisors for other physicians on the wards during the project. They were responsible for follow-up, and supported treating physicians with clinical/treatment implications of the laboratory results. The first author, a medical doctor, was present at JUSH during the project period and followed up data collection. Sample analyses, reporting of results and clinical decisions about treatment were done by local JUSH staff.

Clinical data, treatment, routine investigations and outcome

Patient data were collected on a structured case record form. The treating physician collected the consent and clinical data at admission while microbiological analysis and results were documented by laboratory staff. Laboratory results were, according to routine at JUSH bacteriology laboratory, collected by the treating physician and the paper transcript of the laboratory result was kept in the patient chart. Results were also intended to be immediately reported to the treating physician by cellular phone. However, the latter additional reporting was not always complied with in practice. Data on treatment, routine investigations and outcome were collected by study investigators (all medical doctors), either at discharge or retrospectively within one month of discharge. Patients with none or incomplete data on treatment, routine investigations and outcome were excluded from the relevant statistical/data analyses, but included in analyses on clinical and laboratory data.

Sample collection

CSF samples were collected in sterile glass tubes for neonates and paediatrics and in sterile plastic tubes (5 ml, Sartstedt, Germany) for adults. They were transported to the laboratory at ambient temperature within ten minutes and laboratory analyses were started within two hours, but usually within 30 min. For patients with suspected concomitant septicemia, blood was collected in blood culture bottles using BD BACTEC Peds Plus (Becton Dickinson (BD), Franklin Lakes, NJ, USA) for paediatric patients and BD BACTEC Plus Aerobic medium (BD) for adult patients.

Conventional laboratory analyses of CSF

CSF samples were processed according to standard procedures at JUSH which include bacteriological culture, macroscopic assessment, protein and glucose measurements, manual WBC count with differential count and Gram staining. India ink staining and rapid cryptococcal antigen testing (CrAg, IMMY, OK, USA) were performed upon request. Gram stain was performed on the primary sample, usually without centrifugation due to lack of equipment and/or consumables. CSF glucose and protein measurements, were performed when reagents were available. CSF samples were cultured onto blood agar (BD) and/or chocolate agar (BD) for 72 h at 35 °C in a CO_2-enriched incubator (candle jar). Routine bacterial identification was based on colony morphology, Gram staining and standard biochemical reactions [17].

Molecular diagnostic of CSF

All CSF samples included in the study were analysed using the meningitis/encephalitis (ME) panel (bioMérieux, Marcy l'Etoile, France) on the FilmArray (bioMérieux,) multiplex PCR system. The closed system performs nucleic acid extraction, reverse transcription and multiplex nested PCR, automatically interprets end-point melting curve data and provides the result. The ME panel tests for genetic targets from *Escherichia coli* K1, *Haemophilus influenzae, Listeria monocytogenes, Neisseria meningitidis, Streptococcus agalactiae, Streptococcus pneumoniae*, cytomegalovirus, enterovirus, herpes simplex virus 1 (HSV-1), herpes simplex virus 2 (HSV-2), human herpesvirus 6 (HHV-6), human parechovirus, varicella zoster virus (VZV) and *Cryptococcus neoformans/gattii*. Analyses were performed according to the manufacturer's instructions [18]. A flow-chart of the sample analysis with the FilmArray is shown in Additional file 1: Figure S1.

Other laboratory analysis

CSF samples from patients with suspected tuberculous meningitis (clinical suspicion, HIV-positivity, or no improvement on conventional antibiotic treatment) were tested for *Mycobacterium tuberculosis* with the GeneXpert MTB/RIF assay (Dx System Version 4.0c, Cepheid Inc., CA, US) [19]. CSF was processed as recommended by the manufacturer: a 2:1 volume of the reagent supplied with the assay was added directly to the sample. The mixture was vortexed and incubated at room temperature for 15 min. Two mL of the reagent-sample mix was then transferred to the Xpert cartridge and analysed.

Blood culture bottles were incubated in an automated blood culture incubator BACTEC FX40 system (BD) for a maximum of five days and flagged as either "negative" or "positive" for bacterial growth. Positive blood cultures were analysed using the FilmArray blood culture identification (BCID) panel (BioMerieux, France) [20], and cultured onto blood agar (BD), MacConkey agar (BD) and chocolate agar (BD), with the same routine bacterial identification as for CSF cultures.

Other investigations, such as malaria testing using peripheral blood smear and May-Grünwald-Giemsa staining, rapid testing for HIV, haematological and biochemical analyses were performed according to routine practice at JUSH.

Data management and statistical analysis

All data were entered into a Microsoft Excel 2013 database. Statistical analyses were performed in Microsoft Excel 2013 or in GraphPad Prism 5. Two-sided tests were used and a p-value < 0.05 was considered statistically significant.

Results

Patient characteristics

During the study period, CSF samples from 220 patients with suspected meningitis were analysed at the laboratory. Of these, 218 patients gave consent and were included in the study; 42% were female. The study population consisted of 117 (54%) neonates (0–29 days), 63 (29%) paediatrics (1 month-15 years) and 38 (17%) adults (≥16 years). Demographic data and the number of samples taken per age group is shown in Fig. 1.

Laboratory results

Conventional laboratory investigations

In 213 (97%) of the 218 CSF samples, the macroscopic appearance was recorded. Glucose was measured in 42 (19%) of the samples and a manual cell count was performed in 201 (92%). In 49% of these samples, no cells were detected, and 18% of the samples contained blood which prohibited the cell count. In the remaining 33% of samples WBC were detected and a differential count was available for 91% of these. Gram stain was performed in 217 samples, but microorganisms were observed in only three (bacteria in two and fungal elements in one). In total, 213 (97%) of the samples were cultured and only one sample was positive (*Klebsiella pneumoniae*) (Table 1). Hence, altogether only four (2%) of the CSF samples included in the study were found to be positive for microorganisms using conventional methods (microscopy and/or culture).

Molecular diagnostics

In 21 (10%) of the CSF samples, pathogens were detected by PCR using the FilmArray ME panel ($n = 20$) and BCID panel ($n = 1$). Using the ME panel, viral agents were detected in 57% (HHV-6, HSV-1, enterovirus, HSV-2, varicella zoster virus), bacteria in 33% (*H. influenzae, S. pneumoniae, E. coli, N. meningitidis*) and fungi in 10% (*C. neoformans/gattii*) (Fig. 2). Only one CSF sample was culture positive, but this sample was negative by FilmArray using the ME-panel. The culture was identified as *K. pneumoniae*, which is not included in the ME panel. The CSF sample was therefore analysed by FilmArray using the BCID panel, which confirmed positivity. A blood culture sample from the same patient was also *K. pneumoniae*-positive by the BCID panel.

The proportion of positive CSF samples increased with age with 4% in neonates, 14% in paediatrics and 18% in adults (Fig. 1). Table 2 shows the results of the CSF analyses and patient outcome for samples where a pathogen was detected.

Thirty two (15%) participants had blood cultures taken. Overall 12 (38%) of these were positive including 1 of 2 samples from adults, 5 of 21 samples from paediatrics and 6 of 9 samples from neonates. Two patients were positive for microorganisms in both CSF and blood culture. One patient had *K. pneumoniae* detected in both samples, CSF by culture and blood by FilmArray, while the other had HSV-1 detected in CSF and *Enterococcus spp.* detected in blood, both by FilmArray. For positive blood cultures, routine culture confirmed bacterial isolates in all samples, although in one individual, only *K. pneumoniae* was identified by culture, while the BCID panel in addition to identifying *K. pneumoniae*

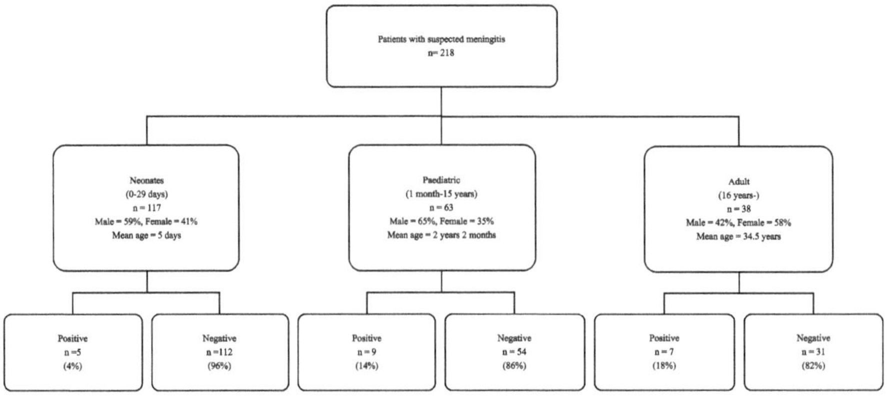

Fig. 1 Study participants and results from analyses of cerebrospinal fluid (CSF) samples using FilmArray and culture with respect to detection of a microorganism (positive) or not (negative). Flow chart of study participants, demographics and CSF samples

Table 1 Laboratory investigations of cerebrospinal fluid (CSF) samples and peripheral blood count of patients with suspected meningitis

	Microorganism detected								No microorganism detected	
	All		Virus		Bacteria		Fungi			
	n	(%)	n	(%)	n	(%)	n	(%)	n	(%)
Macroscopic appearance of CSF										
n	21		12		7		2		192	
Clear	11	(52)	9	(75)	1	(14)	1	(50)	133	(69)
Bloody	2	(10)	2	(17)	0	(0)	0	(0)	48	(25)
Turbid	7	(33)	0	(0)	6	(86)	1	(50)	3	(2)
Xanthochromic	1	(5)	1	(8)	0	(0)	0	(0)	8	(4)
	n	mean	n	mean	n	mean	n	mean	n	mean
Glucose measurement (mg/mL)	5	27	1	47	4	22	0		37	56
Manual cell count using Neubauer chamber	n	(%)	n	(%)	n	(%)	n	(%)	n	(%)
Total	21		12		7		2		180	
Not done due to bloody sample	1	(5)	1	(8)	0	(0)	1	(50)	35	(19)
No cells	5	(24)	5	(42)	0	(0)	0	(0)	94	(52)
Cell count ≥ 10 cells/mm3	12	(57)	4	(33)	7	(100)	1	(50)	11	(6)
Mean cells/mm3		2740		70		7716		9		91
Median cells/mm3		50		5		2500		9		0
Max. cells/mm3		40,000		332		40,000		13		9
Min. cells/mm3		0		0		75		5		0
	n	mean % PMN	n	mean % PMN	n	mean % PMN	n	mean % PMN	n	mean % PMN
Differential count using Neubauer chamber	14	(30)	6	(0)	7	(60)	1	(0)	45	(3)
Gram staining/India ink staining	n	(%)	n	(%)	n	(%)	n	(%)	n	(%)
Total	21		12		7		2		196	
No organisms seen	18	(86)	12	(100)	5	(71)	1	(50)	196	(100)
Positive	3[a]	(14)	0	(0)	2[a]	(29)	1[a]	(50)	0	(0)
Complete blood count (CBC), peripheral blood	n	mean	n	mean	n	mean	n	mean	n	mean
White blood count (× 10^9/L)	16	10.5	9	8.3	6	14.7	1	4.7	134	14.2
Neutrophils (× 10^9/L)	16	6.8	9	3.9	6	11.5	1	3.9	100	7.8
Lymphocyte count (× 10^9/L)	16	2.4	9	3.1	6	1.8	1	0.3	117	3.5

PMN polymorphonuclear leukocytes

[a]The samples positive by Gram strain had Gram-positive cocci (n = 1, CSF positive for *Streptococcus pneumoniae* on rapid molecular diagnostic (RMD), cell count 2500 (5% lymphocytes, 95% neutrophils), Gram-negative coccobacilli (n = 1, CSF positive for *Haemophilus influenzae* on RMD, cell count 40,000 with 90% lymphocytes, 10% neutrophils) and fungal elements (*n* = 1, CSF positive for *Cryptococcus neoformans/gattii* on RMD, cell count 13 with 100% lymphocytes). All three samples were negative on culture

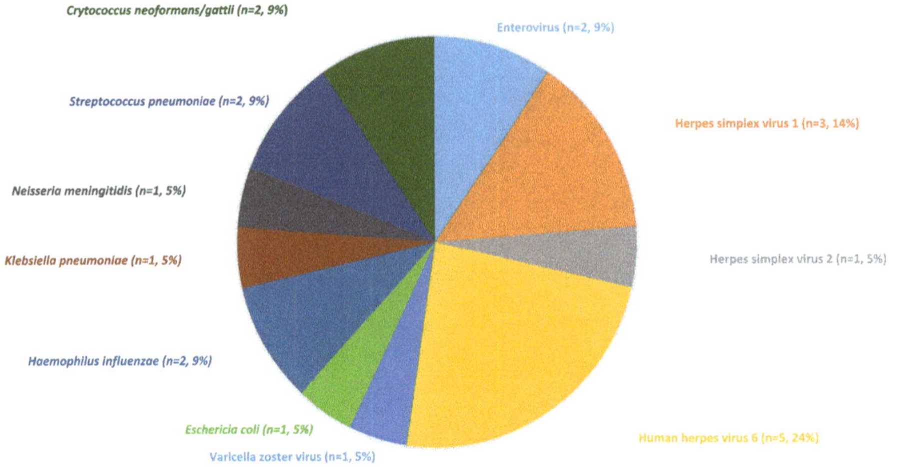

Fig. 2 Etiological agents detected in cerebrospinal fluid (CSF) samples from patients with suspected meningitis using FilmArray and culture. Pie chart of etiological agents detected in CSF samples from patients with suspected meningitis

also detected *Enterobacter cloacae* complex. Three positive blood cultures, in which no agent was detected by FilmArray, were positive by routine culture for *Staphylococcus* spp, *Acinetobacter* spp. and *Salmonella* spp., respectively.

CSF samples from 20 patients, 9 paediatrics and 11 adults, were analysed for *M. tuberculosis* using the GeneXpert system, and all were negative. Three samples were tested using the cryptococcal antigen test, and two of these were positive. These two samples were also positive for *C. neoformans/gattii* by FilmArray (ME panel).

Other diagnostic tests

Data on testing for malaria (tested or not tested) were available for 178 patients. In total, 43 (24%) were tested, all using peripheral blood smear. Only one patient was positive, with a mixed infection of *Plasmodium falciparum* and *Plasmodium vivax*.

HIV status was known for 44 (19%) patients and 12 (27%) of these were HIV positive. Both patients with meningitis caused by *C. neoformans/gattii* had advanced stages of HIV infection.

Laboratory results in samples where microorganisms were detected versus not detected

A comparison was made of laboratory results from analyses of CSF samples where microorganisms were detected and samples where no microorganism was detected (Table 1). There was a significant difference (OR, 28.2; 95%CI 6.4–124.6; $p < 0.0001$) for detecting a pathogen in turbid versus clear samples. In all turbid samples where a pathogen was detected, this was either bacteria or fungi. However, not all samples where bacteria or fungi were detected were turbid.

Glucose measurements were generally lower in samples with bacteria (mean 22 mg/dL) compared to samples where virus (mean 47 mg/dL) or no microorganism (mean 56 mg/dL) were detected, but the number of available measurements was low (Table 1).

For all samples where microorganisms were detected by Gram stain, a pathogen was also detected by FilmArray or culturing. All CSF samples in which bacteria were detected by PCR or culture (Table 3) had a cell count ≥75 cells/mm^3 and/or turbid appearance. In this group of samples (≥75 cells/mm^3 and/or turbid appearance) a bacterial agent was detected in 44%.

The majority of patients had other laboratory investigations performed in addition to CSF analysis. The most common laboratory test was complete blood count in peripheral blood, but no differences were seen in mean WBC count between patients with positive and negative CSF samples (Table 1). However, patients with confirmed bacterial meningitis had a higher mean proportion of polymorphonuclear cells (PMN) in their peripheral blood.

Clinical findings in patients where microorganisms were detected versus not detected in CSF

Table 4 shows the clinical signs and symptoms in patients with or without a microorganism detected in CSF. Fever was the most commonly reported symptom, occurring in 81% of those with a detected microorganism and 74% of those without. Headache, altered consciousness, seizure, neck stiffness, photophobia and Kernig's and Brudzinski's sign were more common in patients where a microorganism was detected although

Table 2 Age, sex, CSF analyses and outcome of patients with microorganism detected in CSF sample

			CSF analyses							
Sex	Age range	Antibiotics prior to sampling	PCR[a]	Appearance	Cell count	% Neutrophils	% Lymphocytes	Gram-stain and microscopy	Culture	Outcome
M	< 1 month	Unknown	Enterovirus	Bloody	No cells			No organism seen	Negative	Improved
F	< 1 month	No	Enterovirus	Clear	25	0	100	No organism seen	Negative	Unknown
M	1–12 months	No	Herpes simplex virus 1	Bloody	N.D[b]			No organism seen	Negative	Improved
M	> 20 years	Yes	Herpes simplex virus 1	Xanthochromic	152	0	100	No organism seen	Negative	Died
F	> 20 years	Yes	Herpes simplex virus 1	Clear	No cells			No organism seen	Negative	Unknown
F	> 20 years	No	Herpes simplex virus 2	Clear	250	0	100	No organism seen	Negative	Unknown
M	< 1 month	Yes	Human herpes virus 6	Clear	5	0	100	No organism seen	Negative	Improved
M	< 1 month	No	Human herpes virus 6	Clear	8	0	100	No organism seen	Negative	Improved
F	1–12 months	No	Human herpes virus 6	Clear	No cells			No organism seen	Negative	Improved
M	1–5 years	No	Human herpes virus 6	Clear	No cells			No organism seen	Negative	Improved
F	6–10 years	Yes	Human herpes virus 6	Clear	332	1	99	No organism seen	Negative	Improved
M	> 20 years	No	Varicella zoster virus	Clear	No cells			No organism seen	Negative	Same condition
F	> 20 years	No	*Escherichia coli*	Clear	75	60	40	No organism seen	Negative	Same condition
M	1–5 years	No	*Haemophilus influenzae*	Turbid	40,000	95	5	Gram negative rods	Negative	Improved
M	10–20 years	No	*Haemophilus influenzae*	Turbid	5200	90	10	No organism seen	Negative	Left hospital against medical advice
M	4 years	Yes	*Neisseria meningitidis*	Turbid	4200	80	20	No organism seen	Negative	Improved
M	1–12 months	No	*Streptococcus pneumoniae*	Turbid	2500	10	90	Gram positive cocci	Negative	Improved
M	10–20 years	No	*Streptococcus pneumoniae*	Turbid	1040	70	30	No organism seen	Negative	Unknown
M	< 1 month	No	Negative	Turbid	1000	10	90	No organism seen	*Klebsiella pneumoniae*	Died
F	> 20 years	No	Cryptococcus[c]	Turbid	13	0	100	Fungal elements	Negative	Died
M	> 20 years	No	Cryptococcus[c]	Clear	5	0	100	No organism seen	Negative	Unknown

N.D. not done
[a] FilmArray system, meningitis-encephalitis panel, from BioMerieux
[b] Cell count not done/not possible due to bloody samples
[c] Sample positive on cryptococcal antigen testing

Table 3 Macroscopic appearance and leucocyte count of cerebrospinal fluid (CSF) with respect to confirmed bacterial meningitis

	CSF appearance[a]			
	Clear/Xanthochromic		Turbid	
	Total	Bacterial meningitis[b]	Total[c]	Bacterial meningitis[b]
Leukocyte count				
< 75 cells/mm3	147	0	1[d]	0
≥ 75 cells/mm3	6	1	8	6

[a]In samples containing blood, cell count was not possible. Among 50 bloody samples, none were confirmed to be bacterial meningitis
[b]Confirmed bacterial meningitis defined as bacterial agent detected on PCR or culture
[c]In one turbid sample, no cell count was performed. No microorganism was detected in this sample
[c]*C. neoformans/gattii* detected on PCR

these characteristics could not reliably distinguish the patients. This trend was even more prominent when only patients with confirmed bacterial meningitis were considered (data not shown). Bulging fontanel was observed only in three patients, none of whom had microorganism detected in their CSF. No patient was reported to have petechiae.

Antibiotic treatment

Ninety-seven percent of patients received one or more antibiotic (Table 5). The most commonly used antibiotic was gentamycin, most often in combination with ampicillin, followed by ceftriaxone (data not shown). The majority (90%) received more than one antibiotic and 39% received three or more antibiotics. Broad spectrum antibiotics were used in 86% of cases (data not shown). No difference in the number of antibiotics received, duration of treatment or cumulative days of antibiotics was seen between patients with a microorganism detected and those with negative CSF (Table 5).

Length of stay and outcome

Data on outcome and duration of hospital stay were available for 161 (74%) and 172 (79%) of the patients, respectively (Table 6). The remaining patients were not documented in the registration book or patient files, and data could not be obtained from the ward or in the medical archive.

For patients where the duration of hospital stay was known (74%), the average length of stay was 9.0 days, and the majority (64%) of patients had improved upon discharge. There was no significant difference in length of hospital stay for patients with a causative agent identified in CSF (mean 10.0 days) versus those who had a negative CSF sample (mean 9.0 days). The overall case fatality rate was 14% and there was a trend towards a higher fatality rate in the group that had microorganisms detected in CSF (18% versus 12%), but this was not statistically significant. About 10% of the patients left the hospital against medical advice and 4% left in the same condition as when they arrived.

Discussion

We analysed clinical and microbiological data from prospectively recruited patients with suspected meningitis in a teaching hospital in Ethiopia. The study was performed within the routine clinical and laboratory settings of a hospital that had very limited prior experience with molecular techniques. In addition to the conventional laboratory investigations used in the hospital, a simple and rapid molecular diagnostic system was introduced to enhance laboratory diagnostics during the study period. To the authors' knowledge, this is the first time a definite etiological diagnosis of viral meningitis has been made in patients in a public health facility in Ethiopia.

Virus were the most common etiological agents of meningitis in this study with HHV-6 being the most common, followed by HSV-1 and HSV-2 and enterovirus. Although the etiology is likely to vary between age groups and local epidemiology, this is in agreement with a study from Finland that found enteroviruses, followed by HSV-2 and VZV to be major causes of aseptic meningitis in adults [21] and a study from Brazil that reported enterovirus as the most common cause of meningitis, followed by HSV-1, cytomegalovirus and dengue virus [22].

Early detection of etiologic agents improves the outcome of meningitis [23] and adequate laboratory diagnostics are imperative. Culturing of bacterial and fungal agents takes time and has low sensitivity, as illustrated by the fact that only one of 9 CSF samples with potentially cultivatable organisms was culture positive. The sensitivity of culture is affected by many factors including prior administration of antibiotics, suboptimal culturing conditions and media, and fastidious nature of some of the bacterial agents. Because of this and the unavailability of viral detection, virtually all patients with suspected meningitis in Ethiopia are treated as bacterial meningitis cases and the diagnosis is rarely re-evaluated over the course of the disease. This over-diagnosis of bacterial meningitis inevitably leads to an overuse of antibiotics. Hence, rapid molecular diagnostics can have a major impact in

Table 4 Signs and symptoms in patients with suspected meningitis with respect to age group and detection of microorganisms in cerebrospinal fluid (CSF)

	Microorganism detected in CSF						No microorganism detected in CSF					
	Neonates		Peadiatrics		Adults		Neonates		Peadiatrics		Adults	
	n	Mean	n	Mean	n	Mean	n	Mean	n	Mean	n	Mean
Total*	5		9		7		112		54		31	
Vital signs												
Temperature	5	38.2	9	38.4	6	36.9	112	37.6	54	38.3	31	37.8
Pulse	5	141	8	126	7	97	111	144	54	137	30	94
Respiratory rate	5	60	8	59	7	27	111	65	53	53	29	25
Glasgow coma scale (GSC) _/15	3	15	7	14	6	15	21	115	21	13	28	15
Symptoms	n	Yes (%)			No (%)		n	Yes (%)			No (%)	
Fever	21	17	(81)		4	(19)	195	145	(74)		50	(26)
Headache[a]	15	9	(60)		6	(40)	85	38	(45)		47	(55)
Nausea[a]	16	6	(38)		10	(63)	81	22	(27)		59	(73)
Vomit	21	11	(52)		10	(48)	195	59	(30)		136	(70)
Fast breathing	21	11	(52)		10	(48)	195	120	(62)		75	(38)
Shortness of breath	20	4	(20)		16	(80)	192	32	(17)		160	(83)
Cough	21	6	(29)		15	(71)	191	26	(14)		165	(86)
Stridor	21	0	(0)		21	(100)	192	3	(2)		189	(98)
Altered consciousness	21	5	(24)		16	(76)	192	31	(16)		161	(84)
Seizure	21	7	(33)		14	(67)	192	23	(12)		169	(88)
Neck stiffness[a]	16	10	(63)		6	(38)	83	26	831)		57	(69)
Photophobia[a]	16	5	(31)		11	(69)	83	11	(13)		72	(87)
Unable to feed	21	7	(33)		14	(67)	193	79	(41)		114	(59)
Abdominal pain[a]	16	1	(6)		15	(94)	84	3	(4)		81	(96)
Rash	21	0	(0)		21	(100)	191	5	(3)		186	(97)
Signs												
Dehydration	21	3	(14)		18	(86)	192	22	811)		170	(89)
Chest in drawing	5	2	(40)		3	(60)	110	43	(39)		67	(61)
Bulging fontanel[b]	5	0	(0)		5	(100)	110	3	(3)		107	(97)
Petecchiae	21	0	(0)		21	(100)	193	1	(1)		192	(99)
Other rash	21	2	(10)		19	(90)	192	5	(3)		187	(97)
Abdominal pain	21	1	(5)		20	(95)	188	5	(3)		183	(97)
Neck stiffness	21	8	(38)		13	(62)	190	32	(17)		158	(83)
Kernig's sign[a]	16	6	(38)		10	(63)	82	13	(16)		69	(84)
Brudzinski's sign[a]	16	5	(31)		11	(69)	82	8	(10)		74	(90)
Reduced consciousness	20	4	(20)		16	(8)	179	25	(14)		154	(86)

*all patients with suspected meningitis and outcome registered, also patient who had only blood culture and no CSF sample taken
[a]only applicable for paediatric and adult patients
[b]only applicable for neonatal patients

low-income settings by increasing the likelihood of reaching a correct diagnosis and enabling correct patient management. This is crucial not only for the outcome of the individual patient, but also for hospital biosecurity measures, public health decisions and both local and global efforts to reduce and improve antimicrobial usage.

The introduction of syndromic testing of infectious diseases and fully automated multiplexed analyses represents a paradigm shift in microbiological diagnostics [24]. Compared to the conventional laboratory investigations performed at JUSH, that detected a microorganism in CSF of only five patients (two by Gram stain, one by Gram stain and cryptococcal antigen-testing, one by

Table 5 Mean duration of antibiotic (ab) treatment and number of different antibiotics received

	Microorganism detected												No microorganism detected		
	All			Virus			Bacteria			Fungi					
	n	%	Mean duration (days)	n	%	Mean duration (days)	n	%	Mean duration (days)	n	%	Mean duration (days)	n	%	Mean duration (days)
Total[a]	16			9			6			1			153		
No. different ab															
0	0	0		0	0		0	0		0	0		5	3	
1	16	100	6	9	100	7	6	100	5	1	100	6	148	9	6
2	15	94	6	9	100	7	5	83	3	1	100	6	136	89	7
3	8	50	4	3	33	3	5	83	5	0	0		54	36	5
4	4	25	7	1	11	5	3	50	7	0	0		15	10	7
5	0	0		0	0		0	0		0	0		5	3	4
6	0	0		0	0		0	0		0	0		2	1	16
Cummulative days of ab	16		15	9		15	6		15	1		12	148		15
	n		Mean no. of antibiotics	n		Mean no. of antibiotics	n		Mean no. of antibiotics	n		Mean no. of antibiotics	n		Mean no. of antibiotics
No of antibiotics received	16		3	9		3	6		3	1		2	148		2

[a]all patients with full record of treatment and duration

Table 6 Duration of hospital stay and outcome for patients with suspected meningitis

	Neonates						Paediatrics						Adults					
	All		Microorg. detected		No microorg. Detected		All		Microorg. detected		No microorg. Detected		All		Microorg. detected		No microorg. Detected	
Duration of illness and length of stay	n	Mean	n	Mean	n	Mean	n	Mean	n	Mean	n	Mean	n	Mean	n	Mean	n	Mean
Days in hospital	99	9.0	4	6.8	95	9.1	50	9.0	9	12.8	41	8.2	23	9.0	4	9.3	19	10.0
	n	%	n	%	n	%	n	%	n	%	n	%	n	%	n	%	n	%
Outcome	92		4		88		49		8		41		20		4		16	
Improved	66	72	3	75	63	67	39	78	7	78	32	78	10	50	0	0	10	63
Same condition	0	0	0	0	0	0	2	4	0	0	2	5	4	20	2	50	2	13
Left hospital against medical advice	12	13	0	0	12	13	3	6	1	11	2	5	2	10	0	0	2	13
Died	14	15	1	25	13	14	5	10	0	0	5	12	3	15	2	50	1	6
Patient not admitted	0	0	0	0	0	0	0	0	0	0	0	0	1	5	0	0	1	6

cryptococcal antigen only and one by culture), the FilmArray was able to detect microorganisms in 20 samples using the ME panel. Hence, such systems can improve patient management in settings with limited laboratory facilities. The FilmArray system was very easily implemented into a modestly equipped laboratory where personnel had little prior experience with molecular diagnostics. The laboratory personnel were able to take on the extra task without disrupting their regular working schedule, while the machine operates.

However, there are a number of limitations to the sustained use of such automated systems in low-income countries. In Ethiopia, procurement of the necessary consumables is a complicated and lengthy process. The main obstacle, however, is the cost. Currently, the reagents needed for the analysis of one sample exceed 100 USD. Needless to say this is not sustainable in a public health system that is already financially constrained. On the other hand, a full course of treatment for suspected bacterial meningitis for 10–14 days [25], including only direct expenses for a hospital stay, routine investigations and antibiotic treatment, is likely to amount to more than 100 USD, even in Ethiopia. Another possible limitation of the system is the predefined selection of the pathogens in the panels. The panels were developed for an American market and may not be equally suited for Africa where other pathogens including *M. tuberculosis* and malaria are major causes of infections. It is also important that clinicians have a good understanding of test characteristics, interpretation of results and test limitations. Although lower than for conventional PCR, there is still a potential for sample contamination when using the FilmArray and the assay may detect latent or reactivated viruses [26]. The assays should be used with care and the positivity rates should be monitored.

Molecular diagnostics should not replace conventional methods. Simple investigations like WBC, Gram stain, and glucose and protein measurements provide valuable diagnostic information, helping distinguish between bacterial and non-bacterial meningitis and guiding treatment [7, 23, 27–30]. These simple methods, however, which are defined as routine investigations at JUSH, were not available for most of the study period. No patients in this study had blood/CSF glucose ratio measured, mainly because of challenges in procurement and finances leading to a lack of basic reagents. Nevertheless, the study did confirm that manual cell counts were useful and could be used more actively to influence patient management.

A combination of laboratory diagnostics and clinical examination have been shown to provide the best prediction of bacterial meningitis, with 100% sensitivity and 52% specificity [28], but even CSF cell count alone can be a good predictor. A cut-off value of 321 leukocytes/mm^3 showed a sensitivity and specificity for bacterial meningitis of 81% in a paediatric population in Portugal [27] and all patients with bacterial meningitis in a mixed-age population in Egypt were found to have > 100 leukocytes/mm^3 [29]. In our study, all confirmed cases of bacterial meningitis had ≥75 leukocytes/mm^3. Thus the use of a cut-off value of ≥75 leukocytes/mm^3 and/or a turbid appearance of CSF to indicate bacterial meningitis and the need for antibiotic treatment would have reduced the number of patients treated with antibiotics by almost 75% in this study.

The high number of patients with no cells or microorganisms detected in the CSF samples indicates that meningitis may be overestimated, especially in children and neonates. Detection of microorganisms in CSF of only 4% of neonates, might suggest that lumbar puncture, an invasive procedure, is overused. In contrast, the high proportion of positive blood cultures in this study (38%), particularly in neonates (67%) suggests that this diagnostic procedure is underused in the hospital.

A limitation of the study is that, despite close follow-up, medical files with treatment and outcome data were not traceable for a considerable proportion (27%) of the patients. This may have introduced a bias with regards to evaluating outcome. However, the proportion of patients where a microorganism was detected in CSF was the same for the overall study population (9.9%) as for the population where outcome was recorded (9.6%).

No differences were observed in this study with respect to prescription of antibiotics to patients with bacterial/fungal agents detected in CSF versus those with viral meningitis or no microorganism detected. This could be due to a lack of clinical treatment guidelines, but a contributing factor might have been poor communication of test results to responsible clinicians due to lack of electronic reporting systems, operational hospital telephones and internal post delivery systems. We acknowledge that changes in prescription habits will require long lasting interventions and coordinated stewardships in order to be successful, and that the short duration of the study was a limitation, in this respect. A recent publication from India observed a target specific escalation and evidence based de-escalation of the use of antimicrobials when a syndromic based molecular diagnostic system for meningitis was used over a period of 4 years [31].

The prescription of antibiotics is far higher in Ethiopia than WHO recommendations [32]. There is no formal antimicrobial stewardship program at JUSH, nor restrictions or specific guidelines on antimicrobials use. In Ethiopia, there is no national policy or guidelines on antimicrobials use, neither do most hospitals have their own systems to ensure correct use of antimicrobials [15]. A study from JUSH also showed that the national guidelines did not cover the management of 20% of diagnosed infectious diseases [15]. Ensuring stable access to simple CSF investigations, including protein and glucose measurements, and developing and implementing treatment guidelines for meningitis based on laboratory results might be a first and important step to improve treatment and reduce the misuse of antibiotics.

Conclusions

In this study we diagnosed viral meningitis in a routine clinical practice for the first time in Ethiopia, and in the study population viral agents were the most common cause of meningitis. A simple, rapid molecular diagnostic system was successfully implemented in a laboratory with little experience in molecular diagnostics, and significantly increased the likelihood of detecting a microorganism in CSF samples. The lack of laboratory methods to effectively distinguish bacterial from non-bacterial causes is an important reason for the overuse of antibiotics in patients with suspected meningitis in Ethiopia. Improved diagnostics together with development of treatment guidelines, based on local epidemiology and laboratory findings, could reduce antibiotic usage and hospitalization without negatively affecting patient outcome in the study hospital.

Abbreviations

BCID: Blood Culture Identification; CSF: Cerebrospinal fluid; JUSH: Jimma University Specialized Hospital; ME: Meningitis/encephalitis; PMN: Plymorphonuclear leukocytes cells; USD: US Dollar; WBC: White blood cells

Acknowledgments

We thank all the study participants and the clinical staff at Jimma University Specialized Hospital, particularly in the paediatric and internal medicine wards. We are very grateful to Dawit Abera, Amanuel Teferi, Wossen Abay and Sara Jemal for performing the PCR and the routine analysis of CSF samples and blood cultures. We are also grateful to Mulualem Tadesse, Zegeye Bonsa, Nefiza Negash and Getu Belay for running the geneXpert analysis of CSF samples.

Funding

This project was supported by the Research Council of Norway grant 220829 to DAC. The funding body has not been involved in the design of the study and collection, analysis, and interpretation of data or in writing the manuscript.

Authors' contributions

GKB, EKG, HJJ, MB, SLF, AA and DAC participated in the study design. GKB, EKG, MB and GT were responsible for recruitment and sampling. GKB, GT, AA and GA were responsible for the laboratory analyses. GKB, EKG, HJJ and SLF analysed the data. GKB, HJJ and SLF drafted the manuscript. All the authors have contributed to the manuscript and approved the final version.

Competing interest

The authors declare that they have no competing interests.

Consent for publication

Not applicable. This manuscript does not contain any individual persons' data.

Author details

[1]Division for Infection Control and Environmental Health, Norwegian Institute of Public Health, Oslo, Norway. [2]Faculty of Medicine, University of Oslo, Oslo, Norway. [3]Institute of Health, Jimma University, Jimma, Ethiopia. [4]Norwegian Veterinary Institute, Oslo, Norway. [5]Mycobacteriology Research Center, Jimma University, Jimma, Ethiopia.

References

1. Institute of Health Metrics and Evaluation. Leading causes of premature death (YLLs) in 2015 and Leading causes of DALYs in 2015. Website: healthdata.org/ethiopia. Accessed 10 July 2017.
2. Colombini A, Bationo F, Zongo S, Ouattara F, Badolo O, Jaillard P, et al. Costs for households and community perception of meningitis epidemics in Burkina Faso. Clin Infect Dis. 2009;49:1520–5.
3. Barquet N, Domingo P, Cayla JA, Gonzalez J, Rodrigo C, Fernandez-Viladrich P, et al. Prognostic factors in meningococcal disease. Development of a bedside predictive model and scoring system. JAMA. 1997;278:491–6.
4. Shah SS, Aronson PL, Mohamad Z, Lorch SA. Delayed acyclovir therapy and death among neonates with herpes simplex virus infection. Pediatrics. 2011; 128:1153–60.
5. Tunkel AR, Hartman BJ, Kaplan SL, Kaufman BA, Roos KL, Scheld WM, et al. Practice guidelines for the management of bacterial meningitis. Clin Infect Dis. 2004;39:1267–84.
6. Biondi EA, Byington CL. Evaluation and management of febrile, well-appearing young infants. Infect Dis Clin N Am. 2015;29:575–85.
7. Dubos F, Lamotte B, Bibi-Triki F, Moulin F, Raymond J, Gendrel D, et al. Clinical decision rules to distinguish between bacterial and aseptic meningitis. Arch Dis Child. 2006;91:647–50.
8. Neuman MI, Tolford S, Harper MB. Test characteristics and interpretation of cerebrospinal fluid gram stain in children. Pediatr Infect Dis J. 2008;27:309–13.
9. Hornik CP, Benjamin DK, Becker KC, Benjamin DK, Li J, Clark RH, et al. use of the complete blood cell count in early-onset neonatal sepsis. Pediatr Infect Dis J. 2012;31:799–802.
10. Jaffe DM, Fleisher GR. Temperature and total white blood cell count as indicators of bacteremia. Pediatrics. 1991;87:670–4.
11. The World Bank. Overview Ethiopia. Website: worldbank.org/en/country/ethiopia/overview#1. Accessed: 01 11 2017.
12. Gudina EK, Tesfaye M, Adane A, Lemma K, Shibiru T, Pfister HW, Klein M. Challenges of bacterial meningitis case management in low income settings: an experience from Ethiopia. Tropical Med Int Health. 2016;21:870–8.
13. Thomas KE, Hasbun R, Jekel J, Quagliarello VJ. The diagnostic accuracy of Kernig's sign, Brudzinski's sign, and nuchal rigidity in adults with suspected meningitis. Clin Infect Dis. 2002;35:46–52.
14. Oostenbrink R, Moons KG, Theunissen CC, Derksen-Lubsen G, Grobbee DE, Moll HA. Signs of meningeal irritation at the emergency department: how often bacterial meningitis? Pediatr Emerg Care. 2001;17:161–4.
15. Yadesa TM, Gudina EK, Angamo MT. Antimicrobial use-related problems and predictors among hospitalized medical in-patients in Southwest Ethiopia: prospective observational study. PLoS One. 2015;10:e0138385.
16. Moges F, Endris M, Mulu A, Tessema B, Belyhun Y, Shiferaw Y, et al. The growing challenges of antibacterial drug resistance in Ethiopia. J Glob Antimicrob Resist. 2014;2:148–54.
17. Cheesbrough M. District laboratory practice in tropical countries. 2nd ed. Cambridge: Cambridge University press; 2006.
18. Leber AL, Everhart K, Balada-Llasat JM, Cullison J, Daly J, Holt S, et al. Multicenter evaluation of BioFire FilmArray meningitis/encephalitis panel for detection of bacteria, viruses, and yeast in cerebrospinal fluid specimens. J Clin Microbiol. 2016;54:2251–61.
19. Helb D, Jones M, Story E, Boehme C, Wallace E, Ho K, et al. Rapid detection of *Mycobacterium tuberculosis* and rifampin resistance by use of on-demand, near-patient technology. J Clin Microbiol. 2010;48:229–37.

20. Blaschke AJ, Heyrend C, Byington CL, Fisher MA, Barker E, Garrone NF, et al. Rapid identification of pathogens from positive blood cultures by multiplex polymerase chain reaction using the FilmArray system. Diagn Microbiol Infect Disease. 2012;74:349–55.
21. Kupila L, Vuorinen T, Vainionpaa R, Hukkanen V, Marttila RJ, Kotilainen P. Etiology of aseptic meningitis and encephalitis in an adult population. Neurology. 2006;66:75–80.
22. Soares CN, Cabral-Castro MJ, Peralta JM, de Freitas MR, Zalis M, Puccioni-Sohler M. Review of the etiologies of viral meningitis and encephalitis in a dengue endemic region. J Neurol Sci. 2011;303:75–9.
23. Bahr NC, Boulware DR. Methods of rapid diagnosis for the etiology of meningitis in adults. Biomark Med. 2014;8:1085–103.
24. Abbott AN, Fang FC. Clinical impact of multiplex syndromic panels in the diagnosis of bloodstream, gastrointestinal, respiratory. and central nervous system infections Clin Microbiol Newsl. 2017;39:133–42.
25. Food, Medicine and Healthcare Administration and Control Authority of Ethiopia (FMHACA). Standard treatment guideline for general hospital. In: 3rd edition; 2014.
26. Hanson KE. The first fully automated molecular diagnostic panel for meningitis and encephalitis: how well does it perform, and when should it be used? J Clin Microbiol. 2016;54:2222–4.
27. Agueda S, Campos T, Maia A. Prediction of bacterial meningitis based on cerebrospinal fluid pleocytosis in children. Braz J Infect Dis. 2013;17:401–4.
28. Dubos F, Korczowski B, Aygun DA, Martinot A, Prat C, Galetto-Lacour A, et al. Distinguishing between bacterial and aseptic meningitis in children: European comparison of two clinical decision rules. Arch Dis Child. 2010;95: 963–7.
29. Fouad R, Khairy M, Fathalah W, Gad T, El-Kholy B, Yosry A. Role of clinical presentations and routine CSF analysis in the rapid diagnosis of acute bacterial meningitis in cases of negative gram stained smears. J Trop Med. 2014:213762.
30. Spanos A, Harrell FE Jr, Durack DT. Differential diagnosis of acute meningitis. An analysis of the predictive value of initial observations. JAMA. 1989;262: 2700–7.
31. Javali M, Acharya P, Mehta A, John AA, Mahale R, Srinivasa R. Use of multiplex PCR based molecular diagnostics in diagnosis of suspected CNS infections in tertiary care setting-a retrospective study. Clin Neurol Neurosurg. 2017;161:110–6.
32. Kebede HK, Gesesew HA, Woldehaimanot TE, Goro KK. Antimicrobial use in paediatric patients in a teaching hospital in Ethiopia. PLoS One. 2017;12: e0173290.

23

Trichosporon inkin meningitis in Northeast Brazil

Eveline Pipolo Milan[1], Walicyranison Plinio Silva-Rocha[2], Jéssica Jacinto Salviano de Almeida[1], Tatiane Uetti Gomes Fernandes[1], André Luciano de Araújo Prudente[1], Matheus Firmino de Azevedo[2], Elaine Cristina Francisco[3], Analy Salles de Azevedo Melo[3], Arnaldo Lopes Colombo[3] and Guilherme Maranhão Chaves[2*]

Abstract

Background: *Trichosporon* species may colonize the skin, respiratory tract and gastrointestinal tract of human beings. The yeast is recognized as etiological agent of *white piedra*, a superficial mycosis. Nevertheless, immunocompromised hosts may develop invasive Trichosporonosis. Central nervous system trichosporonosis is a very rare clinical manifestation. In fact, only a few cases have been published in the literature and none of them was caused by *Trichosporon inkin*.

Case presentation: Here we report the first clinical case of meningoencephalitis due to this species in a female previously healthy patient under corticosteroids and antibiotics therapy for several months. She was submitted to an invasive procedure to remove a left sided acoustic neuroma and further developed a cerebrospinal fistula. After some days of the procedure, she presented a predominantly and intensive occipital holocranial headache, followed by vomiting, hyporexia, weight loss, asthenia, irritability, difficulty to concentrate and rotator vertigo. The patient further developed a cerebrospinal fistula in the occipital region and was submitted to a surgical correction. After several months of clinical interventions, she was diagnosed with CNS Trichosporonosis, after Magnetic Resonance Imaging and positive microbiological cultures obtained within two different occasions (2 weeks apart). Despite the antifungal therapy with Amphotericin B and Voriconazole, the patient did not survive.

Conclusions: Despite CNS Fungal infections are mostly due to *Cryptococcus* spp., other emergent yeasts, such as *T. inkin* may be considered as a likely etiological agent. This is the first case report of CNS Trichosporonosis, where species identification was performed with rDNA sequencing.

Keywords: Invasive Trichosporonosis, Meningoencephalitis, *Trichosporon inkin*, Virulence factors, Antifungal susceptibility testing, Northeast Brazil

Background

Trichosporon species are basidiomycetous yeast-like fungi widely distributed in nature, predominantly found in tropical and temperate areas [1]. *Trichosporon* spp. may be found in substrates such as soil, decomposing wood, air, rivers, lakes, seawater, cheese, scarab beetles, bird droppings, bats, pigeons and cattle [1]. These organisms also are present in the human microbiota of skin and gastrointestinal tract [2]. *Trichosporon* spp. are phenotypically characterized by colonies of white or cream coloring, with dry appearance, cerebriform or radiated surface [3] and microscopically by the presence of blastoconidia, arthroconidia, pseudophyphae and true hyphae [4].

Trichosporon spp. are usually associated with superficial mycosis such as white *piedra* [1, 4, 5], onychomycosis [1, 5–7] interdigital and inguinocrural lesions [5, 7]. Invasive trichosporonosis is a deep-seated infection which

* Correspondence: guilherme.chaves@ufrnet.br
[2]Centro de Ciências da Saúde, Laboratório de Micologia Médica e Molecular, Departamento de Análises Clínicas e Toxicológicas, Universidade Federal do Rio Grande do Norte, Rua Gal. Gustavo Cordeiro de Faria S/N, Petrópolis, Natal, Rio Grande do Norte, Brazil
Full list of author information is available at the end of the article

may be observed in leukemia or lymphoma patients who developed severe neutropenia, associated with broad spectrum antibiotic therapy [2, 4]. *Trichosporon asahii* and *T. mucoides* are the most frequently isolated species in invasive trichosporonosis [4, 8]. Pubmed searches using the terms "*Trichosporon inkin*", "invasive" and "infection" only retrieved six publications [9–14].

The establishment of fungal infection is associated with host immune conditions as well as virulence attributes of the microorganism involved. For instance, adhesion to epithelial cells [15], the production and secretion of hydrolytic enzymes such as phospholipases and hemolysins [16] and the capacity of biofilm formation [17] contribute to yeasts pathogenicity and have been demonstrated in *Trichosporon* spp.

Central nervous system (CNS) trichosporonosis is a rare clinical manifestation associated with immunocompromised patients [18]. In fact, only a few clinical cases of this medical condition have been reported in the literature [2, 4, 18–25] and none of them was due to *T. inkin*.

The gold standard diagnosis of CNS trichosporonosis is the isolation of *Trichosporon* in culture of tissue samples or cerebrospinal fluid (CSF) [1, 19]. The reference method for *Trichosporon* species identification is based on Intergenic Spacer 1 (IGS1) region of the ribosomal DNA sequencing [8, 26]. However, Matrix-Assisted Laser Desorption/ Ionization Time-of-Flight (MALDI-TOF) Mass Spectrometry has been shown to be a valuable alternative to *Trichosporon* species identification [1, 27].

Despite some controversies, triazoles appear to be the best first line antifungal therapy for invasive trichosporonosis, especially when *T. asahii* is involved [1, 10, 18, 19, 27]. In vitro studies suggest that voriconazole exhibits the best antifungal activity against different *Trichosporon* species, when compared to amphotericin B and fluconazole [10]. Echinocandins are associated with high MIC values [19, 28] and indicates no action on *Trichosporon* cells. Therefore, they are not indicated in clinical practice [19, 27].

To the best of our knowledge, we describe the first case of meningoencephalitis due to *T. inkin* in a previously healthy female patient under corticosteroids regimen after having undergonea microsurgery of neuroma in Natal, Rio Grande do Norte State, Northeast Brazil. We also describe theantifungal susceptibility profiling and characterization of the expression of virulence factors in vitro of two *T. inkin* isolates sequentially obtained from the CSF of this patient and also a review of meningoencephalitis clinical cases due to *Trichosporon* spp. reported in the literature.

Case presentation

MECM, a 49-years-old previously healthy woman, married and childless, was admitted at a private hospital in Natal City, Rio Grande do Norte State, Brazil, in June, 2014 for a microsurgery of neuroma. She used to live in a flat with a parrot who had an unknown disease that caused loss of feathers. The microsurgery was performed via the cranial middle fossa to remove a left sided acoustic neuroma. After 40 days of the procedure, she presented a predominantly and intensive occipital holocranial headache, followed by vomiting. She was managed with analgesia and prednisone 20 mg/day for 5 days. The patient also had hyporexia that was accentuated with the worsening of headache, 12 kg of weight loss, asthenia, irritability, difficulty to concentrate and rotator vertigo. She did not have a fever. On physical examination, the patient presented classic signs of irritability of meningeal inflammation.

On the 50th postoperative day, she was diagnosed with a cerebrospinal fistula in the occipital region and submitted to a surgical correction. The CSF analysis revealed 126 cells/mm^3, composed by 63% of lymphomonocytes, 13 mg/dl of glucose levels (89 mg/dl of glycemia) and 189 mg/dL of proteins. Direct examination and CSF microbiological culturing (including common bacterial, mycobacterial and fungal procedures) did not detect any pathogen. Hemogram and biochemical examination of blood were normal. Vancomycin and ceftriaxone were prescribed for 14 days, dexamethasone, 16 mg/day, for 10 days, followed by 15 days of prednisone weaning. She was discharged with partial improvement of headache, without vomiting and presenting normal CSF. After 3 weeks, the headache intensified and vomiting returned. Prednisone 80 mg/day, for 7 days, followed by 30 days of weaning was prescribed, resulting in mild improvement of headache, but with persistent vomiting and return of rotational vertigo. Therefore, cinnarizine, esomeprazole, bromopride and paracetamol/codeine were prescribed. As no relief was obtained after 30 days, the patient was re-hospitalized and CSF analysis revealed: 245 cells/mm^3, 88% of lymphomonocytes, 23 mg/dL of glucose levels and proteins of 324 mg/dL. Microbiological cultures for bacteria and fungi were negative. Hemogram and biochemical examination of blood were still normal. She was diagnosed again with occipital liquoric fistula and submitted to clinical treatment. She was under the same antimicrobial and corticoid regimen of the last hospitalization and was discharged with mild headache. Dexamethasone 16 mg/day, for 10 days, followed by 30 days of weaning with prednisone was prescribed. At that moment, the CSF still had 68 cells/mm^3, with 100% of lymphomonocytes, 56 mg/dL of glucose levels and 78 mg/dL of proteins. Prednisone was prescribed for 30 days.

When the corticoid was discontinued, headache worsened and vomiting returned. After 5 months of the onset of the disease, a new computed tomography (CT) scan of the skull showed a CSF fistula on the same topography. She was hospitalized and submitted to a surgery to correct the fistula. She had leukocytosis on admission (16,000 leukocytes/mm^3, with 88% segmented cells) and CSF analysis showed 280 cells/mm^3, being 88% of lymphomonocytes cells, 12 mg/dL of glucose levels and 312 mg/dL of proteins. Bacterial and fungal cultures were negative. Empirical treatment with vancomycin and cefepime was introduced for 21 days and dexamethasone 16 mg/day for 10 days, followed by 20 days of weaning with prednisone. As the headache worsened, she was again hospitalized and submitted to surgical correction of the fistula. New CSF showed 184 cells, 63% of lymphomonocytes, 41 mg/dL of glucose levels and 285 mg/dL of proteins. Vancomycin, meropenem and dexamethasone, 10 mg/day were initiated. On the 5th day of treatment, headache remained intense and frequent vomiting. A new CT suggested hydrocephalus and the patient was submitted to a ventriculoperitoneal (VP) shunt. After 3 days of VP, the patient continued to present with vomiting and leukocytosis and the CSF pressure was above 300 mmH_2O. She was admitted to the intensive care unit. A magnetic resonance imaging (MRI) of the skull suggested meningeal thickening, spinal cord compression at the level of C5-C6 and the alteration of the CSF signal was compatible with viral or fungal disease (Fig. 1). The initial suspicion was cryptococcosis. Liposomal amphotericin B (300 mg/day) and acyclovir therapy were empirically initiated. After several invasive procedures, broad spectrum antibiotics and corticosteroids, CSF culture showed growth of *Trichosporon* spp. After 2 weeks, another *Trichosporon* CSF positive culture was obtained. As there was progressive worsening of the clinical condition, voriconazole (200 mg/every 12 h) was added to the previous prescription. On the 20th day of hospitalization, the patient died (Table 1).

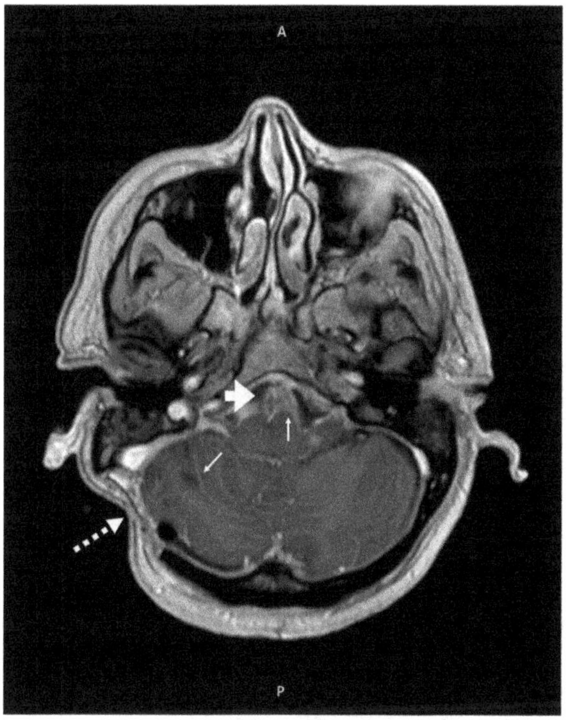

Fig. 1 Axial Magnetic Resonance Imaging (MRI) at the posterior fossa level, showing extensive leptomeningeal enhancement near the anterior bulb contour and cerebellar folds (thin arrows). Heterogeneous material with enhancement near the pre-pontine cistern (thick arrow). Note the signs of surgical manipulation of the extra-cranial soft parts in the right occipital region (dashed arrow)

Culturing procedures and molecular identification of the pathogen

The CSF was centrifuged at 2500 rpm for 10 min and the sediment was used for direct examination and culture. Direct examination was performed with India ink which revealed no encapsulated blastoconidia. The sediment of 2 CSF samples collected at different days (14th and 28th of April, 2015) were plated on Sabouraud Dextrose Agar at room temperature (28 + 2 °C) and yielded positive yeast cultures after 72 h of incubation. The two cultures were send to the Medical and Molecular Mycology Laboratory, Clinical and Toxicological Analyses Department, Federal University of Rio Grande do Norte State for further molecular identification. Of note, both colonies had a mucoid aspect. Besides, because *Cryptococcus* spp. are the main etiological fungal agents obtained from meningitis, that was the first suspicion. Yeast isolates from original cultures were plated onto CHROMagar *Candida* (CHROMagar Microbiology, Paris, France) and corn meal-Tween 80 (to induce sporulation). Surprisingly, both isolates had a macroscopic wrinkled appearance, were able to produce arthroconidia, as revealed by their micromorphology, and to hydrolyze urea (Fig. 2a to d). Therefore, they were considered to belong to the genus *Trichosporon* and named HGT198 and HGT914, respectively. Both strains were further identified by molecular techniques.

Molecular identification

A single colony of each strain was used for DNA extraction with PrepMan Ultra sample preparation reagent (Applied Biosystems, Foster City, CA) according to the manufacturer's instructions. Genomic DNA concentration and purity were checked with a NanoDrop instrument (Thermo Scientific; Amersham Pharmacia Biotech, Wilmington, DE, USA). Both strains were further identified by a molecular method as detailed elsewhere [29]. DNA amplification was obtained by using the primer pair TRF (5′-AGAGGCCTA CCATGGTATCA-3′) and TRR (5′-TAAGACCCAATAGA GCCCTA-3′) [26]. Nucleotide sequences were submitted for BLAST analysis at the NCBI site (http://www.ncbi.nlm.nih.gov) for species identification. Only sequences deposited in GenBank showing high similarities with our query sequences and an *E*-value of lower than 10^{-5} were used in this study. BLAST searches showed the best match with *T. inkin* (FJ153608.1), 100% identity (619 of 619 bp without gap sites) for both strains (HGT198 and HGT914). IGS1

Table 1 Timeline of exposition to multiple risk conditions of a patient submitted to an acoustic neuroma surgery and further developed meningitis in Natal city, Rio Grande do Norte State, Northeast Brazil

Period of time	Acoustic neuroma surgery	Corticosteroids usage	Appearence of the fistula	Antibiotics usage	CSF[a] analisys performing	Surgical fistula correction	VP[b] shunt	Antifungal therapy	*Trichosporon* positive culture	Death
Week 1	X									
Week 6		X								
Week 8		X	X	X	X					
Week 9		X		X						
Week 13		X								
Week 17		X	X	X	X					
Week 18		X		X						
Week 19		X		X						
Week 20		X	X	X	X	X				
Week 21		X		X						
Week 22		X		X						
Week 23		X		X	X	X	X	X	X	
Week 24		X		X				X		
Week 25								X	X	
Week 26								X		X

[a]*CSF* Cerebrospinal fluid, [b]*VP* Ventriculoperitoneal

rDNA sequences of these strains have been deposited in GenBank under accession numbers KY807052 and KY807053, respectively. Of note, both strains were considered of 100% identity, after blastn analysis (all the 641 bp compared among them), with an *E*-value of 0 and no gaps found between the two IGS1 rDNA sequences.

Characterization of virulence factors and in vitro antifungal susceptibility

Strains HGT198 and HGT914 were evaluated according to their ability to adhere to human buccal epithelial cells, biofilm formation, hemolysins and phospholipase production by using the methods described by Zuza-Alves [30]. DNAse production was determined according to Montoya [16].

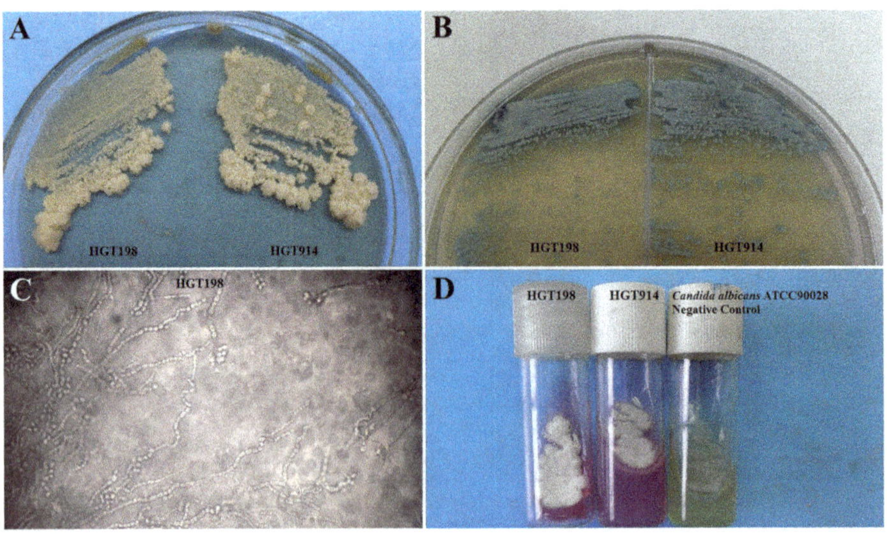

Fig. 2 **a** Cream-colored, dull, wrinkled cerebriform colonies, after 48 h of incubation at 30 °C on Sabouraud dextrose agar. **b** Colonies with typical "dirty" grey-blue color on CHROMagar *Candida*® medium after 72 h of incubation at 35 °C. **c** Micromorphological aspects after incubation in cornmeal agar containing Tween 80 for 72 h at 30 °C, showing long true hyphae e artroconidia. **d** Urease test of yeast cells grown in Cristensen's urea Agar containing phenol red, showing positive results after incubation at 30 °C for 72 h

Both strains did not produce phospholipase or DNAse. However, they showed high biofilm formation capability as compared to *C. albicans* ATCC90028 and *T. asahii* CBS2630 and similar levels of hemolysin production of the two reference strains. In addition, they were able to adhere to epithelial cells to the same extension of *T. asahii* reference strain (Table 2).

Both strains were tested against fluconazole, itraconazole and amphotericin Bby using the CLSI protocol [31–33]. As illustrated on Table 3, they exhibited very low MIC values against all antifungal drugs tested.

Discussion and conclusions

Trichosporon species are present in the environment and may belong to the human microbiota butmay associated with both superficial and deep infections [1, 18]. Infections associated with CNS due *Trichosporon* are rare in immunocompromised patients and extremely rare in immunocompetent patients [20].

The number of cases of invasive trichosporonosis reported worldwide may be still considered restrict once a limited number of publications may be found in the literature [27]. A recent epidemiological study conducted by De Almeida Júnior et al. [27] reviewing global cases of invasive trichosporonosis retrieved from PubMed from 1994 and 2015 only found a total of 203 cases of invasive trichosporonosis, where *T. asahii* accounted for 95 (47.6%) of all cases [27].

The first case of SNC infection due *Trichosporon* was described by Watson and Kallichurum in 1970 [25] in a 39-year-old African woman diagnosed with underlying bronchial adenocarcinoma and brain abscess due *T. cutaneum* [25]. It is important to mention that no molecular techniques were available at this time. Therefore, this could have led to an unreliable species identification. Since then, only other few case reports of *Trichosporon* meningitis have been published in the literature, but none of them was due to *T. inkin* (Table 4).

The geographic distribution of invasive trichosporonosis with CNS complications is higher in Asia (seven cases) [2, 18–22, 24]. There are cases described in Europe [23], Africa [25] and Central America (one case each) [4]. Clinical series with patients' demographic data and underlying conditions may be found in Table 4.

There is only a single study reporting *Trichosporon* meningitis in an immunocompetent patient [22]. In this study, Rastoji et al. [22] reported a case of invasive trichosporonosis with CNS complications in a 18-years-old male, who presented fever, chills and rigor associated with headache, nausea, vomiting and altered sensorium. *T. asahii* was isolated from CSF and sputum of this patient [22].

Several clinical conditions are considered to be risk factors for invasive trichosporonosis including the history of intensive chemotherapy, high dose of corticosteroids, burns, neutropenia, broad spectrum antibiotics usage and hematological malignancies [8, 20, 27]. In fact, the patient described in this study was previously immunocompetent but further submitted to long periods of corticosteroids and broad-spectrum antibiotics, besides suffering the invasive medical procedure to remove an acoustic neuroma. Of note, the CSF fistula probably had an important role for local *Trichosporon* contamination. In addition, the fact that she had a parrot could have led to yeasts skin colonization, once these birds may harbor *Trichosporon* in their gastrointestinal tract [34]. A limitation of our study is that we did not perform her parrot's droppings culture, trying to isolate *Trichosporon* and further checked with molecular techniques to determine the probable source of infection.

Our isolates were as able to adhere to epithelial cells as *T. asahii* CBS2630 that is considered the most virulent and frequently isolated species of the genus *Trichosporon*, as demonstrated by virulence studies with *Galleria mellonella* and murine models of systemic infection [35]. Of note, all *Trichosporon* isolates were less adherent than *Candida albicans* ATCC90028. This was expected, because *C. albicans* is widely recognized as the more adherent *Candida* species [36], but it was used as a reference strain for adhesion assay.

Both isolates (HGT198 and HGT914) had stronger hemolytic activities than reference strain *T. asahii* CBS2630. Our isolates were considered highly hemolytic according

Table 2 Evaluation of attributes of virulence factors in vitro of *Trichosporon inkin* isolates HGT198 and HGT914 obtained from a patient submitted to an acoustic neuroma surgery and further developed meningitis in Natal city, Rio Grande do Norte State, Northeast Brazil

	N° of *T. inkin* cells adhered to 150 HBEC	Hemolytic index (*HI*)	Biofilm formation (OD_{595nm})
Candida albicans ATCC90028	179.8 ± 2.05	0.63 ± 0.01	0.24 ± 0.03
Trichosporon asahii CBS2630	34.3 ± 1.70	0.74 ± 0.01	0.40 ± 0.01
Trichosporon inkin HGT198	36.7 ± 1.50[a]	0.68 ± 0.01[a; b, c]	0.77 ± 0.05[a; b, c]
Trichosporon inkin HGT914	37.3 ± 1.50[a]	0.56 ± 0.01[a; b, c]	1.04 ± 0.01[a; b, c]

NT Not Tested
[a]Statistically significant different from *Candida albicans* ATCC90028
[b]Statistically significant different from *Trichosporon asahii* CBS2630
[c]Statistically significant difference between HGT198 and HGT198

Table 3 Determination of antifungal susceptibility testing of *Trichosporon inkin* isolates HGT198 and HGT914 obtained from a patient submitted to an acoustic neuroma surgery and further developed meningitis in Natal city, Rio Grande do Norte State, Northeast Brazil

Strain	Fluconazole (24 h)	Itraconazole (48 h)	Amphotericin B (48 h)
Candida parapsilosis ATCC 22019	1 µg/mL	NT	NT
Candida krusei ATCC6258	16 µg/mL	NT	NT
Trichosporon inkin HGT-198	0.5 µg/mL	0.062 µg/mL	0.5 µg/mL
Trichosporon inkin HGT-914	0.5 µg/mL	0.062 µg/mL	0.5 µg/mL

with the criteria established by Montoya et al. [16]. These authors reported a single strain of *T. asahii* with strong hemolytic activity, while the other 38 isolates did not produce this enzyme. These finding reinforce virulence attributes properties of the isolates from the present study that may have influenced clinical outcome.

Biofilm formation by microorganisms has gained attention within clinical practice because of its ability to increase mortality in patients with systemic infections by yeasts [37]. Studies on biofilm formation in *Trichosporon* have increased in recent years, since this yeast has been considered the second most common etiological agent of systemic infection in patients with hematological malignancies [38]. In the presence of biofilm, structured microbial communities remain embedded within an extracellular polymeric substance, where *Trichosporon* spp. show significantly greater resistance to antifungals, with MICs ranging from 128 to 1.024 µg/mL for Amphotericin B and 512–1.024 µg/mL for Fluconazole, Itraconazole, and Voriconazole [38]. Our isolates showed an optical density of 595 nm (which reflects biofilm biomass stained by crystal violet) at least two-fold higher than the readings found for *T. asahii* CBS6030. Of note, there is a trend of increased virulence attributes expression over time when both strains isolated 2 weeks apart were compared (Table 1). This phenomenon is observed for both hemolysins and biofilm production. This may reflect strain adaptation to the host in the progress of infection.

Our strains were not resistant to any of the antifungal drugs tested. In addition, MICs obtained from *T. inkin* HGT198 and HGT914 did not increase over time. This observation indicates that probably there was not induced antifungal resistance for the strains recovered within 2 weeks of difference. It is important to emphasize that antifungal susceptibility testing was only possible to be performed after patient's death and was not used to drive antifungal therapy.

Table 4 Systematic review of *Trichosporonosis* meningitis cases published in the literature from to 1970 to 2018

Country	Sex/Age	Diagnosis/Underlying diseases	Species isolated	Clinical Sample	Treatment/outcome	Year/Reference
Brazil			*Trichosporon inkin*	CSF		Present study
Singapore	F/50	Disseminated trichosporonosis/ Aplastic Anemia	*T. asahii*	CSF, Blood	AMB, VOR, ITR, POS/ Survived	2016 [24]
India	M/18	Chronic meningo-ventriculitis and intraventricular fungal ball/immunocompetent	*T. asahii*	Intraventricular biopsy and CSF	AMB/died	2015 [20]
Iran	M/34	Brain abscess/ autoimmune hepatitis, hypothyroidism	*T. asahii*	Brain abscess	Surgical resection, AMB and ITC/ survived	2012 [18]
India	NI	Meningitis/Acquired Immunodeficiency Syndrome (AIDS)	*Trichosporon* sp.	CSF	AMB, FLU, survived	2012 [19]
Jamaica	F/44	Meningitis and cerebral abscess/diabetes, burns	*T. asahii*	Facial wounds, sputum, and a meningeal swab	None/died	2011 [4]
Taiwan	NI	Meningitis/NI	*T. montevideense*	CSF	NI	2009 [2]
India	M/18	Disseminated trichosporonosis/ Imunnocompetent	*T. asahii*	CSF	FLU/survived	2007 [22]
India	F/36	Chronic meningitis/ Chronic back pain after fall	*T. beigelii*	CSF	None/died	1995 [21]
Belgium	M/15	Meningitis/acute lymphocytic leukaemia	*T. beigelii*	CSF	AMB, FC and FLU/died	1990 [23]
South Africa	F/39	Brain abscess/adenocarcinoma	*T. cutaneum*	Brain lesions	None/died	1970 [25]

There are some limitations about the interpretations of MIC values in our *Trichosporon* isolates. First of all, there are still no breakpoints established from Clinical & Laboratory Standards Institute (CLSI) and European Committee on Antimicrobial Susceptibility Testing (EUCAST) Antifungal Susceptibility testing to *Trichosporon* species [27], and second, there are no studies which determined MICs of *T. inkin* strains isolated from patients with meningoencephalitis.

Susceptibility testing to the antifungal drugs Amphotericin B, Itraconazole and Fluconazole were performed by Taj-Aldeen et al. [39] with three *T. inkin* clinical isolates obtained from urine and white *piedra*. MIC range was 1–4 μg/mL (Amphotericin B), 0.25–4 μg/mL (Fluconazole) and 0.013–0.125 μg/mL (Itraconazole). *T. inkin* clinical isolates from bone, urine, skin, subcutaneous abscess, peritoneal liquid and blood susceptibility profiling was determined and MIC range was 0.06–1 μg/mL (Amphotericin B), 1–32 μg/mL (Fluconazole) and 0.06–2 μg/mL (Itraconazole) [40]. In the present study, our *T. inkin* isolates had lower MIC values when compared with other publications [39, 40]. We observed that Itraconazole exhibited better in vitro effect against *T. inkin* isolates compared to Fluconazole and Amphotericin B and this finding was also observed by other studies involving *T. inkin* [39, 40] and other *Trichosporon* species [2, 35].

In conclusion, we may say this is the first case report of meningitis caused by *T. inkin* reported in the literature. Our female previously healthy patient was under corticosteroids and antibiotics therapy for a few months. In addition, she was submitted to an invasive procedure to remove a left sided acoustic neuroma and further developed a cerebrospinal fistula. All those factors are consolidated risk conditions for the infection caused by *T inkin*. The certainty of the invasive infection by *T. inkin* was based on the isolation of the pathogen along two different occasions together with brain images and cytological findings suggestive of meningitis. Both strains showed strong ability to express virulence factors in vitro. These findings together with patient's immunological status may have been crucial for the clinical outcome, because the strains were apparently not resistant to the antifungal drugs prescribed during her period of hospitalization. The physicians main suspicion was cryptococcal meningitis. Corroborating this idea, the strains obtained from CNF presented mucoid aspect in the primary isolation. However, the sending of these isolates to a reference Mycology center for accurate phenotypic and molecular identification revealed that the meningitis caused by *Trichsporon inkin*.

Abbreviations

ATCC: American Type Culture Collection; BLAST: Basic Local Alignment Search Tool; CBS: Centraalbureauvoor Schimmel cultures; CLSI: The Clinical & Laboratory Standards Institute; CNS: Central nervous system; CSF: Cerebrospinal fluid; CT: Computed tomography; Fig.: Figure; IGS1: Intergenic Spacer 1; MALDI-TOF: Matrix-Assisted Laser Desorption/Ionization Time-of-Flight; MIC: Minimal Inhibitory Concentration; MRI: Magnetic Resonance Imaging; rpm: Revolutions per minute; VP: Ventriculoperitoneal

Funding

This work was supported by "Conselho Nacional de Desenvolvimento Científico e Tecnológico" (CNPq) Grant number: Edital Universal 484020/2013-7.

Authors' contributions

JJSA, TUGF and ALAP were the attending physicians for the patient and collected medical data of the patient. MFA performed microbiological analysis and in vitro experiments. ECF and ASAM performed strains molecular identification. ALC made a critical review of the manuscript and provided financial support and structure for molecular identification. WPSR performed experiments and wrote the paper. EPM designed and wrote the paper and critically analyzed medical data. GMC designed all the experiments, structured and wrote the paper and critically reviewed the manuscript. All authors read and approved the final manuscript.

Consent for publication

Written informed consent was obtained from the patient's family for publication of this case report and accompanying images. A copy of the written consent is available for review by the Editor of this journal.

Competing interests

The authors declare that they have no competing interests.

Author details

[1]Departamento de Infectologia, Universidade Federal do Rio Grande do Norte, Natal, Rio Grande do Norte, Brazil. [2]Centro de Ciências da Saúde, Laboratório de Micologia Médica e Molecular, Departamento de Análises Clínicas e Toxicológicas, Universidade Federal do Rio Grande do Norte, Rua Gal. Gustavo Cordeiro de Faria S/N, Petrópolis, Natal, Rio Grande do Norte, Brazil. [3]Laboratório Especial de Micologia, Disciplina de Infectologia, Universidade Federal de São Paulo, São Paulo, Brazil.

References

1. Colombo AL, Padovan AC, Chaves GM. Current knowledge of *Trichosporon spp.* and Trichosporonosis. Clin Microbiol Rev. 2011;24(4):682–700.
2. Ruan SY, Chien JY, Hsueh PR. Invasive trichosporonosis caused by Trichosporon asahii and other unusual *Trichosporon species* at a medical center in Taiwan. Clin Infect Dis. 2009;49(1):e11–7.
3. Chagas-Neto TC, Chaves GM, Colombo AL. Update on the genus Trichosporon. Mycopathologia. 2008;166(3):121–32.
4. Heslop OD, Nyi Nyi MP, Abbott SP, Rainford LE, Castle DM, Coard KC. Disseminated trichosporonosis in a burn patient: meningitis and cerebral abscess due to Trichosporon asahii. J Clin Microbiol. 2011;49(12):4405–8.
5. Silva WP, Lemos VL, Milan EP, Chaves GM. Species distribution and phospholipase activity of fungi isolated from children with dermatomycosis from child day care units in Natal, Brazil. J Eur Acad Dermatol Venereol. 2013;27(10):1319–21.

6. Magalhaes AR, Nishikawa MM, Mondino SS, Macedo HW, Rocha EM, Baptista AR. Trichosporon isolation from human ungueal infections: is there a pathogenic role? An Bras Dermatol. 2016;91(2):173–9.
7. Silva-Rocha WP, de Azevedo MF, Chaves GM. Epidemiology and fungal species distribution of superficial mycoses in Northeast Brazil. J Mycol Med. 2017;27(1):57–64.
8. Duarte-Oliveira C, Rodrigues F, Goncalves SM, Goldman GH, Carvalho A, Cunha C. The cell biology of the Trichosporon-host interaction. Front Cell Infect Microbiol. 2017;7:118.
9. Almeida Junior JN, Song AT, Campos SV, Strabelli TM, Del Negro GM, Figueiredo DS, Motta AL, Rossi F, Guitard J, Benard G, et al. Invasive Trichosporon infection in solid organ transplant patients: a report of two cases identified using IGS1 ribosomal DNA sequencing and a review of the literature. Transpl Infect Dis. 2014;16(1):135–40.
10. Arendrup MC, Boekhout T, Akova M, Meis JF, Cornely OA, Lortholary O. ESCMID and ECMM joint clinical guidelines for the diagnosis and management of rare invasive yeast infections. Clin Microbiol Infect. 2014;20(Suppl 3):76–98.
11. Macedo DP, de Oliveira NT, da Silva VK, de Almeida Farias AM, de Lima Neto RG, Wilheim AB, de Oliveira PC, Pedi N, de Andrade SL, Neves RP. Trichosporon inkin esophagitis: an uncommon disease in a patient with pulmonary cancer. Mycopathologia. 2011;171(4):279–83.
12. Moretti-Branchini ML, Fukushima K, Schreiber AZ, Nishimura K, Papaiordanou PM, Trabasso P, Tanaka R, Miyaji M. *Trichosporon species* infection in bone marrow transplanted patients. Diagn Microbiol Infect Dis. 2001;39(3):161–4.
13. Nobrega de Almeida Junior J, Buccheri de Oliveira R, Duarte A, Lopes Motta A, Rossi F, Sachiko Yamamoto de Figueiredo D, Barbaro Del Negro GM, Aoki V, Wakisaka Maruta C, Giuli Santi C, et al. Trichosporon inkin as an emergent pathogen in patients with severe pemphigus. JAMA Dermatol. 2015;151(6):642–5.
14. Wynne SM, Kwon-Chung KJ, Shea YR, Filie AC, Varma A, Lupo P, Holland SM. Invasive infection with Trichosporon inkin in 2 siblings with chronic granulomatous disease. J Allergy Clin Immunol. 2004;114(6):1418–24.
15. Taguti Irie MM, Lopes Consolaro ME, Aparecida Guedes T, Donatti L, Valeria Patussi E, Estivalet Svidzinski TI. A simplified technique for evaluating the adherence of yeasts to human vaginal epithelial cells. J Clin Lab Anal. 2006;20(5):195–203.
16. Montoya AM, Sanchez Gonzalez A, Palma-Nicolas JP, Gomez-Trevino A, Gonzalez JG, Gonzalez GM. Genotyping, extracellular compounds, and antifungal susceptibility testing of Trichosporon asahii isolated from Mexican patients. Med Mycol. 2015;53(5):505–11.
17. de Aguiar Cordeiro R, Serpa R, Flavia Uchoa Alexandre C, de Farias Marques FJ, Vladia Silva de Melo C, da Silva Franco J, Jose de Jesus Evangelista A, Pires de Camargo Z, Samia Nogueira Brilhante R, Fabio Gadelha Rocha M, et al. Trichosporon inkin biofilms produce extracellular proteases and exhibit resistance to antifungals. J Med Microbiol. 2015;64(11):1277–86.
18. Basiri K, Meidani M, Rezaie F, Soheilnader S, Fatehi F. A rare case of Trichosporon brain abscess, successfully treated with surgical excision and antifungal agents. Neurol Neurochir Pol. 2012;46(1):92–5.
19. Badiye A, Patnaik M, Deshpande A, Rajendran C, Chandrashekara KV. Think fungus NOT just a crypto-meningitis in AIDS! J Assoc Physicians India. 2012;60:21–4.
20. Kumar A, Udayakumaran S, Babu R, Rajamma BM, Prakash A, Panikar D, Karim S, Chowdhary A. Trichosporon asahii infection presenting as chronic meningo-ventriculitis and intra ventricular fungal ball: a case report and literature review. Mycoses. 2015;58(2):99–103.
21. Mathews MS, Prabhakar S. Chronic meningitis caused by Trichosporon beigelii in India. Mycoses. 1995;38(3–4):125–6.
22. Rastogi VL, Nirwan PS. Invasive trichosporonosis due to Trichosporon asahii in a non-immunocompromised host: a rare case report. Indian J Med Microbiol. 2007;25(1):59–61.
23. Surmont I, Vergauwen B, Marcelis L, Verbist L, Verhoef G, Boogaerts M. First report of chronic meningitis caused by Trichosporon beigelii. Eur J Clin Microbiol Infect Dis. 1990;9(3):226–9.
24. Thien SY, Chung SJ, Tan AL, Hwang WY, Tan BH, Tan TT. Recurrent trichosporonosis with central nervous system involvement in an allogeneic hematopoietic stem cell transplant recipient. Transpl Infect Dis. 2016;18(5):768–72.
25. Watson KC, Kallichurum S. Brain abscess due to Trichosporon cutaneum. J Med Microbiol. 1970;3(1):191–3.
26. Sugita T, Nakajima M, Ikeda R, Matsushima T, Shinoda T. Sequence analysis of the ribosomal DNA intergenic spacer 1 regions of *Trichosporon species*. J Clin Microbiol. 2002;40(5):1826–30.
27. de Almeida Junior JN, Hennequin C. Invasive Trichosporon infection: a systematic review on a re-emerging fungal pathogen. Front Microbiol. 2016;7:1629.
28. Hrabovsky V, Takacova V, Schreterova E, Pastvova L, Hrabovska Z, Curova K, Siegfried L. Distribution and antifungal susceptibility of yeasts isolates from intensive care unit patients. Folia Microbiol (Praha). 2017;62(6):525-30.
29. Chagas-Neto TC, Chaves GM, Melo AS, Colombo AL. Bloodstream infections due to Trichosporon spp.: species distribution, Trichosporon asahii genotypes determined on the basis of ribosomal DNA intergenic spacer 1 sequencing, and antifungal susceptibility testing. J Clin Microbiol. 2009;47(4):1074–81.
30. Zuza-Alves DL, de Medeiros SS, de Souza LB, Silva-Rocha WP, Francisco EC, de Araujo MC, Lima-Neto RG, Neves RP, Melo AS, Chaves GM. Evaluation of virulence factors in vitro, resistance to osmotic stress and antifungal susceptibility of Candida tropicalis isolated from the coastal environment of Northeast Brazil. Front Microbiol. 2016;7:1783.
31. CLSI: Clinical and Laboratory Standards Institute. Reference method for broth dilution antifungal susceptibility testing of yeasts; Approved standard—third edition (M27-A3). Wayne; 2008.
32. CLSI: Clinical and Laboratory Standards Institute. Reference method for broth dilution antifungal susceptibility testing of yeasts; Approved standard—third informational supplement (M27-S3). Wayne; 2008.
33. CLSI: Clinical and Laboratory Standards Institute. Reference method for broth dilution antifungal susceptibility testing of yeasts; Approved standard—third informational supplement (M27-S4). Wayne; 2012.
34. Middelhoven WJ, Scorzetti G, Fell JW. Systematics of the anamorphic basidiomycetous yeast genus Trichosporon Behrend with the description of five novel species: Trichosporon vadense, T. smithiae, T. dehoogii, T. scarabaeorum and T. gamsii. Int J Syst Evol Microbiol. 2004;54(Pt 3):975–86.
35. Marine M, Bom VL, de Castro PA, Winkelstroter LK, Ramalho LN, Brown NA, Goldman GH. The development of animal infection models and antifungal efficacy assays against clinical isolates of Trichosporon asahii, T. asteroides and T. inkin. Virulence. 2015;6(5):476–86.
36. Chaves GM, Diniz MG, da Silva-Rocha WP, de Souza LB, Gondim LA, Ferreira MA, Svidzinski TI, Milan EP. Species distribution and virulence factors of Candida spp. isolated from the oral cavity of kidney transplant recipients in Brazil. Mycopathologia. 2013;175(3–4):255–63.
37. Tumbarello M, Fiori B, Trecarichi EM, Posteraro P, Losito AR, De Luca A, Sanguinetti M, Fadda G, Cauda R, Posteraro B. Risk factors and outcomes of candidemia caused by biofilm-forming isolates in a tertiary care hospital. PLoS One. 2012;7(3):e33705.
38. Liao Y, Zhao H, Lu X, Yang S, Zhou J, Yang R. Efficacy of ethanol against Trichosporon asahii biofilm in vitro. Med Mycol. 2015;53(4):396–404.
39. Taj-Aldeen SJ, Al-Ansari N, El Shafei S, Meis JF, Curfs-Breuker I, Theelen B, Boekhout T. Molecular identification and susceptibility of *Trichosporon species* isolated from clinical specimens in Qatar: isolation of Trichosporon dohaense Taj-Aldeen, Meis & Boekhout sp. nov. J Clin Microbiol. 2009;47(6):1791–9.
40. Ramos JM, Cuenca-Estrella M, Gutierrez F, Elia M, Rodriguez-Tudela JL. Clinical case of endocarditis due to Trichosporon inkin and antifungal susceptibility profile of the organism. J Clin Microbiol. 2004;42(5):2341–4.

24

Case report of *Actinomyces turicensis* meningitis as a complication of purulent mastoiditis

Béla Kocsis[1*†], Zoltán Tiszlavicz[2†], Gabriella Jakab[2], Réka Brassay[3], Márton Orbán[3], Ágnes Sárkány[3] and Dóra Szabó[1]

Abstract

Background: Central nervous system (CNS) infections caused by *Actinomyces spp.* including brain abscess, actinomycoma, subdural empyema and epidural abscess are well described, however reports of Actinomyces-associated meningitis are scarcely reported.

Case report: We present the case of a 43-year-old Hungarian male patient with poor socioeconomic status who developed acute bacterial meningitis caused by *Actinomyces turicensis* originating from the left side mastoiditis. The bacterial cultures of both cerebrospinal fluid (CSF) and purulent discharge collected during the mastoid surgery showed slow growing Gram-positive rods that were identified by automated systems (API, VITEK) as *A. turicensis* The bacterial identification was confirmed by 16S rRNA PCR and subsequent nucleic acid sequencing. No bacterial growth was detected in blood culture bottles after 5 days of incubation. Hence, multiple antibacterial treatments and surgical intervention the patient passed away.

Conclusions: Anaerobes are rarely involved in CNS infections therefore anaerobic culture of CSF samples is routinely not performed. However, anaerobic bacteria should be considered as potential pathogens when certain risk factors are present, such as paranasal sinusitis, mastoiditis in patients with poor socioeconomic condition. To the best of our knowledge, our case report is the first description of *A. turicensis* meningitis that has been diagnosed as consequence of purulent mastoiditis.

Keywords: *Actinomyces turicensis*, Anaerobic culture, Cerebrospinal fluid, Mastoiditis, Meningitis, Poor socioeconomic condition

Background

Meningitis caused by anaerobic bacteria is a rare disease therefore anaerobic culture of the cerebrospinal fluid (CSF) samples is not generally recommended. However, by these sparse cases of anaerobic meningitis certain conditions present risk factors namely, recurrent or chronic otitis media, brain abscess, necrotizing bowel lesions or peritonitis [1]. In cases of identifiable risk factors anaerobic meningitis should be kept in mind and the CSF specimen should be cultured both aerobically and anaerobically. The routine CSF sample processing lacks the anaerobic incubation that can lead to false-negative results and as a consequence to misdiagnose and therapy failure.

Actinomyces genus contains strictly anaerobic and aerotolerant, non-acid-fast, Gram-positive organisms with variable morphology, ranging from characteristic branching rods to coccobacilli arranged singly or in pairs. The most well-known species is *Actinomyces israelii*, however altogether 25 published Actinomyces species from human samples have been described [2]. Among these species *Actinomyces turicensis* was first reported in 1995 [3] and has been emerging as an important cause of infections [4]. *A. turicensis* is a non-pigment producing, aerotolerant member of Actinomyces genus. Its biochemical characteristics include negative reactions for the production of catalase, urease, β-N-acetyl-glucosaminidase and β-galactosidase, nitrate reduction, esculin hydrolysis, CAMP test and the fermentation of mannitol additionally, it produces α-glucosidase and

* Correspondence: kocsis.bela@med.semmelweis-univ.hu
†Béla Kocsis and Zoltán Tiszlavicz contributed equally to this work.
[1]Semmelweis University, Institute of Medical Microbiology, Budapest, Hungary
Full list of author information is available at the end of the article

ferments maltose and sucrose. Variable reactions are raffinose and trehalose fermentation [3].

Actinomyces spp. belong to the normal bacterial flora in the oral cavity, pharynx, gut and genitourinary tract [5–10]. Actinomycosis is an uncommon infection caused by *Actinomyces spp.* It is characterized by an indolent, slow growing, granulomatosus disease and categorized based on the anatomical sites as orocervicofacial, thoracic and abdominopelvic forms, or in some other cases it appears as cutaneous or musculoskeletal [11–14]. Actinomyces infections of central nervous system (CNS) such as brain abscess and meningitis are rarely diagnosed [15–18]. To date no published reports of *A. turicensis* meningitis were found on online databases. We herein report the first case of *A. turicensis* meningitis that originated from the left mastoiditis and it was diagnosed in a patient with poor socioeconomic status.

Case presentation

A 43-year-old Hungarian man with poor socioeconomic living conditions was found lying on the floor unresponsively by a family member. He was taken to a regional hospital "Szent György" University Teaching Hospital, Székesfehérvár, Hungary. On admission he had low level of consciousness accompanied by stiff neck, constricted pupils and fever (38.6 °C). Alcohol abuse, smoking and epileptic seizures were found in his past medical records. Urgent skull CT scan was performed revealing left side mastoiditis but neither brain abscess nor vascular disorders were described. Blood was drawn for clinical chemistry and for bacterial culture. Relevant parameters of the blood test showed elevated white blood cell (WBC) count 24.1 10^9/L (87.5% Neutrophils), increased C-reactive protein and procalcitonin levels (211.4 mg/L and 0.46 ng/ml, respectively). Laboratory parameters of blood and liquor are shown in Table 1. The results of the urine tests were normal.

Lumbar puncture was carried out and the CSF sample was taken to the laboratory immediately. The slightly xanthochromic CSF was cloudy showing increased WBC count (7400 cells/μl), elevated protein level (12.4 g/L), and low glucose level (< 0.6 mmol/L) compared to the elevated serum glucose level (8.1 mmol/L).

After taking blood and CSF specimens for culture Ceftriaxone (2 × 2 g), Vancomycin (2 × 1 g) and Ampicillin (6 × 2 g) were started and completed with supportive treatment.

The patient's CSF sample was processed routinely in our Microbiology laboratory (SYNLAB Székesfehérvár, Hungary) on arrival. The Pastorex Meningitis agglutination kit (Bio-Rad) testing the CSF sample for the presence of soluble antigens of *Streptococcus pneumoniae, Haemophilus influenzae* type b, *Neisseria meningitidis* group A, group B/ *E.coli* K1, group C, group Y/W135, and *Streptococcus* group B was negative. Microscopic examination showed several neutrophil granulocytes and a very few number of hardly

Table 1 Laboratory parameters of blood and cerebrospinal fluid

Blood results		
White blood cells	24.1×10^9/L	+
Red blood cells	4.7×10^{12}/L	normal
Hemoglobin	140 g/L	normal
Neutrophil	87.5%	+
Glucose	8.1 mmol/L	+
Total protein	74 g/L	normal
GOT	101 U/L	+
GPT	122 U/L	+
GGT	257 U/L	+
ALP	221 U/L	+
LDH	719 U/L	+
CRP	211.4 mg/L	normal
Procalcitonin	0.46 ng/L	normal
Liquor results		
Liquor glucose	0.6 mmol/L	–
Liquor protein	12.4 g/L	+

dyed short rods or elongated cocci that seemed to be Gram-negatively stained at first examination. To exclude tuberculous meningitis Ziehl-Neelsen staining was performed, but no acid-fast bacilli were detected. At the 18–24-h and 48 h readings bacterial growth was negative both on the blood and on the chocolate culture media. Only the enrichment broth was slightly cloudy, indicating bacterial growth. On the next day, after 72 h of incubation tiny grey pinhead colonies were found on both blood and chocolate agar plates that were catalase and oxidase negative. Similar colonies were seen on the anaerobic plates. Irregular small Gram-positive bacilli and coccobacilli were observed in the microscope. The bacterium was identified as *A. turicensis* by VITEK 2 ANC ID Card (Biomerieux) and API Coryne (Biomerieux). The identification was verified by molecular method. PCR was performed with primers that amplified 1343 bp fragment of bacterial 16 s rRNA coding sequence [19]. PCR thermal profile was as follows: 5 min at 94 °C, 40 cycles of 94 °C for 1 min, 55 °C for 1 min and 72 °C for 1 min and a final extension at 72 °C for 2 min [20]. PCR amplicons have been purified by Qiagen PCR Purification Kit (Qiagen, GmbH, Hilden, Germany) and have been sequenced (BIOMI Kft., Gödöllő, Hungary). Analysis of nucleic acid sequence was done based on online tools of NCBI GenBank thus, the strain was identified as *A. turicensis.*

Antibiotic susceptibility of tested strain was performed by E-test after the European Committee on Antimicrobial Susceptibility Testing (EUCAST) recommendations. The isolated strain was susceptible to penicillin, ampicillin, imipenem, meropenem and vancomycin at concentrations ranging from 0.125 to 0. 5 mg/L.

As the patient's condition did not improve a left side mastoid surgery was performed. During the mastoidectomy intraoperatively removed purulent discharge was sent to our Microbiology laboratory. After two days of incubation colonies grew on the agar plates that were similar to those isolated from the CSF sample. Identification both by biochemical reactions of automated systems and by 16S rRNA PCR and sequencing resulted *A. turicensis*. Moreover, the strain presented the same antibiotic MIC values as isolate of the CSF sample.

Postoperative bleeding occurred leading to the necessity of reoperation. On the third day of postoperative period severe polyuria was presented with dilated pupils insensible to light. The skull CT scan revealed cerebral herniation, intensifying oedema and sinus thrombosis. (Figures 1 and 2). Unfortunately, there was no chance of reoperation because the patient passed away.

After 5 days of aerobic and anaerobic incubation of the blood cultures no bacterial growth was detected. Autopsy was performed that confirmed the clinical diagnosis of cerebral herniation due to the purulent meningitis and the consequent oedema in the CNS. Moreover, a greenish-yellow discharge accumulated at the brain stem and in the lateral ventricules. During histopathology an infiltration of granulocytes at the meninges was seen and suspected signs of actinomycosis was also observed.

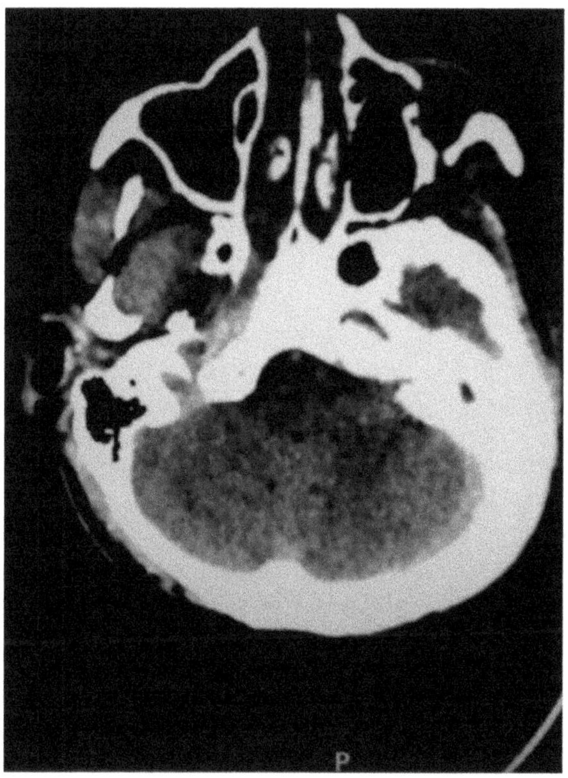

Fig. 1 Skull CT: horizontal slice of brain with left side mastoiditis

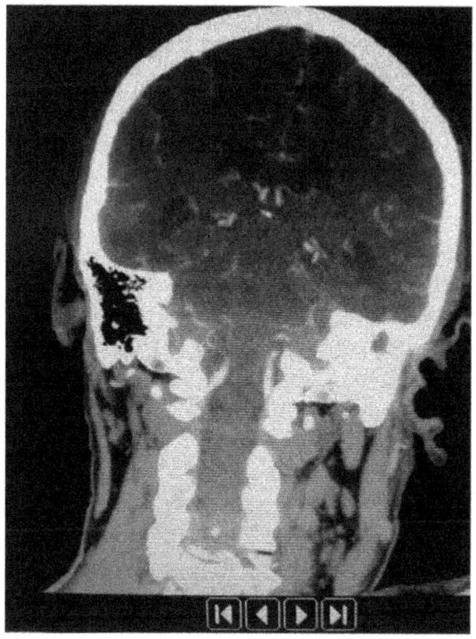

Fig. 2 Skull CT: coronal slice of brain with left side mastoiditis

Discussion and conclusions

Actinomyces spp. resides on mucous surfaces typically in the alimentary and genital tracts. On the other hand, *Actinomyces* spp. can rarely cause CNS infections due to the contiguous extension of neighbouring foci, such as paranasal sinusitis, or hematogenous seeding from a distant infected site such as a dental abscess, lungs and cervicofacial region although no such apparent foci are observed in one-third of cases. The typical manifestation of Actinomyces CNS infection is brain abscess, but Smego reported that 13% of CNS lesions of actinomycosis involve meningitis [17]. *A. turicensis* has been described as a potential pathogen mostly in genital and skin-related infections, however here we presented a case of CNS infection, namely *A. turicensis* meningitis as a complication of purulent mastoiditis with fatal outcome. In our patient an identical *A. turicensis* strain has been identified from a purulent mastoiditis and in meningitis, indicating the invasion of the pathogen from the infectious focus to CNS. There were no signs or symptoms of lung or skin actinomycosis. Anaerobes are found to be rare causative agents of meningitis but as our case report has shown it is worth to keep it in mind as possible pathogens of CNS. It may occur in patients living in poor socioeconomic conditions (e.g: homeless and alcohol abuse) and suffering from paranasal sinusitis or inflammation of other neighbouring foci. Here, we propose the need for anaerobic cultures of CSF specimens that is essential to identify *Actinomyces spp.* as well as other anaerob bacteria in CNS infections.

Abbreviations

16S rRNA: 16S ribosomal subunit ribonucleic acid; CAMP test: Christie-Atkins-Munch-Petersen synergistic heamolysis test; CNS: central nervous system; CSF: cerebrospinal fluid; CT: computer tomograph; EUCAST: European Committee on Antimicrobial Susceptibility Testing; MIC: minimum inhibitory concentration; NCBI: National Center for Biotechnology Information; PCR: polymerase chain reaction; WBC: white blood cell count

Acknowledgements

Not applicable.

Funding

This study was financially supported by OTKA Hungarian Research Fund, Grant No: 108481. The molecular biological analyses of tested strains was financially supported by funding body.

Authors' contributions

RB, MO, ÁS managed the patient and participated in study design. ZT, GJ performed microbiology diagnostics, analysed and interpreted data. BK, DSZ performed molecular identification and handled the manuscript. All authors have been involved in drafting the manuscript as well as revising it. All authors read and approved the final version of the manuscript.

Consent for publication

Consent to publish was obtained from a next-of-kin after the patient's death.

Competing interests

The authors declare that they have no competing interests.

Author details

[1]Semmelweis University, Institute of Medical Microbiology, Budapest, Hungary. [2]SYNLAB Székesfehérvár Microbiology Laboratory, Székesfehérvár, Hungary. [3]"Szent György" University Teaching Hospital, Székesfehérvár, Hungary.

References

1. Hawkey PM, Jewes LA. How common is meningitis caused by anaerobic bacteria? J Clin Microbiol. 1985;22:325.
2. Könönen E, Wade WG. Actinomyces and related organisms in human infections. Clin Microbiol Rev. 2015;28:419–42.
3. Wüst J, Stubbs S, Weiss N, Funke G, Collins MD. Assignment of*Actinomyces pyogenes*-like (CDC coryneform group E) bacteria to the genus *Actinomyces* as *Actinomyces radingae* sp. nov. and *ctinomyces turicensis*sp. Nov. Lett Appl Microbiol. 1995;20:76–81.
4. Sabbe LJ, Van De Merwe D, Schouls L, Bergmans A, Vaneechoutte M, Vandamme P. Clinical spectrum of infections due to the newly described *Actinomyces* species *A. turicensis*, *A. radingae*, and *A. europaeus*. J Clin Microbiol. 1999;37:8–13.
5. Dewhirst FE, Chen T, Izard J, Paster BJ, Tanner ACR, Yu W-H, et al. The human oral microbiome. J Bacteriol. 2010;192:5002–17.
6. Sarkonen N, Könönen E, Summanen P, Kanervo A, Takala A, Jousimies-Somer H. Oral colonization with *Actinomyces* species in infants by two years of age. J Dent Res. 2000;79:864–7.
7. Hoyles L, Clear JA, McCartney AL. Use of denaturing gradient gel electrophoresis to detect *Actinobacteria* associated with the human faecal microbiota. Anaerobe. 2013;22:90–6.
8. El Aila NA, Tency I, Claeys G, Verstraelen H, Saerens B, Santiago GLDS, et al. Identification and genotyping of bacteria from paired vaginal and rectal samples from pregnant women indicates similarity between vaginal and rectal microflora. BMC Infect Dis. 2009;9:167.
9. Nikolaitchouk N, Hoyles L, Falsen E, Grainger JM, Collins MD. Characterization of *Actinomyces* isolates from samples from the human urogenital tract: description of *Actinomyces urogenitalis* sp. nov. Int J Syst Evol Microbiol. 2000;50:1649–54.
10. Lu H, Qian G, Ren Z, Zhang C, Zhang H, Xu W, et al. Alterations of *Bacteroides sp., Neisseria sp., Actinomyces sp.*, and *Streptococcus sp.* populations in the oropharyngeal microbiome are associated with liver cirrhosis and pneumonia. BMC Infect Dis. 2015;15:239.
11. Smego RA, Foglia G. Actinomycosis. Clin Infect Dis. 1998;26:1255–61.
12. Wong VK, Turmezei TD, Weston VC. Actinomycosis. BMJ. 2011;343:d6099.
13. Sama CB, Mbarga NF, Oben CE, Mbarga JA, Nfor EK, Angwafo Iii FF. Massive paediatric cervicofacial actinomycoses masquerading as an ulcerative malignancy. BMC Infect Dis. 2016;16:417.
14. Endo S, Mishima E, Takeuchi Y, Ohi T, Ishida M, Yanai M, et al. Periodontitis-associated septic pulmonary embolism caused by Actinomyces species identified by anaerobic culture of bronchoalveolar lavage fluid: a case report. BMC Infect Dis. 2015 Dec;15(1):552.
15. Chotmongkol V, Panthavasit J, Chuesakoolvanich K. Actinomycotic meningitis: report of a case. J Med Assoc Thail. 2002;85:739–41.
16. Imamura K, Kamitani H, Nakayasu H, Asai Y, Nakashima K. Purulent meningitis caused by Actinomyces successfully treated with rifampicin: a case report. Intern Med. 2011;50:1121–5.
17. Smego RA Jr. Actinomycosis of the central nervous system. Rev Infect Dis. 1987;9:855–65.
18. Koda Y, Seto Y, Takeichi S, Kimura H. Fatal subarachnoid haemorrhage complicating actinomycotic meningitis. Forensic Sci Int. 2003;134:169–71.
19. Woo PCY, Cheung EYL, Leung K, Yuen K. Identification by 16S ribosomal RNA gene sequenceing of an Enterobacteriaceae species with ambiguous biochemical profile from renal transplant recipient. Diagn Microbiol Infect Dis. 2001;39:85–93.
20. Jenkins C, Ling CL, Ciesielczuk HL, Lockwood J, Hopkins S, McHugh TD, et al. Detection and identification of bacteria in clinical samples by 16S rRNA gene sequencing: comparison of two different approaches in clinical practice. J Med Microbiol. 2012;61:483–8.

Evaluation of the enhanced meningitis surveillance system, Yendi municipality, northern Ghana, 2010–2015

Basil Benduri Kaburi[1], Chrysantus Kubio[1,2], Ernest Kenu[1*], Kofi Mensah Nyarko[1], Jacob Yakubu Mahama[3], Samuel Oko Sackey[1] and Edwin Andrew Afari[1]

Abstract

Background: Meningitis is the inflammation of the meninges of the brain and or spinal cord. Global mortality rates vary from 2% to 30%. Epidemic meningitis remains a public health concern along the meningitis belt of Africa. Despite the operation of an enhanced meningitis surveillance system in Ghana, institutional mortality rates are estimated to range from 36% to 50%. In 2014, Yendi recorded 83 confirmed cases; with focal epidemics in some sub-municipals. We evaluated the system over a five-year period to find out whether it was achieving its objectives of systematic collection and analyses of data for the prevention or early detection of meningitis epidemics.

Methods: We used cross-sectional design. Both qualitative and quantitative data from Yendi Municipality between January 2010 and December 2015 were collected and analyzed. The updated guidelines for evaluating surveillance systems from Centers for Disease Control and Prevention were used. Content analysis was performed on the responses of key informants. Surveillance data was analyzed using MS-Excel.

Results: Fifteen healthcare workers were interviewed. For the period under evaluation, the annual incidence of meningitis ranged from 1.6/100,000 in 2012 to 62.6/100,000 in 2014. The average case fatality rate for the period was 8.3%. The system was sensitive, representative, and acceptable. The predictive value positive was 100% from 2010 to 2014 and 63.3% in 2015. Data quality was good, but timeliness of reporting was poor.

Conclusions: The enhanced meningitis surveillance system in Yendi Municipality is achieving most of its objectives. However, financial constraints and poor personnel motivation pose threats to the sustainability of the system.

Keywords: Meningitis, Epidemics, Surveillance, Evaluation, Yendi, Ghana

Background

Meningitis is the inflammation of the meninges of the brain. If the meninges of the spinal cord are involved, the disease state is termed Cerebrospinal Meningitis (CSM). Meningitis contributes significantly to morbidity and mortality in many regions of the world [1, 2]. There have been advancements in the diagnosis and treatment of meningitis over the years. These advances notwithstanding, mortality rates are still high.

Meningitis has both infectious and non-infectious causes. Infectious causes include: bacteria, viruses, fungi, parasites, and rickettsiae [3]. Non-infectious causes range from drugs as common as non-steroidal anti-inflammatory drugs (NSAIDs), to systemic diseases such as sarcoidosis and a host of collagen vascular disorders [3]. Neoplastic disorders, and post-vaccination complications from common vaccines such as those against rubella, rabies, and yellow fever can also cause non- infectious meningitis [3]. Viruses, non-pus producing bacteria, and some non-infectious aetiologies can cause aseptic meningitis; a unique type of meningitis with clear cerebrospinal fluid (CSF) [3].

* Correspondence: ernest_kenu@yahoo.com
[1]Field Epidemiology and Laboratory Training Programme, Department of Epidemiology and Disease Control, School of Public Health, College of Health Sciences, University of Ghana, Legon, Accra, Ghana
Full list of author information is available at the end of the article

A number of bacterial species are implicated in meningitis during the neonatal period, but about 9 in every 10 cases in the post-neonatal period are caused by *Streptococcus pneumoniae, Haemophilus influenzae,* and *Neisseria meningitides* [4]. All the three regions of northern Ghana lie completely in the meningitis belt of sub-Saharan Africa. In areas within this belt, epidemics of acute bacterial meningitis are commonly caused by different subtypes of *N. meningitides* and *S. pneumonia* [5, 6].

As at 1997, the annual non-epidemic cases of acute bacterial meningitis was estimated at 1.2 million globally with 135,000 fatalities [7]. By February 2012, WHO reported a rise in the estimated global annual fatalities to 170,000 [8]. Global mortality rates vary from 2% to 30% [9, 10]. Studies in Ghana estimate institutional mortality rates at 36 to 50% [11]. About 10 to 20% of patients who recover from acute bacterial meningitis suffer grave sequelae such as: epilepsy, mental retardation, hearing impairment, and several related neurological deficits [4]. The estimated risk of suffering at least one complication of acute bacterial meningitis after recovery can be as bad as nearly 4 of every 10 patients; with a median risk of about 20% of such patients [4]. As would be anticipated, acute bacterial meningitis is more prevalent in developing countries and ranks as the fourth leading cause of disability in these countries [4].

Epidemic meningococcal meningitis is characterized by a sudden onset of severe headache, fever, nausea, vomiting, neck rigidity, and photophobia [12]. These primary symptoms are commonly accompanied by one or more observable neurological signs such as delirium, lethargy, coma, and convulsions [12]. These signs may not be marked in infants and a high index of suspicion would then be required for prompt diagnosis [13].

Humans are the only known natural reservoir of *N.* meningitides [14]. About one in every 10 adolescents and adults are transient carriers of many strains of *N. meningitidis*. Fortunately, most of these colonise the nasophayrnx as commensals [14]. Risk factors for contracting an infection are broadly categorized into four: environmental, demographic, socioeconomic, and host-related factors.

Environmental risk factors include hot temperatures, dusty winds, and low absolute humidity; as found in the long dry seasons of countries in the meningitis belt [14, 15]. Such conditions lead to breaks in nasopharyngeal mucosal linings and opportunistic invasion of the blood stream by *N. meningitidis* may then ensue.

Demographic factors such as mass gathering as in the cases of refugee camps, military communities, and pilgrimages promote the circulation of infectious strains among individuals. In recent history, the 1987 meningococcal outbreak at the end of a pilgrimage in Mecca illustrates the reality of this risk category [14].

Poor socioeconomic conditions result in inadequate housing and poor living standards. Overcrowding is common in these situations especially during the cold and dry harmattan season. These conditions are associated with higher incidence meningococcal disease in general [14].

Host-related factors such as compromised immunity [13] from chronic diseases such Acquired Immunodeficiency Syndrome (AIDS) and diabetes mellitus carry increased risk of contracting infection. These diseases by themselves do not pose unique threats for epidemics, except when other conducive conditions exist to initiate and facilitate spread from primary cases. Non-vaccination of susceptible populations is a serious risk factor for epidemics. A low heard immunity also poses a risk for epidemics [14]. Poorly managed respiratory tract infections can complicate into meningococcal disease epidemics [14].

The mode of spread is by droplet infection from diseased persons. Consequently, epidemics flourish in conditions where overcrowding of people is inevitable as seen in pilgrimages and refugee camps. The typical meningitis season occurs during the dry and windy harmattan season because these conditions are pertinent for the spread of the infection.

The World Health Organization (WHO) in its determination to eliminate CSM, has joined forces with other stakeholders, at the international and country level to advocate and support an enhanced surveillance system [16]. To this end, the Ghana Health Service (GHS) has in collaboration with 13 other African countries, developed a Standard Operating Procedures (SOPs) in 2004 for meningitis surveillance. An updated version was published in December 2010 by the Public Health Division of GHS to cater for lessons learnt in the 2009/2010 CSM outbreak in the country [16]. This revised SOP manual further underscores the crucial role of: the laboratory for case confirmation, readily available supplies, health personnel capacity strengthening, as well as clear operating procedures for the effective implementation of an enhanced meningitis surveillance.

From 2010 to 2013, Yendi municipality recorded a total of 19 confirmed cases of acute bacterial meningitis. Thus, an average of about five cases for each of these years. However, in 2014 alone, the municipality recorded a total of 83 confirmed cases of acute bacterial meningitis with focal epidemics in some sub-municipals. This trend of events attracts interest regarding the operation of the meningitis surveillance system in the municipality. We evaluated the system and its attributes over a six-year period to find out whether it was achieving its objectives of systematic collection and analyses of both epidemiological and laboratory data for the prevention or early detection of meningitis epidemics.

Methods

Study area

The Yendi Municipality is located in the eastern corridor of the Northern Region of the Republic of Ghana between Latitude 9° – 35° North and Longitude 0° – 30° West and 0° – 15° East (Fig 1). The Greenwich Meridian thus passes through Yendi and other settlements in the municipality. The population of the Municipality in 2015 was about 136,434. The Dagomba ethnic group constitutes the majority. The other ethnic groups include Konkomba, Akan, Ewe, Basare, Chokosi, Hausa and Moshie.

The municipality has one hospital situated in Yendi, four (4) health centres, one (1) clinic owned by the Church of Christ, and fifteen functional Community-based Health Planning and Services (CHPS) zones. Of these CHPS zones, six (6) do not have compounds. There are five (5) main private pharmacy shops and several small chemical shops in the municipality. Drug peddling is common in the municipality.

The entire municipality lies within the African meningitis belt. Mean annual rainfall (January to December) for the Municipality is 1125 mm. Mean dry season rainfall (November to March) is 75 mm. Temperatures range between 21 °C and 36 °C and accompanied by low humidities. The vegetation is of the tree savannah type. The degraded savannah type of vegetation is found around settlements. Rampant and extensive bush burning is a significant contributor to the hot and dry climate. Such a climate is very conducive for triggering meningococcal epidemics.

Study design

The evaluation was cross-sectional design; involving the collection of both qualitative and quantitative data. Qualitative data was collected by means of semi-structured interviewer-administered questionnaires. The following documents were used to guide the surveillance system evaluation process: the updated guidelines of the Centers for Disease Control and Prevention (CDC), for evaluating public health systems (2001), the WHO practical guidelines on the control of epidemic meningococcal disease [17], and the GHS standard operating procedures (SOPs) manual on meningitis [16]. The period under evaluation was January 2010 to December 2015.The study was conducted between December 2015 and January 2016.

Data collection

All four Yendi sub-municipal health centers, municipal hospital, and municipal health directorate were visited. Various categories of healthcare workers were interviewed using the aforementioned questionnaires. Overall, the staff categories actively involved in the operation of the surveillance were interviewed: Technical Officers (disease control), Disease Control Officers (DCO), Physician Assistants (PA), Health Information Officers (HIO), and Biomedical Scientists (BMS). A cross section of Community-based Surveillance Volunteers (CBSVs) were also engaged in a discussion on their roles in the operation of the surveillance system. The data flow of the surveillance system was assessed and described.

Records at the four sub-Municipal health centers, Municipal Health Directorate, Regional Health Directorate, and the National Disease Surveillance Department

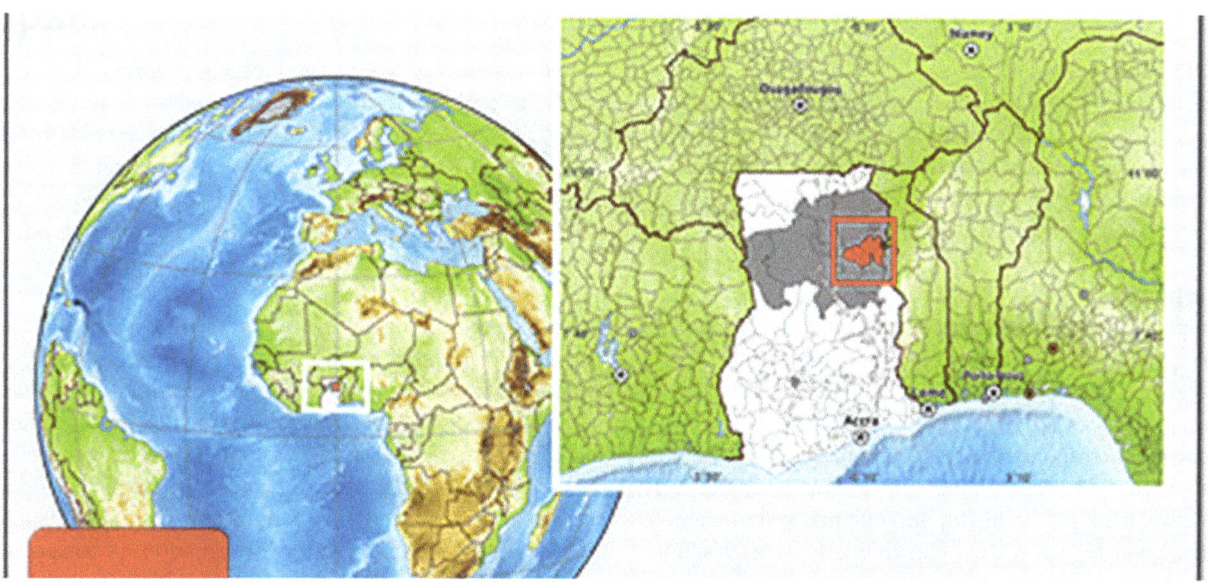

Fig. 1 Geographical location of Yendi Municipality, Ghana. Source: google maps

(NDSD) of the Ghana Health Service were reviewed. These included Integrated Disease Surveillance and Response (IDSR) 1 weekly report forms, IDSR 2 monthly report forms, laboratory register of the municipal hospital, and the Zonal Public Health Reference Laboratory (ZPHRL). IDSR immediate case-based report forms, line listing forms, clinical case notes of cases captured on line listing forms, case notification forms, community based surveillance summary report forms, monitoring charts and community register for vital events were also reviewed. The reviewed records were all part of the surveillance system and spanned the period from January 2010 to December 2015.

The inspection of standard meningitis protocols supposed to be in use was done to assess their availability and ready visibility. Pieces of laboratory equipment and other relevant logistics pertinent to the meningitis surveillance system were also inspected.

Case definitions

The following case definitions for meningitis were used: suspected, probable, and confirmed [16].

Suspected meningitis case

Any person with sudden onset of fever (>38.5 °C rectal or ≥ 38.0 °C axillary) and one of the following signs: neck stiffness, bulging fontanelle, convulsions, altered consciousness or other meningeal signs.

Probable meningitis case

Any suspected case with macroscopic aspect of cerebrospinal fluid turbid, cloudy or purulent or with microscopic test showing Gram negative diplococci, Gram positive diplococci, Gram negative bacilli; or leukocyte count of more than 10 cells/mm^3.

Confirmed meningitis case

Isolation or identification of causal pathogen (Neisseria meningitides, Streptococcus pneumoniae, Haemophilus influenzae b) from the Cerebrospinal fluid of a suspected or probable case by culture, Polymerase Chain Reaction or agglutination test.

Data analysis

We performed both qualitative and quantitative analyses. The qualitative data gathered by means of the interviewer-administered questionnaire were analysed by directed content analysis approach [18, 19]. By this approach, the participants' responses were systematically analysed along themes that were in keeping with the updated guidelines for evaluating public health surveillance systems as recommended by the CDC. The thematic areas included: the purpose and objectives of the system, components of the system, operational resource requirements, and the nine (9) system attributes. For each of the six years, we estimated the incidence and case fatality ratio (CFR) of acute bacterial meningitis using quantitative surveillance data retrieved from line lists.

An estimate of the amount of money spent on each suspected case of meningitis picked in the municipality was obtained by summing the personnel cost of officers involved to the costs of transport, stationary, communication, and laboratory services. The direct personnel cost was computed by summing the products of the hourly salary rates of officers involved and their respective person-hours spent on meningitis surveillance.

Ethical considerations

Approval for this study was granted by the Ghana Field Epidemiology and Laboratory Training Programme (GFELTP); run by both the Ghana Health Service and the School of Public Health - University of Ghana. Permission was officially sought from the Regional and the Municipal Directors of Health Services to assess the surveillance system and for the use of the data. Verbal consent was obtained from interviewees without any form of coercion. Data held on computers were encrypted with a password which was made available only on a need to know basis.

Results

Overview

A total of 15 officers who are directly involved in the operation of the meningitis surveillance system at the various levels from the sub-municipal level to the regional level granted detailed interviews. Of these, two (2) were females. The mean age of respondents was 39.1 ± 10.7 years. For each of the four sub-municipal health facilities, there was one technical officer and one physician assistant who were in charge of the surveillance system. In all, a total of eight interviews were done at that level. At the municipal level, there were two Disease Control Officer (DCO), one Health Information Officer (HIO), and one Biomedical Scientist (BMS). Each of them was also interviewed. From the Regional level: one DCO, one BMS, and one HIO; bringing the total number of respondents to 15.

Respondents at all levels had a clear knowledge and understanding of the purpose and objectives of the system. All respondents were able to produce copies of the *standard operating procedures for surveillance and management of epidemic cerebrospinal meningitis in Ghana* as their source of written documentation of the objectives of the meningitis surveillance system. They underscored the non-negotiable role of enhanced surveillance in the early detection and confirmation of suspected cases in order that swift public health interventions would be taken to prevent outbreaks.

All respondents referred to the 1992 constitution of Ghana (Act 525 of 1996) that established the Ghana Health Service as their legal authority for data collection. They understood that the data collected would be useful if only it is analysed to produce trends. They also understood the availability of quality data as a means of providing evidence to stakeholders for purposes of obtaining support in forms such as: human resource capacity building, provision of logistics, and funds. Stakeholders as identified by respondents included: Ministry of Health, Ghana Health Service, National Health Insurance Authority (NHIA), Expanded Programme on Immunisation (EPI), GFELTP, CDC, WHO, Coalition of NGOs into Health, CBSV, Health Care Workers (HCW), traditional authorities, and opinion leaders.

The list of case definitions were available at all levels. Whereas these were boldly displayed in the form of posters at the municipal health directorate, the same was not observed at the sub-municipal health centers.

Data communication in meningitis surveillance system

At all the levels, respondents were conversant with the flow of information for meningitis surveillance as shown in Fig. 2. However, no separate printed communication flow chart was available for meningitis. A general flow chart for all the diseases under surveillance in Ghana was available and covered meningitis as well.

The meningitis information flow started with the epidemiological reports from the community level, to laboratory reports from the municipal hospital laboratory and the Zonal Public Health Reference Laboratory

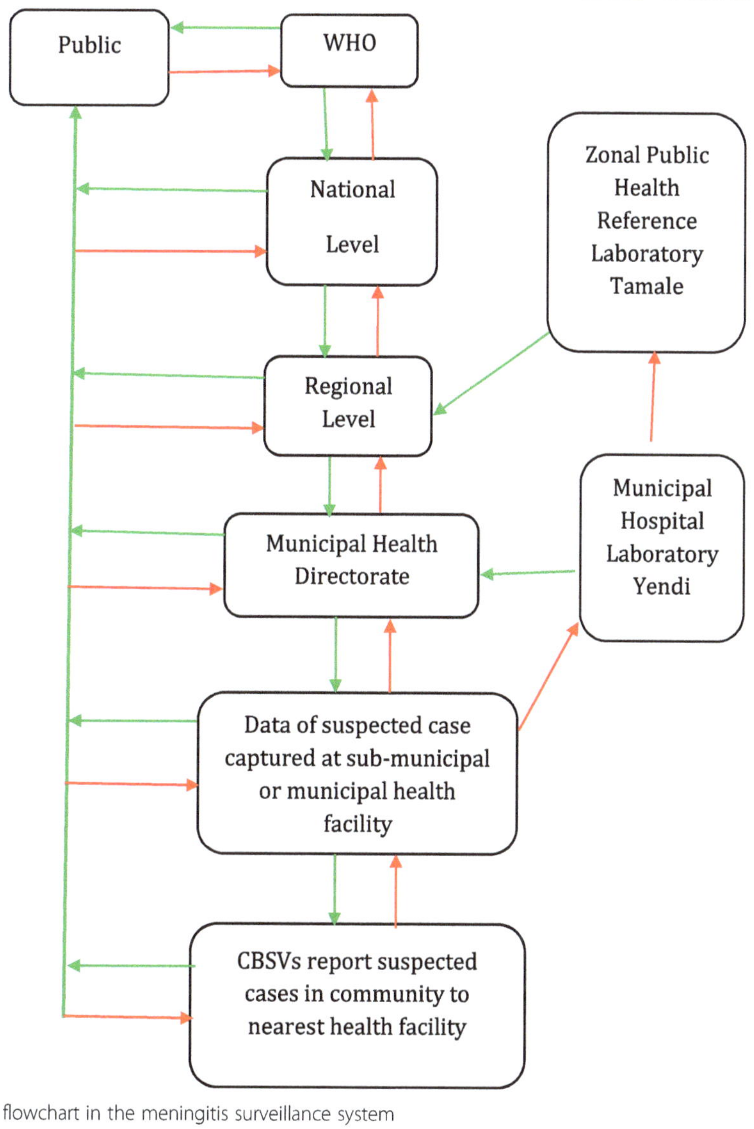

Fig. 2 Data communication flowchart in the meningitis surveillance system

(ZPHRL). Sick individuals from the community sought healthcare in a sub-municipal health facility where they could be suspected of meningitis. Other adequately informed members on health matters such as CBSVs could reported suspected cases to the facility. Sub-municipal health staff notified DCOs at the municipal level and referred suspected cases to the municipal hospital. At the municipal hospital, a Medical Officer (MO) or a nurse anaesthetist performed a lumbar puncture (LP) to sample cerebrospinal fluid (CSF). The municipal hospital laboratory, could perform the following tests: CSF glucose, cell count, Gram staining and agglutination tests. A portion of the specimen was sent to the ZPHRL for polymerase chain reaction (PCR), and culture & sensitivity tests. At the same time, the information about the case was relayed to the municipal health directorate for onward transmission to the Northern Regional Health Directorate (NRHD) and the disease surveillance department (DSD). Feedback reports from the ZPHRL were sent in the reverse direction through NRHD, YMHD, sub-municipal health facilities and finally back to the community. The NRHD fed the national DSD with information, which in turn fed WHO. During outbreaks or suspected outbreaks, the public and key stakeholders received updates of information at every stage of the investigation.

Components of the meningitis surveillance system

The entire population of the municipality; males and females of all ages, was under surveillance. DCOs and HIOs were responsible for collecting primary data on suspected cases. They collected and reported these data on daily, weekly, and monthly bases. For any given suspected case, the sub-municipal DCO completed a case notification form to notify municipal officers. Staff of sub-municipal health centers did not have the capacity to perform lumbar punctures (LPs). Suspected cases were therefore referred to the municipal hospital at Yendi where LPs were performed to sample CSF. Each specimen was accompanied by a completed meningitis case investigation form. Line listing forms were available for capturing multiple cases. Additionally, contact tracing and follow-up forms were available for tracing patient contacts in the communities.

A functional data validation team was in place at the municipal health directorate. This ensured that quality data is generated. Data quality validation was done by cross examining all hard copies of reporting tools for completeness and consistency before entering them onto the District Health Information Management System-2 (DHIMS-2) database. Upon entry of data onto the DHIMS-2, care was taken to ensure completeness and consistency of information before logging out. At the regional level, data was entered into Epi-info7 and check codes put in place to ensure proper validation. Physical checks were done and phone calls made to reporting districts whose data had inconsistencies for reconciliation. The northern regional weekly epidemiological bulletins also served to assist in data validation.

Hard copies of surveillance data were kept in files. Soft copies were saved in office computers and the DHIMS-2 under passwords. Additionally, data was stored on external hard drives. The DCOs and HIOs analysed the data using MS-Excel, Epi-info, and SPSS. Graphs, tables, and spot maps were generated.

Surveillance system resource requirements

The meningitis surveillance system has no separate budgetary allocation for its operation. It is part of the integrated disease surveillance system. It therefore shared resources allocated to all surveillance activities.

At the municipal level, six persons were directly involved in the meningitis surveillance system. For the year 2015, 30 suspected cases of meningitis were reported. The total personnel cost was estimated at GHC 137.48 per case. Table 1 shows a summary of estimations of the cost of handling each case.

Estimated costs of laboratory services (CSF glucose, cell count, Gram staining, and pastorex) at the municipal hospital was GH¢ 26.00 per case. Estimates of other routine costs were: communication - GH¢ 7.0, stationary - GH¢ 2.5, and the transportation of samples to the ZPHRL- GH¢ 23.00. These non-personnel costs summed up to GH¢ 58.50 per case. A grand total of GH¢ 195.98 (USD 52.96) was spent on each suspected case that underwent investigation.

Other resources required for meningitis surveillance activities included costs of training, logistics, and allowances of health personnel working on this system. Costs of Medical supplies, routine travel, information management, and case management were however excluded from the above estimates.

Usefulness of the meningitis surveillance system

The operation of the meningitis surveillance system in Yendi municipality was found to be very useful. From

Table 1 Personnel Cost Estimation for Meningitis Surveillance, Yendi Municipal Health Directorate, 2015

Designation of officer	Hourly salary rate (GH¢)	Person-hours per case	Cost of service per officer (GH¢)
MDHS	36.25	0.75	27.19
MO	22.50	0.50	11.25
BMS	11.25	1.00	11.25
DDCO	10.62	2.50	26.55
STO	8.75	4.00	35.00
TO	6.56	4.00	26.24

epidemiological and laboroatory data generated over the period, the overall case fatality rate was 8.3%. Table 2 depicts the annual CFR for the period evaluated. In 2014, some sub-municipal areas exceeded their epidemic thresholds even though the municipal as a whole was at the alert stage. Focal epidemics were therefore picked up by the system. As a result, reactive vaccinations within those affected areas and their neighbouring communities were carried out.

The meningitis surveillance data are also used to help prepare annual meningitis epidemic preparedness plans. These data were also useful in making realistic estimations of resource requirements for prevention and containment of any epidemic. Stakeholders also depended on these data to make decisions on the nature and quantum of support that should be given for the operation of the system.

System attributes

Simplicity

The system was rated as simple because of the clarity of its case definitions and the ease with which cases could be captured using easily detectable symptoms and observable signs. It took less than 30 min to collect data required to fill the new and separate meningitis case investigation form. The demographic and exposure information were easy to understand and record. Though there were multiple levels of reporting, all the 15 respondents demonstrated a good understanding of the scope of their respective roles in the system. Sequential relay of information from the sub-municipal through the YMHD and NRHD to the national level was effective.

Flexibility

The system was found to be flexible because it was well integrated with other surveillance systems. Additionally, modifications in its operations did not cause any setbacks. For example, the meningitis case investigation form was introduced in 2012 to replace the case based surveillance reporting form which catered for 5 other diseases under surveillance namely: cholera, diarrhoea with blood/shigella, measles, viral haemorrhagic fever, and yellow fever.

Stability

The systems was seen to be fairly stable partly because it is fully integrated with the other diseases under surveillance. The energy crisis that hit the country for the past 3 years posed challenges to the information management systems and communication due to rampant and unscheduled power outages. This notwithstanding, surveillance activities went on satisfactorily because on some occasions, power backups such as generators were used to mitigate the crisis. Other routine challenges with logistics, transport, and communication were also apparent during the evaluation.

Representativeness

The surveillance system was representative in person and place over the time period evaluated. The surveillance system collected data all year round with intensification of active case searches during the dry season and epidemics. It was noted that for the period under evaluation, 89.4% of the cases were recorded in the first quarter of the year; and none in the last quarter. The latest recorded case was in week-36 of 2015.

Over the six-year period all persons were under surveillance. Cases were reported from: both sexes, all ages, ethnicities, religions, occupations, and socioeconomic backgrounds. Cumulatively, 61.4% of cases were females.

In the four (4) years that preceded the epidemic, a total of 19 cases were recorded. These cases originated from all sub-municipals, they included males and females, and their ages ranged from one (1) year to 45 years. This representative distribution of cases was still true when individual years within the pre-epidemic period were considered. For example in 2011, when eight (8) cases were recorded, these were distributed across seven different sub-municipalities, with five females, and ages ranging from one (1) to 45. Similarly, with only three recorded cases in 2013, three sub-municipalities were represented, two of the three cases were females, and their ages were 2, 8, and 30 years.

Acceptability

The meningitis surveillance system was very acceptable among all stakeholders. All 17 reporting units of the Yendi municipality reported to the municipal health

Table 2 Incidence and Case Fatality Rate of meningitis, Yendi Municipality, 2010–2015

Year	Mid-Year Population	No. of Cases	No. of Deaths	Incidence/100,000	Case Fatality Rate (%)
2010	118,260	6	2	5.1	33.3
2011	121,690	8	1	6.6	12.5
2012	125,220	2	0	1.6	0.0
2013	128,850	3	1	2.3	33.3
2014	132,589	83	5	62.6	6.0
2015	136,434	19	1	13.9	5.3

directorate. All 26 districts of the northern region also submit reports to the regional health directorate as evidenced in the weekly epidemiological bulletins. Community members, CBSVs, health care professional of all categories, and patients all cooperated in the reporting and investigation of suspected cases. At the municipal level, LP rates have been consistently100% over the 6 year period under evaluation. The participation of CBSVs was however passive. They attributed this development to poor motivation.

Predictive value positive (PVP)

At the level of case detection, the predictive value positive was100% for each of the five (5) years from 2010 to 2014. Thus, all the suspected cases turned out to be confirmed as positive cases. However, in 2015, 19 of the 30 reported suspected cases turned out to be positive. This gave PVP of (19/30)*100% = 63.3%.

At the level of epidemic detection, the PVP was also 100%; as the only epidemic identified by the surveillance system within the study period (in 2014) turned out to be a true epidemic.

Sensitivity

The system was assessed qualitatively and found not to be very sensitive at the level of case detection because it was not able to detect many cases from 2010 to 2014. However, at the level of outbreak detection, it was sensitive enough to detect focal outbreaks in some sub-municipal areas in 2014.

Timeliness

Timeliness was assessed to be poor. It was assessed at three stages: timeliness of patient reporting to health facilities, timeliness of delivery of CSF to ZPHRL, and timeliness of the feedback from ZPHRL to municipal hospital and other stakeholders.

It took an average of three days (3 ± 0.8 days) for symptomatic patients to report to the nearest health facility within the municipality. Delivery of CSF samples from YMHD to the ZPHRL took three days on the average (3.0 ± 1.6 days). Sometimes samples could delay up to seven days. It took an average of five days (4.7 ± 2 days) to receive feedback from the ZPHRL.

Data quality

The quality of data generated in the municipality did not have major issues. On cross examination, information on hard copies of line listing forms and case investigation forms from the reporting units were mostly consistent with that found at the sub-municipal records. A few data reconciliations had to be done on the geographical origin of some suspected cases.

Case investigation forms were largely complete. However, in about 24% (32/132) of cases, the immunisation histories could not be obtained. The LP rate was 100% and all such cases had records of laboratory investigations performed on CSF samples. The municipal data as captured in their records and DHIMS-2 were also largely consistent with those available at the NRHD. A feedback of five additional confirmed cases were yet to reach the YMHD. The NRHD was also yet to update the number of suspected cases for 2015, from 23 to 30 as at the time we reviewed their records.

Discussion

The enhanced meningitis surveillance system, as run in the Yendi Municipality is largely effective despite human resource and financial constraints. It is achieving the key surveillance objectives of early detection and prevention of epidemics. Even in the case of the focal epidemics within the municipality in 2014, the response was early enough to avert a major epidemic. The response took the forms of sensitization and health education of the general public, and a reactive vaccination exercise. The public was educated on how to recognise signs and symptoms of meningitis, the facilities to report to, and how to avoid the spread of the disease. This was done by the epidemic response teams of the municipal and region using the mass media, community durbars, schools, and places of worship. Confirmatory PCR results from the ZPHRL indicated the causative organism was Nm W. Residents of the municipality were encouraged to patronise the reactive vaccination exercise against Nm W. This exercise started within a week of the outbreak detection. These interventions helped to contain the spread of the outbreak.

The system was found to be simple, flexible, and highly acceptable to all stakeholders. It was fairly stable despite the energy and economic crisis the country had experienced over the period under review. The multiple storage forms of data that were in place provided backups should one storage form get lost or corrupted. The attainment of the remaining system attributes is largely contingent on performance of these preceding four surveillance system attributes. This assertion is very much in keeping with findings of similar evaluation studies of dengue fever in Taiwan [20] and of meningitis in the Talensi district in the Upper East Region of Ghana [21].

The high level of acceptability had a positive influence on data quality. Any evidence of effective operation of the system will be demonstrated by the reliability of the data generated. This in turn is not possible if the system is not very representative in time, person, and place. Cases of meningitis were reported from all sub-municipals and these covered both males and females of all age groups. Of the 132 reported suspected cases for the period under review, majority (61.4%) were females. This finding is also consistent with the general literature that espouses a higher prevalence among females. Females are thought to be at a higher risk of secondary attack because they mostly take care of family members who become primary cases. This was observed in the evaluation of the meningitis surveillance systems of Burkina Faso and Mali [22]. Two in every three cases were aged 29 years and younger. This gives further credence to the ascription of the most at-risk age group to those between 2 to 29 years [22]. All persons from neighbouring communities outside the municipality, and temporary residents who are in transit for socioeconomic reasons were also considered as part of the target population. These were captured as imported cases. They accounted for nearly a quarter (23.1%) of the 121 confirmed cases within the period under evaluation.

The PVP of 100% could be attributed to a strict adherence to the standard case definition for a suspected case. Thus, meeting the criteria for a suspected case invariably led to the confirmation of acute bacterial meningitis. However, the system could have been missing cases as a result of this strict adherence to the case definition. The PVP reduced to 63.3% in 2015 because a broader case definition was adopted. This broader case definition differed only in one respect from the standard one: it did not require all suspected cases to present with fever or honestly disclose a history of fever. The reason was that, it is common practice in Ghana for patients to resort to NSAIDs for self-medication as a first option when they develop a fever. They would also try treating themselves for malaria because it is still the commonest cause of fever among Ghanaian patients. As a result, they may subsequently present to the health facility without fever. Some may also fail to disclose a history of fever for which they self-medicated for fear of being reprimanded by clinicians. The recognition of these common patient behaviours informed the reduced importance placed on fever in suspecting a meningitis case in 2015. Furthermore, a higher index of suspicion within the population and among clinicians, informed by the focal epidemics that hit parts of the municipality in 2014, also contributed to increased reporting of suspected cases and hence the reduced PVP. The relatively high prevalence of endemic meningitis in this municipal probably contributed to these findings which stand in contrast to those of the Talensi district as reported by Apanga and Awoonor-Williams [21].

Even though the YMHD promptly alerted the NRHD of suspected meningitis cases, this did not translate to prompt laboratory investigation of CSF specimen for a number of reasons. Firstly, the YMHD had some difficulties delivering specimen of CSF to the ZPHRL due to transportation challenges. Secondly, investigation and feedback from the ZPHRL could delay up to a week on some occasions. Unlike the challenge of distance cited by Apanga and Awoonor-Williams [21] as mainly responsible for delays in feedback, Yendi Municipality is about one hour drive from the ZPHRL in Tamale. Thus, apart from distance, other challenges to do with personnel and logistics are at play as indicated by some of the managers interviewed. Delays in feedbacks tend to undermine the whole essence of the surveillance system. The reason being that, prompt public health actions that are key to averting epidemics may be delayed as a result.

The Nm W was the causative organism identified by the ZPHRL at Tamale. In 2012, the same organism was responsible for causing outbreaks first in the Upper West region [23] and then in the Upper East region [24]. Given that this same organism had caused two successive outbreaks in two of the neighbouring regions, the public health community in Ghana was not surprised because routine laboratory surveillance kept recording increasing numbers of this organism across the three northern regions of the country. However, delays in laboratory confirmation of cases during non-epidemic periods contribute to delays in outbreak detection. This situation could be improved by tackling two main problems: ensuring readily available means of transport to deliver specimen speedily to the ZPHRL, and boosting the logistic capacity of this laboratory to perform investigations speedily. Equipment breakdown is one recurring reason for laboratory delays and so the culture of plan preventive maintenance should be enforced particularly at the ZPHRL.

The importance of the laboratory in the operation of the enhanced meningitis surveillance has been demonstrated severally [25]. Analyses of laboratory data before 2010 indicated that *N. meningitides* strain A was mostly responsible for large meningococcal outbreaks in Ghana. Similar findings were made in countries along the African meningitis belt [16]. This necessitated a policy change by which Men A vaccines were substituted for previous ones in mass vaccinations. Consequently, the prevalence of this strain has reduced. No Meningitis A epidemics have occurred in Ghana since the mass vaccination was carried out 2012.

Unlike funded programmes such as Tuberculosis, HIV/AIDS, Malaria, and Maternal health, meningitis surveillance has no dedicated budgetary allocation to ensure unfettered execution of its activities. Its reliance on the common budget allocated for the integrated surveillance activities poses difficulties of motivating non-salaried players in the chain of reporting such as the CBSVs. Their place at the very beginning of the reporting pathway is crucial to early detection of suspected cases for subsequent investigations at our health facilities. Our interaction with a cross-section of 17 CBSVs of Gnani sub- municipality revealed that they no longer feel a part of the system as they did about eight years before. Hitherto, they had opportunities of attending regular training workshops and earning some allowances. They also indicated that, they and their families no longer enjoy express services at health facilities. In the absence of all these incentives, a good number of them have abandoned their duties, and the remaining ones do not do any more than passive reporting. Passive reporting on the part of these CBSV contributed to the poor timeliness of case reporting from the community to health facilities. This is a worrying development because, the foundation of the surveillance hinges on these CBSVs.

Study limitations

Some limitations of the study include the following; Clinical case notes for periods when there were no outbreaks, were sampled and reviewed. As such, it is possible some cases were missed due to the sampling process.

Also the review required the interviewees recalling events over the past five years, there is therefore likely to be a recall bias, however, this was minimized since frontline workers were interviewed.

Conclusions

The meningitis surveillance system operated by the Yendi municipality is achieving most of its objectives even in the face of systemic challenges that border largely on inadequate finances. The system was found to be simple, flexible, and acceptable. It was fairly sensitive, representative, and stable. The data quality was good and the PVP was high. However, timeliness of case reporting from communities to health facilities and specimen collection at municipal hospital were poor. There was low morale among CBSVs resulting in passive case reporting.

The WHO, coalition of NGOs into health, and other donor partners should consider increasing the funding support for the integrated surveillance activities in order to consolidate the gains made this far. The low morale of our indispensable CBSVs could be improved if managements of the health centers and municipal hospital could renew their commitment to engage them regularly, and also assist them access health care services speedily for themselves and immediate family members. GHS should also consider training physician assistants on how to perform lumbar puncture in order to improve timeliness of CSF collection.

Abbreviations

AIDS: Acquired Immunodeficiency Syndrome; BMS: Biomedical Scientist; CBSVs: Community Based Surveillance Volunteers; CDC: Centers for Disease Control and Prevention; CHPS: Community-based Health Planning and Services; CSF: Cerebrospinal Fluid; CSM: Cerebrospinal Meningitis; DCO: Disease Control Officers; DHIMS: District Health Information Management Systems; EPI: Expanded Programme on Immunization; GFELTP: Ghana Field Epidemiology and Laboratory Training Programme; HCW: Health Care Workers; HIO: Health Information Officers; IDSR: Integrated Disease Surveillance and Response; LP: Lumbar Puncture; MO: Medical Officer; NDSD: National Disease Surveillance Department; NRHD: Northern Regional Health Directorate; NSAIDs: Non-Steroidal Anti-inflammatory Drugs; PA: Physician Assistant; SOPs: Standard Operating Procedures; WHO: World Health Organization; YMHD: Yendi Municipal Health Directorate; ZPHRL: Zonal Public Health Reference Laboratory.

Acknowledgements

We would like to acknowledge the Yendi Municipal Health Directortate, Ghana Health Service for assisting with the data evaluation.

Funding

Funding was by the Ghana Field Epidemiology and Laboratory Training Programme.

Authors' contributions

Conceptualization of idea – BBK, KMN, EK, SOS, EAA. Data collection – BBK, CK, JYM. Data analyses – BBK. Draft manuscript – BBK, CK, EK, KMN, SOS and EAA. Review of manuscript – CK, EK, KMN, SOS and EAA. All authors read and approved the final manuscript.

Competing interests

The authors declare that they have no competing interests.

Consent for publication

Not applicable.

Author details

[1]Field Epidemiology and Laboratory Training Programme, Department of Epidemiology and Disease Control, School of Public Health, College of Health Sciences, University of Ghana, Legon, Accra, Ghana. [2]Ghana Health Service, West Gonja District Health Directorate, Damongo, Ghana. [3]Ghana Health Service, Northern Regional Health Directorate, Tamale, Ghana.

References

1. Theodoridou M, Vasilopoulou V, Atsali E, Pangalis A, Mostrou G, Syriopoulou V, et al. Meningitis registry of hospitalized cases in children: epidemiological patterns of acute bacterial meningitis throughout a 32-year period. BMC Infect Dis. 2007;7:101.
2. Dash N, Panigrahi D, Al Khusaiby S, Al Awaidy S, Bawikar S. Acute bacterial meningitis among children < 5 years of age in Oman: a retrospective study during 2000-2005. J Infect Dev Ctries. 2008;2(2):112–5.
3. Kumar R. Aseptic meningitis: diagnosis and management. Indian J Pediatr. 2005;72:57–63.
4. Edmond K, Clark A, Korczak V, Sanderson C, Griffiths U, Rudan I. Global and regional risk of disabling sequelae from bacterial meningitis: a systematic review and meta-analysis. Lancet Infect Dis. 2010;10(5):317–28.
5. Greenwood B. Editorial: 100 years of epidemic meningitis in West Africa - has anything changed? Tropical Med Int Health. 2006;11(6):773–80.
6. World Health Organization. Meningitis in Burkina Faso, Chad, Niger, Nigeria and Ghana: 2010 epidemic season. Wkly Epidemiol Rec. 2011;86(15):143–51.
7. Tikhomirov E, Santamaria M, Esteves K. Meningococcal disease: public health burden and control. World Health Stat Q. 1997;50(3–4):170–77.
8. World Health Organisation. New and under-utilized vaccines implementation (NUVI): bacterial meningitis (online). Available from: http://www.who.int/immunization/global_vaccine_action_plan/GVAP_Guiding_Principles_Measures_of_Success_and_Goals.pdf. Accessed 21 Apr 2017.

9. Chavez-Bueno S, McCracken G Jr. Bacterial meningitis in children. Pediatr Clin N Am. 2005;52(3):795–810.
10. Perez A, Dickinson F, Rodriguez M. Community acquired bacterial meningitis in Cuba: a follow up of a decade. BMC Infect Dis. 2010;10:130.
11. Holliman R, Liddy H, Johnson J. Ohene Adjei. Epidemiology of invasive pneumococcal disease in Kumasi, Ghana. Trans R Soc Trop Med Hyg. 2007;101(4):405–13.
12. Fitch M, van de Beek D. Emergency diagnosis and treatment of adult meningitis. Lancet Infect Dis. 2007;7(3):191–200.
13. Dubos F, Martinot A, Gendrel D, Bréart G, Chalumeau M. Clinical decision rules for evaluating meningitis in children. Curr Opin Neurol. 2009;22(3):288–93.
14. Control of epidemic meningococcal meningitis. Risk factors for epidemics. WHO practical guidelines, 2nd edition, 1998; p 12. Available at: www.who.int › publications ›meningitis [Accessed March 9, 2017].
15. Harrison L, Pass M, Mendelsohn A, Egri M, Rosenstein N, Bustamante A, et al. Invasive meningococcal disease in adolescents and young adults. JAMA. 2001;286:694–9.
16. Ministry of Health: Ghana Health Service. Standard operating procedures for surveillance and management of epidemic cerebro-spinal meningitis in Ghana. Accra; 2011.
17 Centers for Disease Control and Prevention. Updated guidelines for evaluating public health surveillance systems: recommendations from the guidelines working group. MMWR. 2001;50(RR-13):1–35.
18 Control of epidemic meningococcal disease. WHO practical guidelines. 2nd edition. Available:1998; pp12–16. Available at: http://www.who.int/csr/disease/meningococcal/en/. Accessed 9 Mar 2017.
19 Blignault I, Ritchie J. Revealing the wood and the trees: reporting qualitative research. Health Promot J Austr. 2009;20(2):140–5.
20 Carter S, Richie J, Sainsbury P. Doing good qualitative research in public health: not as easy as it looks. NSW Public Health Bull. 2009;20(7–8):105–11.
21 McKerr C, Lo Y, Edeghere O, Bracebridge S. Evaluation of the national notifiable disease surveillance system for dengue fever in Taiwan, 2010-2012. PLoS Negl Trop Dis. 2015;9(3):e0003639.
22 Apanga P, Awoonor-Williams J. An evaluation of the meningitis surveillance in northern Ghana. International Journal of Tropical diseases and Health. 2016;12(2):1–10; IJTDH. 22489
23 Centres for Disease Control and Prevention (CDC). Evaluation of the meningitis surveillance before introduction of serogroup a menningococcal conjugate vaccine in Burkina Faso and Mali. MMWR Morb Mortal Wkly Rep. 2012;21(50):1025–8.
24 Afifi S, Wasfy MO, Azab MA, Youssef FG, Pimentel TW, Graham H, et al. Laboratory-based surveillance of patients with bacterial meningitis in Egypt (1998-2004). Eur J Clin Microbiol Infect Dis. 2007;7(26):5. 331-340.
25 Annual Health Performance Review Report, 2010. Upper West regional health directorate; 2010.

Molecular characterization of an outbreak of enterovirus-associated meningitis in Mossel Bay, South Africa, December 2015–January 2016

Heidi Smuts[1*], Sarah Cronje[2], Juno Thomas[3], Delene Brink[4], Stephen Korsman[1] and Diana Hardie[1]

Abstract

Background: Human enteroviruses (HEVs) are common causal agents of aseptic meningitis in young children. Laboratory and syndromic surveillance during December 2015 and January 2016 noted an unusually high number of paediatric aseptic meningitis cases at a hospital in Mossel Bay, Western Cape Province, South Africa. HEV was detected in clinical samples, prompting an outbreak investigation.

Methods: Epidemiological investigations were conducted to ascertain possible linkage between cases. Amplification, sequencing and phylogenetic analysis of the 5'UTR and VP1 regions was undertaken to determine the HEV serotype associated with the outbreak as well as other cases of aseptic meningitis in the area in the preceding 6 weeks.

Results: Over the 2-month period, 63 CSF samples were available for testing. A total of 43 outbreak cases (68.3%) were observed, and the 26 (60.5%) that could be typed were coxsackie virus A9 (CVA9). Children attending three crèche facilities were epidemiologically linked, accounting for 60.5% (26/43) of the CVA9 cases. The majority of patients were under 10 years of age (55/63, 87.3%) and there was a male predominance (66%). Nucleotide sequence analysis of the 5'UTR and VP1 regions identified 2 lineages of CVA9 co-circulating during the outbreak, although the VP1 capsid protein sequence was identical as all nucleotide differences were synonymous. There was a unique isoleucine at position 64 and all outbreak viruses had a valine to threonine change in the hypervariable BC loop of VP1. Other HEV types circulating in the preceding period were echovirus 30 ($n = 4$), echovirus 5 ($n = 3$) and 1 each of echovirus 6, echovirus 9 and echovirus 15.

Conclusion: CVA9 was identified as the pathogen responsible for the large outbreak of aseptic meningitis, with 2 distinct co-circulating lineages.

Keywords: Aseptic meningitis, Coxsackie virus A9, Outbreak, South Africa

Background

Human enteroviruses (HEVs) are ubiquitous and cause an array of clinical syndromes ranging from asymptomatic infections, in about 80% of cases, to more severe illnesses including respiratory infection, acute haemorrhagic conjunctivitis, hand- foot-and-mouth disease, neonatal sepsis, myocarditis, paralytic disease, encephalitis and aseptic meningitis [1, 2]. The virus is spread from person to person most commonly via the faecal-oral route and less frequently through respiratory droplets [3, 4]. Transmission often occurs within the family, in schools, hostels and chronic care facilities [1, 4]. Community and nosocomial spread is also reported, particularly where there is overcrowding [3, 5].

Most HEV infections occur in the summer/autumn months in temperate climates and throughout the year in tropical regions [4, 6]. Usually only a few serotypes

* Correspondence: Heidi.Smuts@uct.ac.za
[1]Division of Medical Virology, Department of Pathology, Faculty of Health Sciences, University of Cape Town, South Africa and the National Health Laboratory Service, Anzio Road, Observatory, Cape Town 7925, South Africa
Full list of author information is available at the end of the article

predominate in each HEV season and these can lead to outbreaks of a localised or more widespread nature.

HEVs belong to the family *Picornaviridae*, genus *Enterovirus* and are classified into 4 species (A, B, C and D) based on neutralizing assays, sequence data and analysis of the virus capsid VP1 gene [7–9]. The VP1 capsid protein is exposed on the outer surface of the virion, has specific epitopes, particularly in the BC loop, that elicit type-specific neutralising antibodies and are primarily responsible for defining the serotype [1, 6, 10–12]. Laboratory diagnosis using molecular technologies enables rapid detection of HEV and has largely replaced the more labour intensive virus culture and isolation methods. Reverse transcription PCR (RT-PCR) diagnostic methodologies target the most conserved region of the HEV genome, 5′ untranslated region (5'UTR), while typing for the investigation of outbreak and clinical disease associations usually targets the VP1 gene.

Aseptic meningitis is a self-limiting illness occurring in adults and children, with neonates most at risk of severe systemic illness. HEVs are the most common causal agent and association is inferred by the detection or isolation of virus from the cerebrospinal fluid [13].

Numerous viral meningitis outbreaks associated with HEVs have been reported in South Africa. The most comprehensive study from Cape Town during 1981–1989 identified 5 major episodes involving over 1400 cases with echovirus 4, echovirus 9 and coxsackie virus A9 (CVA9) most commonly identified [14]. Other reports include an outbreak of echovirus 3 at a summer camp in 2001 involving 15 children [15], 9 cases of enterovirus 84 in the small town of Ladismith in 2009 [16] and an outbreak of echovirus 4 in 23 children from the Tshwane region in 2010–2011 [17].

This study reports the epidemiology of a large outbreak of aseptic meningitis associated with enteroviruses in Mossel Bay, Western Cape Province, South Africa from December 2015–January 2016.

Objectives

The objective of this study was to determine the molecular epidemiology of HEVs in the CSF of patients presenting with aseptic meningitis in Mossel Bay, South Africa, over a 2-month period.

Methods

Patients and samples

Mossel Bay is coastal town in the Western Cape Province, South Africa, located midway between Cape Town and Port Elizabeth. There is one municipal and one private hospital and numerous educational and crèche facilities. During the study period schools closed on 12th December 2015 for annual summer vacation and reopened on 13th January 2016.

In mid-January 2016 local healthcare workers noticed an increase in young children presenting at a private sector hospital (Life Bay View Private Hospital) with clinical manifestations and laboratory findings suggestive of aseptic meningitis. The increase was from 3 to 7 cases weekly preceding the outbreak to 4–6 cases daily during the outbreak period. Cerebrospinal fluid (CSF) samples were collected from hospitalised patients and tested at a private laboratory (PathCare, in George), where an HEV was identified as the causative pathogen. The Western Cape Department of Health was notified of the suspected outbreak, prompting an epidemiological investigation to ascertain possible links between cases, implementation of control measures, and health promotion activities. Demographic data was collected on all HEV-positive patients hospitalised with symptoms of aseptic meningitis from 1st December 2015 to the first week in February 2016 in order to place the outbreak in context.

CSF samples from aseptic meningitis cases were referred to the PathCare George laboratory and screened using the Meningitis/Encephalitis (ME) Panel (BIOFIRE® FILMARRAY®) which detects 14 relevant bacterial, viral and yeast pathogens. Samples that were positive for HEV and still stored at the PathCare George laboratory were sent to the NHLS Molecular Virology diagnostic laboratory in Cape Town for HEV typing.

Case definitions

A confirmed case of aseptic meningitis was defined as any person admitted to the Life Bay View Private Hospital in Mossel Bay between 1st December 2015 and 3rd February 2016 with a history of acute onset of severe headache, nausea and/or vomiting and fever with compatible laboratory findings on CSF analysis.

RNA extraction

Total nucleic acid was extracted from 500 μl CSF using the NucliSENS easyMag (bioMerieux SA, Lyon, France) and eluted in 50 μl elution buffer.

HEV typing by VP1, VP2 and 5'UTR amplification

cDNA was generated with random primers using the RevertAid First Strand cDNA synthesis kit (Thermo Scientific, Lithuania), as per manufacturer's instructions.

Species-specific nested PCRs were used to amplify a region of the VP1 gene of EV-A and EV-B using primers from McWillliam Leitch et al. [18], while the VP2 gene was used to detect EV-C [19], generating PCR fragments of 784 bp, 1085 bp and 406 bp, respectively. Samples that were still negative after species- specific amplification were investigated by amplification of a 498 bp fragment of the 5'UTR region [18]. The PCR was performed in a 50 μl reaction containing 5 μl cDNA, 15 mM Tris-HCL (pH 8), 50 mM KCl, 1.5 mM $MgCl_2$, 0.2 mM dNTPs

(ABgene, Epsom, UK), 50 pmol of primers and 1.5 U Supertherm Taq polymerase (JMR Holdings, Kent, UK). Amplification was as follows: 95 °C for 3 min, 40 cycles of 95 °C for 15 s, 50 °C for 25 s and 72 °C for 35 s followed by 72 °C elongation for 7 min. Nested amplification was the same, but with an annealing temperature of 55 °C. PCR products were visualised by electrophoresis through a 2% agarose gel, ethidium bromide staining and UV illumination.

Sequencing

PCR products were cleaned up using the Zymoclean Gel DNA Recovery kit (Zymo Research Corp. Irvine, California, USA) and sequenced directly with the BigDye terminator cycle sequencing kit (Applied Biosystems, Foster City CA, USA) using PCR-specific primers. Sequences were confirmed to be of HEV origin using BLASTn [20] and the Enterovirus Genotyping Tool Version 0.1 [21]. Sequences obtained were aligned with reference sequences obtained from the GenBank database and the NIAID Virus Pathogen Database and Analysis Resource (ViPR) [22] through the website "http://www.viprbrc.org/" using BioEdit version 7.2.5 [23]. Additional HEV sequences from Cape Town (NHLS Virology Molecular Diagnostic Laboratory) and Johannesburg (National Institute for Communicable Diseases, NICD) were also included. Neighbour-joining phylogenetic trees were constructed in MEGA 6.06 using the maximum-likelihood algorithm with 1000 bootstrap re-sampling [24]. Highlighter plots were generated by Highlighter [25] using 5' UTR and VP1 aligned nucleotide and amino acid sequences to visualize individual sequence polymorphisms.

Nucleotide accession numbers

The 5'UTR and VP1 sequences reported in this study were deposited in the GenBank sequence database under accession numbers MH558061 - MH558083 and MH558084 - MH558112, respectively. The raw nucleotide data is also available (Additional files 1 and 2).

Results

Epidemiological investigation during the 2-month period (1st December 2015 to 3rd February 2016) identified 63 laboratory-confirmed cases of HEV meningitis (Table 1). Forty-three (68.3%) cases were associated with the outbreak as these could either be epidemiologically linked, and/or occurred after the reopening of schools on 13th January 2016. In addition, where typing was successful, CVA9 was linked to these outbreak cases (26/43, 60.5%) (see below). Accordingly, it was presumed that the 43 cases of the outbreak were caused by CVA9. In the remaining 20 cases no epidemiologically linkage could be established. These cases probably represented sporadic cases of aseptic meningitis, with different HEV types, occurring during the summer season when aseptic meningitis caused by HEVs is common. All patients were admitted to hospital. The demographic features of the laboratory-confirmed cases are shown in Table 1.

Epidemiological investigations showed that 3 crèches (A, B and C) were linked to 26 outbreak cases: 6 cases from crèche A, 16 cases from crèche B and 4 cases from crèche C. Of the remaining 17 cases, two were family members of crèche-related cases, and no definitive link to a crèche could be established for 15 cases. The epidemiological curve illustrating the background sporadic cases and progression of the outbreak is shown in Fig. 1.

The age of confirmed HEV-positive cases ranged from 10 days to 37 years with a median age of 3 years 9 months (Fig. 2). There was a predominance of males affected (66.7%; 42/63).

HEV typing

VP1/VP2 typing

CSF was available for typing in 51/63 cases (81%), of which the VP1 or VP2 region could be successfully amplified in 29 samples (56.9%), with 24/29 (82.8%) identified as HEV species B. The PCR products of the remaining samples were too weak to sequence. No HEV species A and C were detected. The Enterovirus Typing Tool and BLASTn analysis identified the majority of samples to be CVA9 (n = 19; 79.2%) followed by echovirus 5 (n = 3; 12.5%) and one case each of echovirus 30 and echovirus 9 (4.2%).

5'UTR typing

The 5'UTR primers were used to amplify samples negative for HEV species amplification (n = 22). Thirteen of the 22 (59.1%) cases were successfully amplified, sequenced, and BLASTn analysis identified 6 CVB3 cases, 3 echovirus 16 cases, 2 echovirus 30 cases and one each of echovirus 15 and echovirus 6 (Table 1 and Fig. 1). Interestingly, 8/9 CVB3 and echovirus 16 positives were detected during the outbreak period. Further amplification and sequencing of the 5'UTR region from known CVA9 samples (typing based on VP1/VP2 analysis) and associated with the outbreak, showed that these samples either had a CVB3-like or echovirus 16-like 5'UTR suggesting that these may be recombinant viruses. The assumption was therefore made that the samples identified as CVB3 and echovirus 16 by 5'UTR sequencing were in fact CVA9. This is supported by phylogenetic analysis of the VP1 and 5'UTR (Fig. 3A and B).

Phylogenetic analysis

Phylogenetic analysis of the VP1 gene of CVA9 cases showed that the South African sequences clustered together and formed 2 lineages with a bootstrap value of 99%. Lineage 1 clustered with sequences from contemporaneous

Table 1 Demographics of the HEV-positive aseptic meningitis cases

Patient	Age Range (years)	Place of permanent residence	Epidemiological link	HEV serotype
1501	0–4	NK	No school involvement	
9525	0–4	Mossel Bay	No school involvement	
9365	0–4	Mossel Bay	Unknown	E9
0784	0–4	Pretoria	No school involvement	E30*
0780	0–4	Mossel Bay	No school involvement	
0785	0–4	Mossel Bay	Unknown	E6*
1502	0–4	NK	No school involvement	
0838	10–14	Witbank	No school involvement	E5
0847	5–9	Pretoria	No school involvement	E5
0864	0–4	Mossel Bay	No school involvement	
1503	10–14	NK	No school involvement	
1104	0–4	Middelburg	No school involvement	E5
0947	5–9	Pretoria	Unknown	
2083	5–9	Riversdal	Unknown	CVA9
2149	10–14	Kimberley	Unknown	E30*
2314	0-4	Mossel Bay	Unknown	CVA9/CVB3*
2319	0-4	Mossel Bay	Unknown	
2446	5–9	Douglas	Unknown	E15*
2572	5-9	Jan Kempdorp	Unknown	
2407	5–9	Bloemfontein	Unknown	E30
3965	10–14	Mossel Bay	Unknown	CVA9
4103	0–4	Mossel Bay	Unknown	
4751	0–4	Mossel Bay	Unknown	CVA9
5012	0–4	Mossel Bay	A crèche	CVA9
5018	0–4	Mossel Bay	Unknown	CVA9
4809	0–4	Mossel Bay	A crèche	CVA9
1601	0–4	Mossel Bay	A crèche	
4969	0–4	Mossel Bay	Unknown	CVA9/E16*
5081	5-9	Mossel Bay	Unknown	CVA9
5084	0–4	Mossel Bay	Unknown	CVA9
1602	10–14	Mossel Bay	C crèche	
5114	0–4	Mossel Bay	B crèche	CVA9
5146	0–4	Mossel Bay	B crèche Sibling of 4938	CVA9
5064	0–4	Mossel Bay	B crèche	CVA9/E16*
1603	0–4	NK	A crèche	
5088	0–4	Mossel Bay	B crèche	CVA9
5100	0–4	Mossel Bay	B crèche	
5112	0–4	Mossel Bay	B crèche	CVA9/CVB3*
5145	0–4	Mossel Bay	B crèche	CVA9
5157	0–4	Mossel Bay	B crèche	
1604	0–4	Mossel bay	B crèche	
5110	0–4	Mossel Bay	B crèche Child of 5470	CVA9

Table 1 Demographics of the HEV-positive aseptic meningitis cases *(Continued)*

Patient	Age Range (years)	Place of permanent residence	Epidemiological link	HEV serotype
4929	0–4	Mossel Bay	B crèche	CVA9
4938	0–4	Mossel Bay	Sibling of 5146	CVA9
4962	0–4	Mossel Bay	B crèche	CVA9/CVB3*
4965	0–4	Mossel Bay	C crèche	CVA9
1605	5–9	Mossel Bay	C crèche	
5408	10–14	Mossel Bay	Unknown	CVA9/ E16*
5411	10–14	Mossel Bay	Unknown	
5433	0–4	Mossel Bay	Unknown	CVA9/CVB3*
5470	30-40	Mossel Bay	Parent of 5110	CVA9/CVB3*
5575	0–4	Mossel Bay	Unknown	CVA9/ CVB3*
5486	5–9	Mossel Bay	Unknown	
5557	0–4	Mossel Bay	A crèche Sibling of 5488	
5578	0–4	Mossel Bay	Unknown	CVA9
4886	5–9	Mossel Bay	B crèche	CVA9
4876	5–9	Mossel Bay	Unknown	
4869	0–4	Mossel Bay	Unknown	CVA9
5488	5–9	Mossel Bay	A crèche Sibling of 5557	
1606	0–4	Mossel Bay	C crèche	
1607	5–9	Mossel Bay	B crèche	
1608	0–4	Mossel Bay	B crèche	
1609	0–4	Mossel Bay	B crèche	

*typing by 5'UTR sequencing and BLASTn analysis; E5- echovirus 5; E6- echovirus 6; E9- echovirus 9; E15- echovirus 15; E16- echovirus 16; E30-echovirus 30; CVA9-coxsackie virus A9; CVB3- coxsackie virus B3

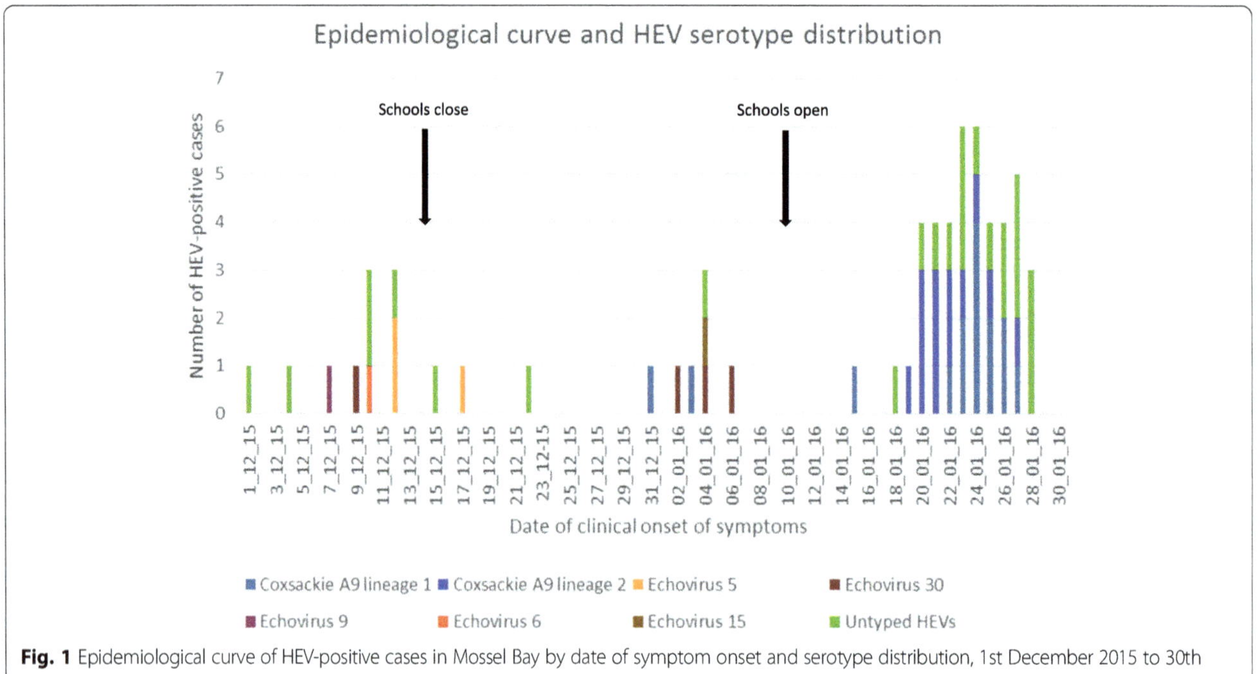

Fig. 1 Epidemiological curve of HEV-positive cases in Mossel Bay by date of symptom onset and serotype distribution, 1st December 2015 to 30th January 2016 (*n* = 63)

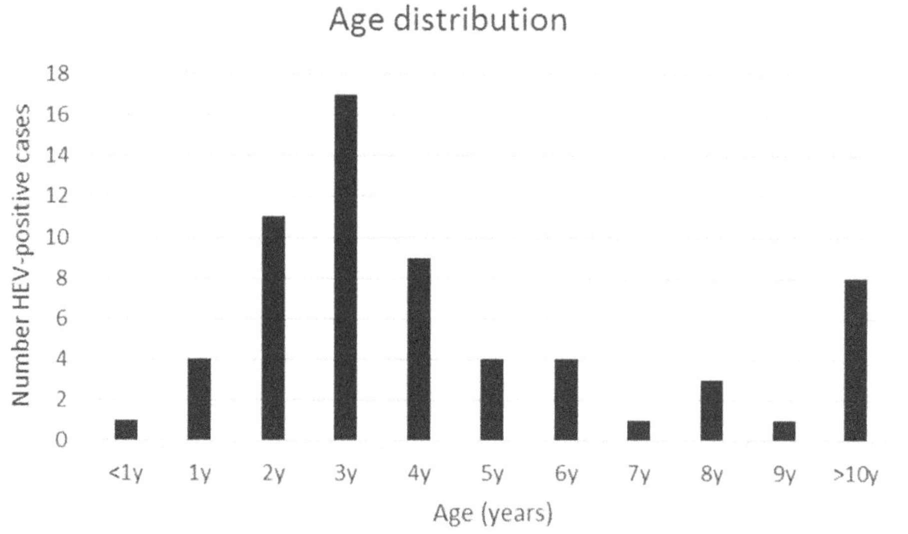

Fig. 2 Age distribution of HEV- positive aseptic meningitis cases (n = 63)

infections from Cape Town and Johannesburg. However, 7/9 Mossel Bay sequences formed a distinct cluster. These included 6 cases from the crèche B and 1 case with an unknown epidemiological link.

Lineage 2 contained only Mossel Bay sequences. They were from cases from crèches A and B, as well as patients with unknown epidemiological links (Fig. 3A). Both lineages co-circulated during the outbreak (Fig. 1 and Fig. 3A). Interestingly, 2 siblings, one who attended B crèche and the other a 10 day-old baby, had CVA9 that clustered with lineage 1 and lineage 2, respectively (Fig. 3A with asterisk).

The phylogenetic tree of the 5'UTR region (Fig. 3B) also showed 2 lineages, as found in the VP1 phylogenetic tree (Fig. 3A). Lineage 1 samples had a CVB3-like 5'UTR, while lineage 2 had an echovirus 16-like 5'UTR (as determined by Blastn analysis).

Sequence analysis of Coxsackie virus A9 lineages

5' UTR and VP1 nucleotide sequences

The 5'UTR and VP1 nucleotide differences between the two lineages of CVA9 were compared using Highlighter plot. Lineage 2 had 8/417 (1.9%) and 13/289 (4.5%) nucleotide differences in the 5'UTR and VP1 region, respectively compared to lineage 1 (Fig. 4A and B). All nucleotide changes in the VP1 region were synonymous.

VP1 amino acid sequences

The VP1 amino acid sequences were identical for both lineages 1 and 2 and were also identical to the isolates from Cape Town (Fig. 5). All Mossel Bay sequences had a unique isoleucine at position 64, while valine was present at this position in all other reference sequences, including the Griggs prototype (Fig. 5). A threonine replaced a valine within the BC loop (Fig. 5). The BC loop is one of them most exposed regions of the VP1 capsid protein.

Discussion

In this study we describe the molecular epidemiology of HEV associated with a large outbreak of aseptic meningitis in a small coastal town in the Western Cape Province, South Africa which occurred in the summer of 2015/2016. During the 2-month period (December 2015 and January 2016) numerous cases presented to hospital with aseptic meningitis, of which 63 were confirmed by a private diagnostic laboratory to be caused by an HEV. Enterovirus typing of CSF samples collected over this period showed the presence of multiple circulating HEV species, including echovirus 5, 6, 9, 15 and 30 in the weeks preceding the outbreak. As 60% of the cases that occurred during the outbreak period were typed as CVA9, it was presumed that this was the causal agent of the outbreak. The first CVA9 case presented on 31st December 2015 and a further 2 cases with no apparent epidemiological links presented 3 and 15 days later. However, a dramatic increase in cases was noted within a week after crèches and schools reopened (13th January 2016). It can be postulated that the return of children to a crowded environment may have facilitated the spread of the virus.

Crèches and preschool facilities are vulnerable to rapid spread of viruses transmitted via the faecal-oral route, including HEVs [26–28]. The maintenance of good personal and communal hygiene practices with the prompt disposal of faeces and soiled clothing, disinfection of contaminated surfaces and the frequent washing of hands may be challenging in such an environment. In

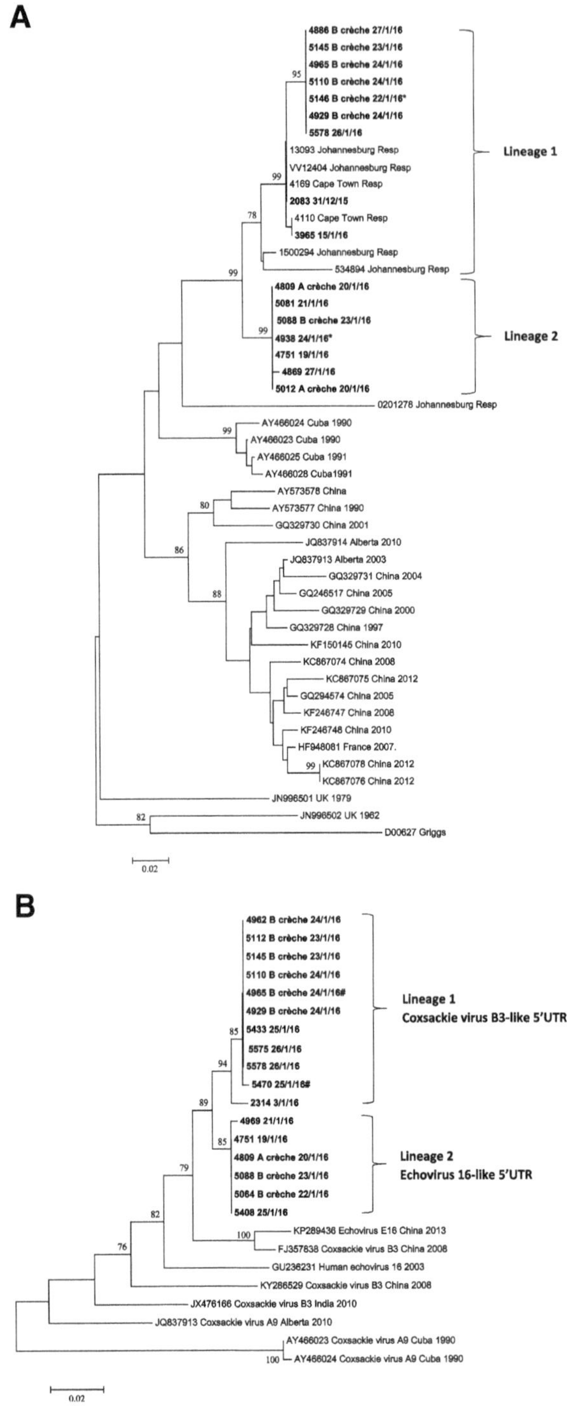

Fig. 3 (**a**) VP1 and (**b**) 5'UTR phylogenetic trees of aseptic meningitis cases associated with CVA9

this outbreak three crèches with aftercare facilities were affected, recording numerous cases of aseptic meningitis. Although these facilities were not closed, in order to contain the outbreak, local health authorities initiated daily hand hygiene practise training for staff and parents, and children suspected of being ill were kept at home. While the primary route of transmission of HEV is via the faecal-oral route, other transmission routes including respiratory droplet spread and indirect spread through water- borne sources could also have played a role, although none of these were investigated in this study [29–31].

There are numerous reports of CVA9 as a significant causal agent of aseptic meningitis from around the world, including Japan (1961) [32], Northern Ireland (1970) [33], Poland (1974) [34, 35], Cuba (1990–1991) [36], Argentina (2007–2008) [37], Switzerland [38], Canada (2010) [39, 40], China (2006–2012) [41] as well South Africa [14]. Consistent with our study, the majority of cases occurred in children under 10 years of age.

Reasons for large outbreaks of specific HEV serotype-associated aseptic meningitis are not clear. Herd immunity plays an important role, and a decline in immunity to a particular serotype is either due to the emergence of a new serotype lineage or the re-emergence of a lineage from the past to which the population is susceptible. In addition, HEVs are subject to recombination and genetic divergence and these events may change the virus antigenicity, thus changing the immune response and also the HEV circulation patterns [42, 43]. Tracking of circulating HEV serotypes in South Africa has only recently recommenced with the growing interest in understanding serotype prevalence over time and clinical association. Hellferscee et al. [44] identified 33 different serotypes circulating over a 3-year period (2012–2014) in respiratory samples with echovirus 30, coxsackie virus B5 and enterovirus D68 most prevalent, and 3 cases of CVA9 detected. Unpublished data from Cape Town from 2014 to 2017 showed 38 different serotypes circulating in respiratory samples with different serotypes predominating in each year (Smuts, unpublished). Similarly, over the same period, more than 10 different serotypes were detected in the CSF of patients with central nervous system disease each year, with echovirus 9, echovirus 30 and CVA9 most commonly found (Smuts, unpublished). As historic sequence data of the VP1 region of CVA9 from South Africa is not available, it is not possible to determine if this outbreak was a result of an increase in the number of susceptible individuals in the population or the emergence of an immune escape mutant. However, it can be speculated that the homology of the outbreak virus with that found in Cape Town and Johannesburg early in 2015 would suggest that the virus had been in circulation for a while and that herd immunity may have dropped to below a critical threshold.

Nucleotide sequence and phylogenetic analysis of the 5'UTR and VP1 regions of CVA9 showed the co-circulation during this outbreak of 2 distinct lineages. Lineage 1 included the earliest aseptic meningitis cases detected on 31st December 2015, 3rd and 15th January 2016. This lineage also clustered with CVA9 from respiratory samples

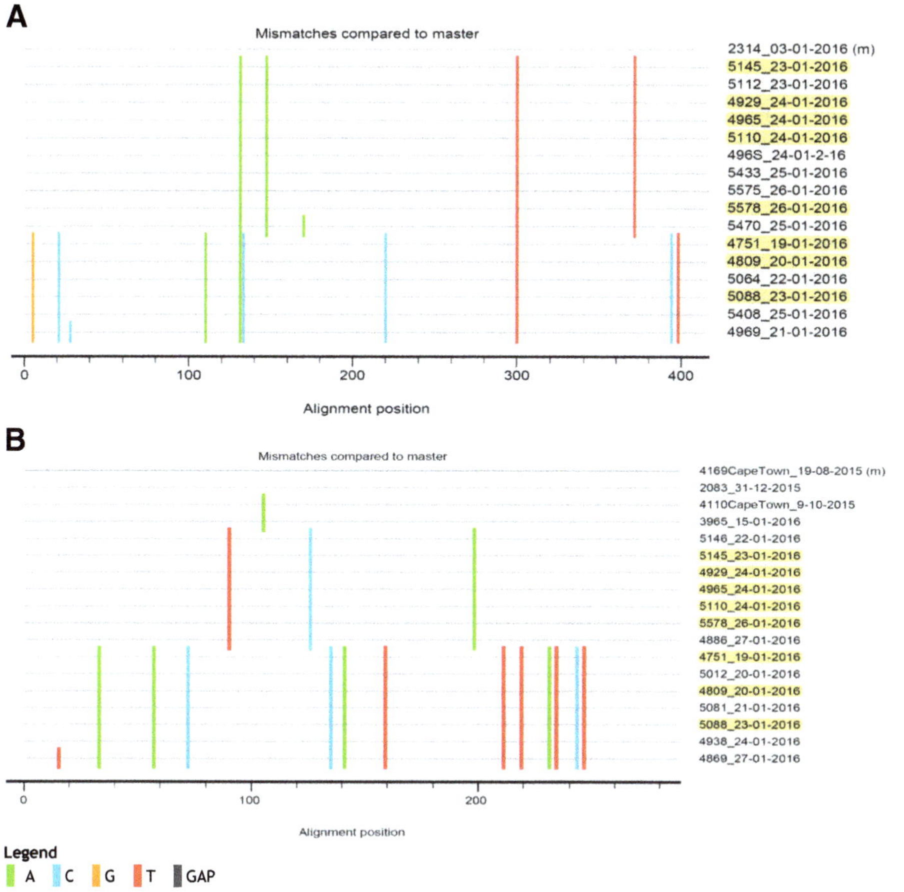

Fig. 4 Highlighter plot of the 5'UTR (**a**) and VP1 (**b**) nucleotide sequences of CVA9-positive aseptic meningitis cases by similarity. Highlighted sequences are common to both data sets

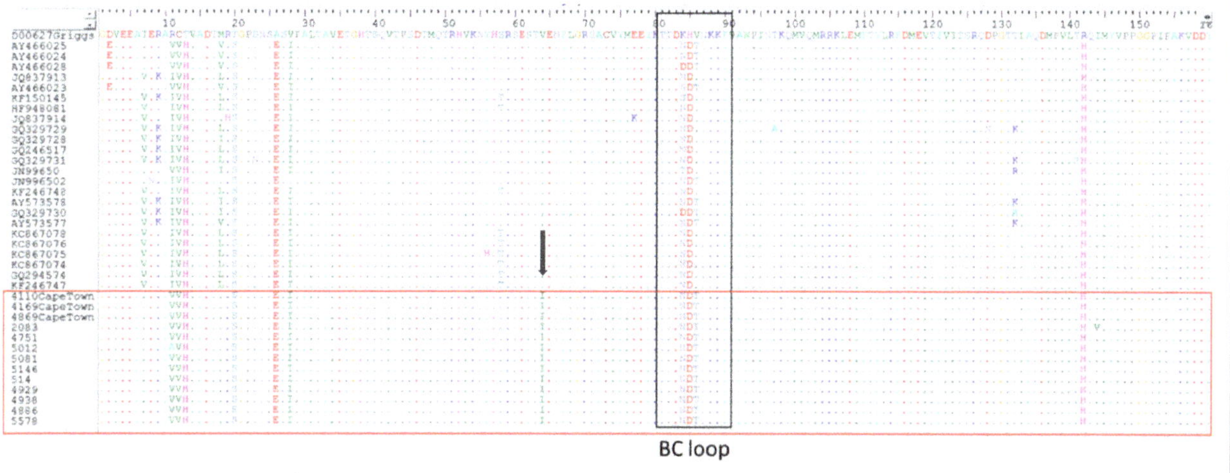

Fig. 5 VP1 amino acid alignment of CVA9 –positive aseptic meningitis cases with other sequences from GenBank. Boxed sequences in black represent the BC loop and red box indicates South African sequences. Grey arrow shows unique amino acid change at position 64

collected in Cape Town and Johannesburg earlier in 2015. The outbreak virus however, formed a distinct cluster within this lineage.

The VP1 amino acid sequence, on the other hand, was identical in both the outbreak viruses as well as viruses from Cape Town earlier in 2015. All had a unique isoleucine at position 64 which was not present in any of the reference sequences from GenBank, including the prototype Griggs strain. There was also an amino acid substitution in the hypervariable BC loop with a threonine replacing a valine. The VP1 capsid protein is 292 amino acids in length with many of the immunodominant serotype-specific epitopes located in the exposed BC loop (amino acid 82–93) [45, 46]. Although valine and threonine are structurally very similar, the substitution at this important neutralizing immunogenic site may have changed the conformation of the BC loop, thus altering the antigenicity. This may account for the increased susceptibility in this population. While the amino acid sequence of the VP1 gene was the same, the 2 lineages had distinct (synonymous) signature nucleotide substitutions in both 5'UTR and VP1 genes.

There are some limitations to this study. Firstly, the number of outbreak-related cases is likely under-reported. In the early stages of the outbreak all children with clinical manifestations suggestive of aseptic meningitis were routinely admitted to hospital where lumbar punctures were performed. However, as news of this outbreak spread it is possible that clinicians were familiar with the syndromic manifestations and opted for out-patient management of milder cases and not subject them to lumbar punctures. Anecdotally it was reported that many adults presented with a similar constellation of symptoms, but no CSF was collected and they were treated symptomatically. In this report CSF was available from only 1 adult, the father of a child attending one of the affected crèches. Attempts were made to obtain stool samples from adults presenting with compatible symptoms where the clinician had opted not to collect CSF, but no samples were received. Secondly, medical history and additional clinical data which would have provided additional information on the clinical course of aseptic meningitis was not available. A third limitation was the use of the 5'UTR for serotyping in some cases. As mentioned previously this is not the ideal target for serotyping, but where VP1 amplification failed, sequencing of this region did provide useful phylogenetic data. The 5'UTR sequence data showed that in the weeks preceding the outbreak echovirus 6, 15 and 30 were circulating in the Mossel Bay area. Further, correlation of the VP1 CVA9 sequence data with the 5'UTR results showed that there were 2 distinct lineages of this virus circulating during the outbreak. However, despite these shortcomings the study identified CVA9 as the causal agent in this large outbreak of aseptic meningitis.

Conclusions

Our study identified CVA9 as the pathogen responsible for a large outbreak of aseptic meningitis, with the co-circulation of 2 distinct lineages.

Abbreviations

5'UTR: 5' untranslated region; CSF: Cerebrospinal fluid; CVA9: Coxsackie virus A9; CVB3: Coxsackie virus B3; E16: Echovirus 16; HEV: Human enterovirus; RT-PCR: Reverse transcription polymerase chain reaction; VP1: Viral capsid protein 1; VP2: Viral capsid protein 2

Acknowledgements

We thank Drs. Orienka Hefferscee and Florette Treurnicht from the National Institute for Communicable Diseases (NICD) for generously allowing us to use their CVA9 sequence data. We also thank the NHLS Virology Molecular Diagnostic staff at Groote Schuur Hospital for RNA extraction of CSF samples.

Author contributions

HS, JT, SK and DH conceived and designed the study. HS performed the experiments, analysed the data and drafted the manuscript. SC and DB participated in the study investigation and provide the samples and clinical data. DH, JT and SK critically revised the manuscript. All authors have read and approved the final manuscript.

Funding

This study was funded by the Poliomyelitis Research Foundation grant number 15/28. The funders had no role in the design of the study and collection, analysis, and interpretation of data and in writing the manuscript.

Consent for publication

Not applicable.

Competing interests

The authors declare that they have no competing interests.

Author details

[1]Division of Medical Virology, Department of Pathology, Faculty of Health Sciences, University of Cape Town, South Africa and the National Health Laboratory Service, Anzio Road, Observatory, Cape Town 7925, South Africa. [2]Life Bay View Private Hospital, Ryk Tulbach Street & Alhof Drive, De Nova, Mossel Bay 6506, South Africa. [3]Centre for Enteric Diseases, National Institute for Communicable Diseases, 1 Modderfontein Road, Sandringham, Johannesburg 2130, South Africa. [4]PathCare George Laboratory, 1 Gloucester Avenue, George 6529, South Africa.

References

1. Pallansch MA, Oberste MS, Whitton JL. Enteroviruses: polioviruses, coxsackieviruses, echoviruses, and newer enteroviruses. In Knipe DM, Howley P, editors. Fields virology 2. 6th ed. Lippincott Williams & Wilkins; 2013.
2. Pons-Salort M, Parker EP, Grassly NC. The epidemiology of non-polio enteroviruses: recent advances and outstanding questions. Curr Opin Infect Dis. 2015;28:479–87.
3. Julbert B and Lipton HL. Enterovirus/Picornavirus infections. Chapter 18 in Handb Clin Neurol, Vol. 123 (3rd series) Neurovirology A.C. Tselis and J. Booss, Editors 2013.
4. Rotbart HA. Viral meningitis. Semin Neurol. 2000;20:277–92.
5. Bailly J-L, Be'Guet A, Chambon M, Henquell C, Lafeuille HP. Nosocomial transmission of echovirus 30: molecular evidence by phylogenetic analysis of the VP1 encoding sequence. J Clin Microbiol. 2000;38:2889–92.

6. Romero JR. Reverse-transcription polymerase chain reaction detection of the enteroviruses. Arch Pathol Lab Med. 1999;123:1161–9.
7. Knowles NJ, Hovi T, Hyypiä T, King AMQ, Lindberg AM, Pallansch MA, Palmenberg AC, Simmonds P, Skern T, Stanway G, Yamashita T, Zell R. Picornaviridae. In: King AMQ, Adams MJ, Carstens EB, Lefkowitz EJ, editors. (ed), virus taxonomy: classification and nomenclature of viruses: ninth report of the international committee on taxonomy of viruses. San Diego, CA: Elsevier; 2012. p. 855–80.
8. Oberste MS, Maher K, Kilpatrick DR, et al. Molecular evolution of the human enteroviruses: correlation of serotype with VP1 sequence and application to picornavirus classification. J Virol. 1999;73:1941–8.
9. Picornaviridae.com. www.picornaviridae.com/enterovirus/enterovirus. Accessed 9 March 2018.
10. Caro V, Guillot S, Delpeyroux F, Crainic R. 2001. Molecular strategy for "serotyping" of human enteroviruses. J Gen Virol. 2001;82:79–91.
11. Ramers C, Billman G, Hartin M, et al. Impact of a diagnostic cerebrospinal fluid enterovirus polymerase chain reaction test on patient management. JAMA. 2000;283:2680–5.
12. Norder H, Bjerregaard L, Magnius L, Lina B, Aymard M, Chomel J-J. Sequencing of "untypeable" enteroviruses reveals two new type, EV-77 and EV-78, within human enteroviruses type B and substitutions in the BC loop of the VP1 protein for known types. J Gen Virol. 2003;84:827–36.
13. Lee BE, Davies HD. Aseptic meningitis. Curr Opin Infect Dis. 2007;20:272–7.
14. McIntyre JP, Keen GA. Laboratory surveillance of viral meningitis by examination of cerebrospinal fluid in Cape Town, 1981-9. Epidemiol Infect. 1993;111(2):357–71.
15. Yeats J, Smuts H, Serfontein CJ, Kannemeyer J. Investigation into a school enterovirus outbreak using PCR detection and serotype identification based on the 5′ non-coding region. Epidemiol Infect. 2005;133(6):1123–30.
16. Smuts H, Hardie D. Phylogenetic identification of human enteroviruses associated with clusters of meningitis in 2009 and 2010. Commun Dis Surv Bull. 2010;8:55–7.
17. Wolfaardt M, Buchner A, Myburgh M, Avenant T, du Plessis NM, Taylor MB. Molecular characterization of enteroviruses and clinical findings from a cluster of paediatric viral meningitis cases in Tshwane, South Africa 2010-2011. J Clin Virol. 2014;61:400–5.
18. McWilliam Leitch EC, Harvala H, Robertson I, Ubillos I, Templeton K, Simmonds P. Direct identification of human enterovirus serotypes in cerebrospinal fluid by amplification and sequencing of the VP1 region. J Clin Virol. 2009;44:119–24.
19. McLeish NJ, Witteveldt J, Clasper L, McIntyre C, McWilliam Leitch EC, Hardie A, et al. Development and assay of RNA transcripts of enterovirus species a to D, rhinovirus species a to C, and human parechovirus: assessment of assay sensitivity and specificity of real-time screening and typing methods. J Clin Microbiol. 2012;50(9):2910–7.
20. Basic Local Alignment Search Tool. https://blast.ncbi.nlm.nih.gov/Blast.cgi. Accessed 15 January 2018.
21. Enterovirus Genotyping Tool Version 0.1. http://www.rivm.nl/mpf/enterovirus/typingtool. Accessed 20 November 2017.
22. Pickett BE, Sadat EL, Zhang Y, Noronha JM, Squires RB, Hunt V, et al. ViPR: an open bioinformatics database and analysis resource for virology research. Nucleic Acids Res. 2012;40(Database issue):D593–8.
23. Hall TA. BioEdit: a user-friendly biological sequence alignment editor and analysis program for windows 95/98/NT. Nucl acids Symp. Ser. 1999;41:95–8.
24. Tamura K, Stecher G, Peterson D, Filipski A, Kumar S. MEGA6: Molecular Evolutionary Genetics Analysis version 6.0 Mol Biol Evol 2013; 30(12): 2725–2729.
25. HIV Database Tools. https://www.hiv.lanl.gov/content/sequence/HIV/HIVTools.html. Accessed 16 March 2018.
26. Chan JH, Law CK, Hamblion E, Fung H, Rudge J. Best practices to prevent transmission and control outbreaks of hand, foot, and mouth disease in childcare facilities: a systematic review Hong Kong Med J. 2017;23(2):177–90.
27. Mohle-Boetani JC, Matkin C, Pallansch M, Helfand R, Fenstersheib M, Blanding JA, Solomon SL. Viral meningitis in child care Centre staff and parents: an outbreak of echovirus 30 infections. Public Health Rep. 1999; 114(3):249–56.
28. Helfand RF, Khan AS, Pallansch MA, Alexander JP, Meyers HB, DeSantis RA, Schonberger LB, Anderson LJ. Echovirus 30 infection and aseptic meningitis in parents of children attending a child care Centre. J Infect Dis. 1994;169(5): 1133–7.
29. Faustini A, Fano V, Muscillo M, Zaniratti S, La Rosa G, Tribuzi L, Carlo A. Perucci CA. 2006. 297 An outbreak of aseptic meningitis due to echovirus 30 associated with attending school and swimming in pools. Intern J of Infect Dis 2006; 10: 291–297.
30. Dente FA, Blanchollun E, Delicnierex A, Flamen P. 1974. Coxsackievirus A16 infection from lake water. JAMA. 1974;228:1370–1.
31. Kee F, McElroy G, Steward D, Coyle P, Watson J. 1994. A community outbreak of echovirus infection associated with an outdoor swimming pool. J Public Health Med. 1994;16:145–8.
32. Nakao T, Nitta T, Miura R, Ogata K, Kume T, Nobuta K, Hinuma Y. Clinical and epidemiological studies on an outbreak of aseptic meningitis caused by Coxsackie B5 and A9 viruses in Aomori in 1961. Tohoku J Exp Med. 1964; 83:94–102.
33. Connolly JH, O'Neill HJ. Coxsackie A9 virus outbreak in Northern Ireland during 1970. Ulster Med J. 1971;40(2):146–50.
34. Kocielska W, Gruszecka A. An epidemic of meningitis caused by Coxsackie A9 virus in the City of Wrocław in 1974. Przegl Epidemiol. 1975;29(4):431–2.
35. Holówka A, Gawron H, Janowicz M, Wysoczyńska H, Zabicka J. An epidemic of meningitis in the Kwidzyń County caused by Coxsackie A9 virus. Przegl Epidemiol. 1975;29(4):433–7.
36. Bello M, Más Lago P, Palomera R, Castillo A, Amín N, Acosta B, et al. Enterovirus meningoencephalitis in the last 5 years. Rev Cubana Med Trop. 1996;48(2):118–22.
37. Farías A, Cabrerizo M, Ré V, Glatstein N, Pisano B, Spinsanti L, et al. Molecular identification of human enteroviruses in children with neurological infections from the central region of Argentina. Arch Virol. 2011;156(1):129–33.
38. Butsch R, Tapparel C, Keller P, Herzog K, Krause M, Wunderli W, et al. Family outbreak of an infection with a recombinant Coxsackie a virus in eastern Switzerland. Infection. 2013;41:231–5.
39. Pabbaraju K, Wong S, Chan EN, Tellier R. Genetic characterization of a Coxsackie A9 virus associated with aseptic meningitis in Alberta, Canada in 2010. Virol J. 2013;10:93–101.
40. Peci A, Winter A-L, Eshaghi A, Marchand-Austin A, Olsha R, Lombardi N, et al. Coxsackie viruses in Ontario, January 2005 to December 2011. International J Infect Dis. 2014;25:136–41.
41. Cui A, Yu D, Zhu Z, Meng L, Li H, Liu J, et al. An outbreak of aseptic meningitis caused by coxsackievirus A9 in Gansu, the People's Republic of China. Virol J. 2010;7:72–80.
42. Santti J, Hyypiä T, Kinnunen L, Salminen M. Evidence of recombination among enteroviruses. J Virol. 1999;73(10):8741–9.
43. Oberste MS, Peñaranda S, Pallansch MA. RNA recombination plays a major role in genomic change during circulation of coxsackie B viruses. J Virol. 2004;78(6):2948–55.
44. Hellferscee O, Tempia S, Walaza S, Variava E, Dawood H, Wolter N, et al. Enterovirus genotypes among patients with severe acute respiratory illness, influenza-like illness, and asymptomatic individuals in South Africa, 2012-2014. J Med Virol. 2017;89(10):1759–67.
45. Norder H, Bjerregaard L, Magnius LO. Homotypic echoviruses share amino terminal VP1 sequence homology applicable for typing. J Med Virol. 2001;63(1):35–44.
46. Reimann BY, Zell R, Kandolf R. Mapping of a neutralizing antigenic site of Coxsackievirus B4 by construction of an antigen chimera. J Virol. 1991;65(7):3475–80.

27

Naïve-pooled pharmacokinetic analysis of pyrazinamide, isoniazid and rifampicin in plasma and cerebrospinal fluid of Vietnamese children with tuberculous meningitis

Thomas Pouplin[1,2*†], Nguyen Duc Bang[3,4†], Pham Van Toi[3], Pham Nguyen Phuong[3], Nguyen Huy Dung[4], Tran Ngoc Duong[4], Maxine Caws[2,3,5], Guy E. Thwaites[2,3], Joel Tarning[1,2] and Jeremy N. Day[2,3]

Abstract

Background: Among the various forms of TB, tuberculous meningitis (TBM) is the most severe, with about 30 % mortality and 50 % of survivors left with neurological sequelae. Children suffer more frequently from TBM than adults and outcomes are often poor due to difficulties in making the diagnosis and uncertainty regarding the best anti-tuberculosis drug regimen. The aim of this prospective study was to describe the pharmacokinetics of pyrazinamide, isoniazid and rifampicin in plasma and cerebrospinal fluid of children with tuberculous meningitis treated with the standard TBM regimen.

Methods: We performed a prospective observational study of 100 consecutively treated children (≤15 years of age) with tuberculous meningitis in Ho Chi Minh City, Vietnam. Children were treated according to the 2006 WHO recommended pediatric treatment regimen consisting of isoniazid (5 mg/kg), rifampicin (10 mg/kg) and ethambutol (15 mg/kg) for 8 months, with the addition of pyrazinamide (25 mg/kg) for the first 3 months and streptomycin (15 mg/kg) for the first 2 months. Pyrazinamide, isoniazid and rifampicin concentrations were measured in plasma at day 14 and in cerebrospinal fluid (CSF) at 1 month by HPLC-UV. A naïve-pooled non-compartmental data analysis was used to describe the pharmacokinetic properties of drugs in the two-age groups of children ≤ 4 years or > 4 years of age.

Results: Younger children, when compared to older children, presented a higher body weight-normalized clearance and volume of distribution, and lower median total plasma exposures for the three studied drugs with −14 %, −22 % and −16 % for Pyrazinamide, Isoniazid and Rifampicin, respectively. In CSF, individual concentrations of isoniazid and pyrazinamide were comparable to that in plasma in both age groups; but rifampicin concentrations were lower than the minimum inhibitory concentration of susceptible bacteria in all but two children.

Conclusions: There is an age-dependent variation in the plasma and cerebrospinal fluid pharmacokinetics of rifampicin, isoniazid and pyrazinamide. The safety and efficacy of higher doses of rifampicin should be investigated for the treatment of childhood tuberculous meningitis.

Keywords: TB, Meningitis, Children, Pharmacokinetics, Rifampicin, Anti-tuberculosis drugs, HPLC

* Correspondence: thomas@tropmedres.ac
†Equal contributors
[1]Mahidol-Oxford Tropical Medicine Research Unit, Faculty of Tropical Medicine, Mahidol University, Bangkok, Thailand
[2]Centre for Tropical Medicine and Global Health, Nuffield Department of Medicine, University of Oxford, Oxford, UK
Full list of author information is available at the end of the article

Background

Tuberculosis (TB) remains one of the major diseases afflicting children. Among the various forms of TB, tuberculous meningitis (TBM) is the most severe, with about 30 % mortality and 50 % of survivors left with neurological sequelae [1, 2]. Children suffer more frequently from TBM than adults and outcomes are often poor due to difficulties in making the diagnosis, which can delay treatment, and uncertainty regarding the best anti-tuberculosis drug regimen. More than 60 years after the development of the first anti-TB drugs, the optimal treatment of childhood TBM is still uncertain and clinical care is almost exclusively extrapolated from studies in adults. The different multiple drug regimens used in TBM are not uniform and mostly extrapolated from those used in pulmonary TB, with very little supportive evidence.

The first line anti-TB drugs are known to have differing cerebrospinal fluid (CSF) penetration. While plasma and CSF exposure tend to be similar for isoniazid and pyrazinamide, the penetration of rifampicin in CSF is poor, as it is for ethambutol [3–6]. The death rate of TBM patients may reflect both the poor penetration of drugs into the brain and the poor antibacterial activity at the current dosages. Whilst the pharmacokinetics of first-line TB drugs has been extensively studied in plasma in adults, only few published data describe exposure of these drugs in plasma and CSF of children. Higher doses and maybe different agents to those used for pulmonary TB may be required to improve outcomes from childhood TBM, but there are scant data to determine the best therapeutic approach. New randomized controlled trials have emerged from the literature, trying to assess experimental regimens in TBM [7–9]. However, evaluating modifications in a multiple drug regimen is complex and complicated trial designs can be required to measure and separate the effect of combination treatment [10].

Our aim was to perform a naïve-pooled data non-compartmental pharmacokinetic analysis of pyrazinamide, isoniazid and rifampicin in plasma and CSF in the treatment of childhood TBM and to determine whether age influenced drug exposure.

Methods

Patients

The study was a prospective observational study of 100 patients under 15 years of age presenting with suspected TBM to the Pham Ngoc Thach Hospital for Tuberculosis and Lung Diseases (PNT) in Ho Chi Minh City. This hospital is the tertiary referral centre for patients with TB from the whole of southern Vietnam (population around 45 million). All patients aged ≤15 years presenting to PNT with meningitis symptoms and signs (e.g. fever, headache, neck stiffness, vomiting, confusion, coma, convulsions, cranial nerve palsies, hemiplegia or paraplegia) and who were suspected to have TBM by their attending physician were eligible to enter the study. Patients were graded for severity at the point of study entry. For children more than 5 years of age severity was graded using the modified UK Medical Research Council (MRC) criteria, based on Glasgow Coma Score (GCS). For children less than 5 years of age, severity was graded according to the Blantyre Coma Score (BCS).

Ethical approval for the study was granted from the ethical review board of Pham Ngoc Thach Hospital, Viet Nam, Health Services of Ho Chi Minh City and the Oxford Tropical Research Ethics Committee (OxTREC), UK. Written informed consent was obtained from the parents or guardians of all participants.

Anti-tuberculosis drug treatment

Children diagnosed with TBM were treated with the standard Vietnamese National TB Programme (NTP) 8-month regimen. At the time the study was initiated, Vietnam had not yet adopted the new doses recommended by WHO [11] in 2011. Therefore, children received once daily treatment with pyrazinamide (25 mg/kg), isoniazid (5 mg/kg), rifampicin (10 mg/kg), ethambutol (15 mg/kg) and streptomycin (15 mg/kg) for the first 2 months; then isoniazid, rifampicin, ethambutol and pyrazinamide for the third month; and then isoniazid, rifampicin and ethambutol for the continuation phase of 5 months. Dexamethasone was used as adjunctive therapy for the first 6 (MRC/BCS grade I disease) or 8 (MRC/BCS grades II or III disease) weeks of treatment in all patients according to standard practice [12].

Locally produced adult fixed dose combination (FDC) tablets were used for treatment (Turbezid® Namha Pharmaceutical Joint-Stock Company). These consisted of film-coated and scored tablets containing 150 mg of rifampicin, 75 mg of isoniazid and 400 mg of pyrazinamide. Each tablet was designed for ≥ 15 kg of body weight and used a drug ratio compatible with the adult TB regimen. Tablets were split in thirds for the lightest patients (<5 kg), halves (5–7.5 kg), 2 thirds (7.5–10 kg) or used as whole plus extra split for over 15 kg. Ethambutol was given orally as a single drug tablet and streptomycin was injected intravenously.

Pharmacokinetic sampling

Each patient enrolled in the study was asked to provide plasma on day 1 (first day of treatment), day 14 (steady-state), and plasma and CSF at months 1 and 3. Enrolled patients were stratified into two groups (below and above 4 years of age) and randomisation of plasma sampling times was stratified by group. Previous admission patterns led us to believe that this age grouping would deliver to groups of approximately equal size. For each patient, two plasma samples were collected at two of ten randomly allocated pre-specified time points (i.e. at 1, 2, 3, 4, 5, 6, 8, 12, 18 or 24 h post-dose) on each of days 1 and 14. One additional plasma sample was collected for each patient at month 1 and 3, again at a randomly allocated time points between 3 to 5 h post-dose. Each child provided a maximum of 6 plasma samples over the trial.

CSF sampling by lumbar puncture (LP) was conformed to standard clinical care with CSF examination executed to assess treatment response. LPs were performed at months 1 and 3 post study entry at randomly allocated time points either 3, 4 or 5 h post-dose. Each LP was followed by a blood draw performed within 15 min. Freshly collected clinical samples were immediately processed and stored at −80 °C pending bioanalysis.

Acetylator genotyping

Acetylator genotype and predicted phenotype for each patient was determined by sequencing the second exon of the arylamine N-acetyltransferase 2 (NAT2) gene which contains the functional polymorphisms [13, 14]. Genomic DNA was extracted from blood using the Nucleon Genomic DNA extraction kit (GE Healthcare, Amersham, United Kingdom). Two primers NAT2F 5′-TGGGCTTAGAGGCTATTT and NAT2R 5′-GAGTT GGGTGATACATACAC were designed using Primer Express version 2.0 software (Applied Biosystems Inc, Foster City, CA, USA) to amplify a 768 bp sequence of the second exon of the NAT2 gene which contains the relevant polymorphisms (G191A, C282T, T341C, C481T, G590A, A803G, G857A). Following purification (QIAgen PCR purification kits, QIAGEN, United Kingdom) amplicons were sequenced (3130xl Genetic Analyzer Applied Biosystem, Hitachi, Singapore) and phenotypes predicted from genotypes previously defined in a cohort of healthy Vietnamese volunteers in a study correlating urinary caffeine metabolites ratios with NAT2 genotypes (data not shown) [15, 16].

Drug bioanalysis

The concentrations of pyrazinamide, isoniazid and rifampicin in plasma and CSF were measured by a fully validated HPLC method with UV detection following the Food and Drug Administration (FDA) and International Conference on Harmonization (ICH) recommendations [17]. Ethambutol is only detectable with mass spectrometry and was not analysed in this study. Thawed samples (plasma or CSF) were mixed for at least 30 s and left undisturbed on the bench for further 10 min. Then, 300 μL of IS solution (Guanosine and Phenacetine in saturated NaCl) were added to 300 μL of sample (plasma or CSF) in a 1.5 mL microcentrifuge tube. The tube was mixed for 15 s and left at room temperature for 10 min followed by a centrifugation at 3000 g for 5 min. The samples were loaded into a conditioned ISOLUTE-C18 50 mg/mL 96 well-plate (Biotage, Uppsala, Sweden) and washed with 0.5 mL of saturated NaCl until dryness. Isoniazid, pyrazinamide and guanosine were eluted with 2 × 250 μL of methanol–water (10:90, v/v). A second elution containing rifampicin and phenacetine was carried out by using 250 μL acetonitrile followed by 250 μL methanol. Ten μL of each eluate were injected into 2 independent equilibrated LC-UV systems (Lachrom Elite – Hitachi – Merck system). Separation was performed on a 5 μm LichroCart 125 × 4.6 mm Purosphere RP-18 end-capped column, equipped with 5 μm guard column LichroCart 4 × 4 mm, RP-18e (Merck, Darmstadt, Germany), and an isocratic flow rate of 1 mL/min of phosphate buffer (pH 4.2, 50 mM) and acetonitrile 0.25 % (v/v) for isoniazid, pyrazinamide and guanosine, and phosphate buffer (pH 4.2, 50 mM) and acetonitrile 36 % (v/v) for rifampicin and phenacetine. The chromatography time for all assays was set to 7 min with detection at 263 nm for isoniazid, pyrazinamide and guanosine and 247 nm for rifampicin and phenacetine, respectively. In plasma, the calibration ranged [lower limit of quantification (LOQ) to upper limit of quantification (ULOQ)] from 0.2 to 80 μg/mL, 0.2 to 32 μg/mL and 0.1 to 20 μg/mL for pyrazinamide, isoniazid and rifampicin, respectively. In CSF, the ranges were 0.2 to 40 μg/mL, 0.2 to 32 μg/mL and 0.1 to 16 μg/mL for pyrazinamide, isoniazid and rifampicin, respectively. Triplicates of quality control samples (low, middle and high) were analyzed within each batch to ensure accuracy and precision throughout the analysis. The precision of all quality control samples were below 15 % CV during routine drug measurements.

Naïve-pooled non-compartmental analysis

The naïve-pooled data analysis was based on plasma and CSF data collected at the first steady-state occasion (i.e. at day 14 for plasma samples and at month 1 for CSF samples). Drugs reach their respective steady-states after a minimum of 5 half-lives. With anti-TB drugs, the steady-state is assumed to be reached after 2 weeks even for RIF and its well described autoinduction metabolism [18, 19]. We also anticipated no significant pharmacokinetic changes between day 14 and month 1. The concentration-time data were pooled dependent on sampling matrix and split into 2 independent age-groups: ≤ 4 years and > 4 years. All concentration-time data were pooled for the following time windows: 0–0.5, 0.5–1, 1–2, 2–3, 3–4, 4–5, 5–6, 6–8, 8–12, 12–18, and 18–24 h post-dose. The 25th percentile (Q1), 50th

percentile (median), and 75th percentile (Q3) of drug concentrations were calculated within each time window. Drug measurements below the LOQ were set to LOQ/2 to avoid bias on account of data censoring. Median concentrations and mid-time intervals were used in the non-compartmental analysis, and Q1 and Q3 were used for graphical representation only.

Naïve-pooled concentration-time data were evaluated using a non-compartmental analysis approach implemented in WinNonlin version 6.3 (Pharsight Corporation, California, USA). Median drug exposure up to the last time point ($AUC_{0\text{-}t}$) was calculated using the linear trapezoidal method for ascending concentrations and the logarithmic trapezoidal method for descending concentrations. The median terminal elimination rate constant (λ_Z) was determined as the slope of the terminal elimination phase by best-fit ordinary linear regression. Drug exposure was extrapolated from the last observed median concentration to time infinity by C_{LAST}/λ_Z for each individual group to compute total drug exposure ($AUC_{0\text{-}\infty}$). The terminal elimination half-life ($t_{1/2}$) was calculated as $\ln(2)/\lambda_Z$. Maximum median concentration (C_{MAX}) and time to C_{MAX} (T_{MAX}) were taken directly from the observed data. Apparent median volume of distribution (V_Z/F) and median oral clearance (CL/F) were computed according to standard procedures. The wild-type minimum inhibitory concentrations (MIC) were arbitrary chosen from reference values from the literature [20, 21]. They were set at 12.5 mg/L, 0.2 mg/L and 1.0 mg/L for pyrazinamide, isoniazid and rifampicin, respectively. These MIC values were implemented in WinNonlin for the calculation of time above MIC (T > MIC) and exposure above MIC (AUC > MIC) as therapeutic indices. Sub-therapeutic thresholds were applied using maximum plasma concentrations (C_{MAX}) associated with poor outcome in adults with pulmonary TB [18, 22–25]. The use of these cut-off concentrations is difficult in the context of a multiple drugs therapy and they are still controversial and debated in the literature. However, although there are no consensus values for sub-therapeutic thresholds associated with TBM, or in children, they can be considered as "biomarkers" of clinical outcome. More importantly even if only used graphically in this study, they are able to visualize under-exposure and compare peak concentrations between observed values in children and an adult reference. The sub-therapeutic thresholds were set at 35 μg/mL, 3 μg/mL and 8 μg/mL for pyrazinamide, isoniazid and rifampicin, respectively. Naïve-pooled pharmacokinetic parameter estimates are summarized in Tables 2 to 5, and the relative differences (%) in individual median parameter estimates were calculated between the two age strata for each drug, using the older age group as a reference.

Results

Clinical study characteristics

One hundred children were enrolled in this study. The overall median age of the studied children was 36 months with the largest proportion of children (64 %) below 4 years of age. Among the 33 children ≥ 5 years of age, 16 (48 %) patients were admitted with stage I TBM according to the MRC criteria, 11 (33 %) with stage II and 6 (18 %) with stage III. Among the remaining 67 children < 5 years of age, 43 (64 %) were admitted with a BCS of 4–5 (BCS I), 12 (18 %) with a BCS of 2–3 (BCS II) and 12 (18 %) with a BCS of 0–1 (BCS III). An important proportion (39 %) of the Vietnamese children in this study were classified as malnourished according to the WHO growth criteria with a body mass index (BMI) Z-score below −2 (negative two) [26]. However, a significant weight gain occurred during the first 3 months of treatment (Table 1). The treatment doses in mg/kg, based on the body weight measured at enrollment, did not show significant differences between the two age-groups (Table 2, 3 and 5 for pyrazinamide, isoniazid and rifampicin, respectively).

Fifteen patients (15 %) died. Ten of 64 children under 4 (16 %) vs 5 of 36 children ≥ 4 years (14 %). The majority of deaths occurred in patients with advanced grades of disease at presentation (MRC grade II or III, or BCS from 0–3), but a single death occurred in a patient presenting with MRC grade-I TBM with concomitant HIV infection. It must be noticed that a higher proportion of older children had definite or probable TBM (30/36: 83 %) compared to younger children (42/64: 66 %) which might influence the respective mortality and morbidity in each group. Eight deaths occurred within the first 6 days, six between 6 and 45 days and the last death occurred at day 92. There were no significant differences in mortality or morbidity between the two age groups. At the end of the treatment, 6 out of 81 children (7 %) had severe symptoms and/or required help day and night, 21 of 81 children (26 %) had intermediate sequelae but independent life (modified Rankin scale from 2–3 [12]), and 54 out of 81 children (67 %) recovered fully (4 children did not complete the final study visit). In this study, AST and ALT levels were measured repeatedly for all patients for 90 days (pre-dose, 30, 60 and 90 days) or at any time the children developed symptoms. Two out of 99 children (2 %) met the criteria for drug-induced liver toxicity (DILI) but no child died due to DILI in this study.

Pharmacokinetic analysis

All pharmacokinetic blood draws were close to the pre-specified protocol sampling times (<10 % CV for both age-groups). The absolute difference between the actual sampling time and mean time in the assigned window

Table 1 Baseline characteristics and outcomes of studied children

	<4 years old[a]	>4 years old[b]	Total
Number of patients enrolled, n	64	36	100
Male/Female, n (male %)	36/65 (56.3)	20/36 (55.6)	56.0
Age (months)	12 (2–48)	96 (48–180)	36 (2–180)
Body weight (kg)	9.0 (4.0–15.0)	19.0 (13.5–43.0)	10.9 (4.0–43.0)
BMI (kg/m^2)	15.4 (11.9–22.0)	13.3 (10.6–20.2)	14.3 (10.6–22.0)
Malnourished, n (%)	18/64 (28.1)	20/36 (55.5)	38.0
Body weight gained (kg)			
after 1 month	0.5 (−0.3–2.5)	0.75 (−7.5–6.0)	0.5 (−7.5–6.0)
after 3 months	1.3 (−0.8–5.3)	2.0 (−9.0–12.5)	1.5 (−9.0–12.5)
Fast/Slow acetylator status, n (%)[c]	35/23 (60 %)	29/5 (85 %)	64/28 (70 %)
HIV positive, n (%)[d]	2/61 (3.3 %)	2/35 (5.7 %)	4/96 (4.2 %)
TBM Grade I, n (%)	43/67 (64 %)	16/33 (48 %)	59/100 (59 %)
TBM Grade II, n (%)	12/67 (18 %)	11/33 (33 %)	23/100 (23 %)
TBM Grade III, n (%)	12/67 (18 %)	6/33 (18 %)	18/100 (18 %)
TB diagnosis: Definite, n (%)	3/64 (4.7 %)	3/36 (8.3 %)	6/100 (6.0 %)
TB diagnosis: Probable, n (%)	39/64 (61 %)	27/36 (75 %)	66/100 (66 %)
TB diagnosis: Possible, n (%)	22/64 (34 %)	6/36 (17 %)	28/100 (28 %)
Death, n (%)	10/64 (16 %)	5/36 (14 %)	15/100 (15 %)
Permanent Sequelae, n (%)[e]	19/51 (37 %)	8/30 (27 %)	27/81 (33 %)

All values are reported as median (range) unless otherwise specified. [a]disease severity grade assessed in children below 5 years old by Blantyre Coma Score; [b]disease severity grade assessed in children over 5 years old by Glasgow Coma Score; [c]8 patients did not complete the NAT2 genotype; [d]4 patients out of 100 did not complete HIV testing; [e]surviving patients were assessed after treatment completion at month 8 (4 were lost to follow-up)

Table 2 Pharmacokinetic non-compartmental results of pyrazinamide in children above and below 4 years of age

Pyrazinamide	<4 years old	>4 years old	% difference
Number of patients enrolled	64	36	
Body Weight (median kg - range)	9.0 (4.0–15.0)	19.0 (13.5–43.0)	
Age (median months - range)	12 (2–48)	96 (48–180)	
Dosage (mean - % CV)	4.70 (12.8)	5.12 (9.18)	*p*-value: 0.0001[a]
C_{MAX} (ug/mL)	30.1	37.4	−19.5
T_{MAX} (hr)	2	3	−33.3
CL/F (L/hr)	1.09	1.88	−42
CL/F/BW (L/hr/kg)	0.12	0.1	20
V/F (L)	7.57	12.2	−37.9
V/F/BW (L/kg)	0.84	0.64	31.3
$T_{1/2}$ (hr)	4.82	4.5	7.11
$AUC_{0-\infty}$ (hr × ug/mL)	245	284	−13.7
$AUC_{0-\infty}$/dosage (hr × ug/mL/(mg/kg))	10.1	10.8	−6.2
T > MIC (hr)	7.28	8.46	−13.9
T > MIC/24 h (%)	30.3	35.2	−13.9
AUC > MIC (hr × ug/mL)	62.3	95.2	−34.6

Apart for dosage with mean and % CV, all values are reported as median (range) or as median estimates for pharmacokinetic parameters. C_{MAX} maximum observed plasma concentration after oral administration, T_{MAX} observed time to reach C_{MAX}, *CL/F* oral elimination clearance, *CL/F/BW* elimination clearance corrected by the median body weight, *V/F* apparent volume of distribution, *V/F/BW* apparent volume of distribution corrected by the median body weight, $T_{1/2}$ terminal elimination half-life, $AUC_{0-\infty}$ predicted area under the plasma concentration-time curve after the last dose from zero time to infinity, *T > MIC* time above the minimum inhibitory concentration, *T > MIC/24 h* percentage of the time above the minimum inhibitory concentration over the 24 h dose interval, *AUC > MIC* observed area under the plasma concentration-time curve above the minimum inhibitory concentration. % difference is calculated with the > 4 years group used as the reference. [a]Mann–Whitney T-test

Table 3 Pharmacokinetic non-compartmental results of isoniazid in children above and below 4 years of age

Isoniazid	<4 years old	>4 years old	% difference
Number of patients enrolled	64	36	
Body Weight (median kg - range)	9.0 (4.0–15.0)	19.0 (13.5–43.0)	
Age (median months - range)	12 (2–48)	96 (48–180)	
Dosage (mean - % CV)	25.0 (12.8)	27.3 (9.17)	*p*-value: 0.0002[a]
C_{MAX} (ug/mL)	4.38	5.11	−14.3
T_{MAX} (hr)	2	3	−33.3
CL/F (L/hr)	2.48	3.88	−36.1
CL/F/BW (L/hr/kg)	0.28	0.2	40
V/F (L)	11.3	14.9	−23.8
V/F/BW (L/kg)	1.26	0.78	61.5
$T_{1/2}$ (hr)	3.17	2.66	19.2
AUC0-∞ (hr × ug/mL)	20.2	25.8	−21.8
$AUC_{0-\infty}$/dosage (hr × ug/mL/(mg/kg))	4.48	5.26	−14.8
T > MIC (hr)	14.2	14.5	−1.8
T > MIC/24 h (%)	59.3	60.3	−1.79
$AUC_{0-24\ h}$ > MIC (hr × ug/mL)	16.3	22	−25.8

Apart for dosage with mean and % CV, all values are reported as median (range) or as median estimates for pharmacokinetic parameters. C_{MAX} maximum observed plasma concentration after oral administration, T_{MAX} observed time to reach C_{MAX}, *CL/F* oral elimination clearance, *CL/F/BW* elimination clearance corrected by the median body weight, *V/F* apparent volume of distribution, *V/F/BW* apparent volume of distribution corrected by the median body weight, $T_{1/2}$ terminal elimination half-life, $AUC_{0-\infty}$ predicted area under the plasma concentration-time curve after the last dose from zero time to infinity, *T > MIC* time above the minimum inhibitory concentration, *T > MIC/24 h* percentage of the time above the minimum inhibitory concentration over the 24 h dose interval, *AUC > MIC* observed area under the plasma concentration-time curve above the minimum inhibitory concentration. % difference is calculated with the > 4 years group used as the reference. [a]Mann–Whitney T-test

ranged between −8.2 min to +6.4 min for children below 4 years of age, and between −6.5 min to +0.3 min for children above 4 years of age. The density of individual data points used in each bin was also comparable between the two age groups (after adjusting for the different sample size).

The median and inter-quartile range of naïve-pooled plasma concentrations represented the central trends and the variability of the measured concentration-time profiles well in both age-groups for all drugs (Figs. 1, 2, 3 and 4). As seen in Tables 2, 3 4 and 5, the dosages were in agreement with the 2006 WHO recommendations at the time of the study. However, significant differences were found between young and old children for all drugs but INH when the dosing of fast and slow acetylators was compared. This is likely an inevitable consequence of larger relative body weight differences for younger children enhanced by the need to fit the weight bands and the lack of uniformity when tablets have to be split [27].

Pyrazinamide

Pooled pharmacokinetic parameters, stratified for children above and below 4 years of age, are presented in Table 2. Young children, as compared to older children, showed a trend of 22 % higher body weight-normalized elimination clearance and 31 % higher volume of distribution, a 20 % lower maximum concentration but a modest decrease of 14 % in total exposure. Total exposure, normalized on dosage (mg/kg), showed a less pronounced decrease with 6.3 %. However, a relatively small decrease of 14 % in the time above MIC was seen while the total exposure above MIC was found lower (35 %) in young children compared to older children. The previously defined sub-therapeutic plasma concentration threshold of 35 μg/mL was only reached by older patients [18, 28]. The distribution and accumulation of pyrazinamide into CSF could only be assessed graphically but showed similar exposure to that in plasma, above the wild-type MIC, in both age groups (Fig. 1).

Isoniazid

Pooled pharmacokinetic parameters, stratified for children above and below 4 years of age, are presented in Table 3. Young children, as compared to older children, showed a higher body weight-normalized elimination clearance (35 %) and volume of distribution (61 %), with a 14 % lower maximum concentration and a 22 % lower total exposure. Total exposure, normalized on dosage (mg/kg), showed a less pronounced decrease of 15 %. Similar time above MIC was seen while the total exposure above MIC was lower (26 %) in young children compared to older children. However, the previously defined sub-therapeutic plasma concentration threshold of 3 μg/mL [18, 23] was reached in both age groups

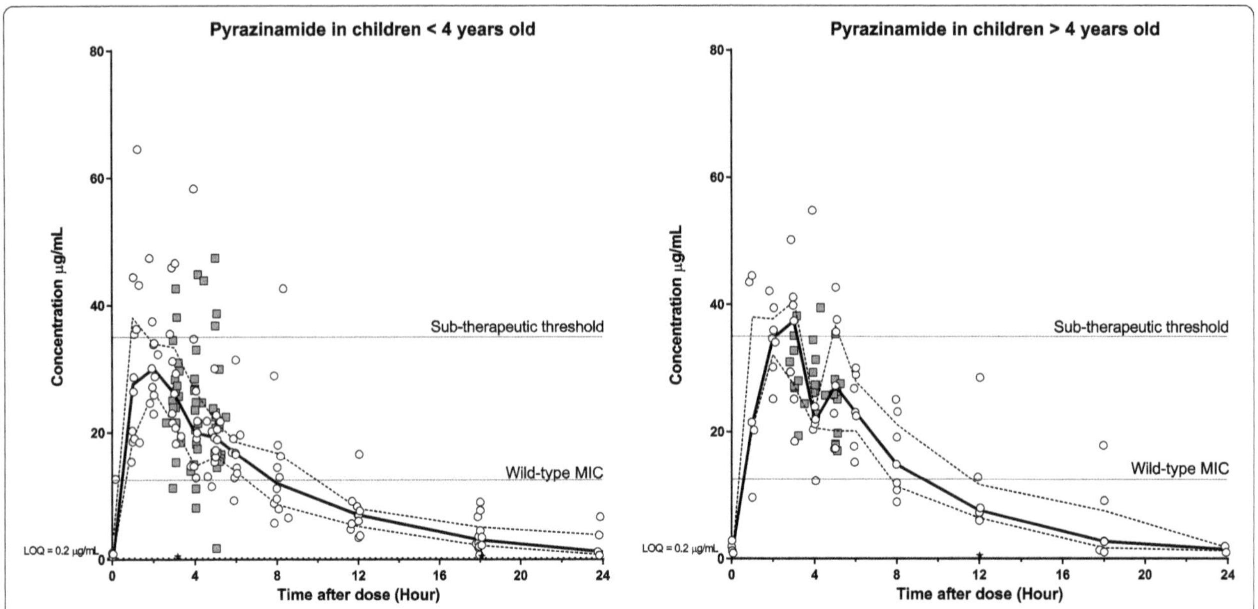

Fig. 1 Plasma (open circles) and CSF (grey squares) concentration-time profiles for pyrazinamide stratified for age (<4 years old [left] and > 4 years old [right]). Continuous lines represent the median plasma concentration and broken lines represent the plasma upper and lower quartiles. Black stars represent plasma samples with concentrations below LOQ. Sub-therapeutic threshold of 35 µg/mL; Minimum Inhibitory Concentration (MIC) of 12.5 µg/mL; and Limit of Quantification (LOQ) of 0.2 µg/mL

with an overall exposure in CSF close to that seen in plasma (Fig. 2).

Isoniazid is known to be affected by acetylator status (fast vs slow phenotype) [29–31]. A stratified analysis was therefore performed to evaluate potential pharmacokinetic differences between these two groups composed by 35 fast and 23 slow acetylators in the young group versus 29 fast and 5 slow for older children (Table 4 and Fig. 3). Surprisingly, there was a higher body weight-normalized clearance (20 %) in patients with a slow acetylator phenotype and we observed a 12 % lower dosage-normalized exposure. A large increase of 124 %

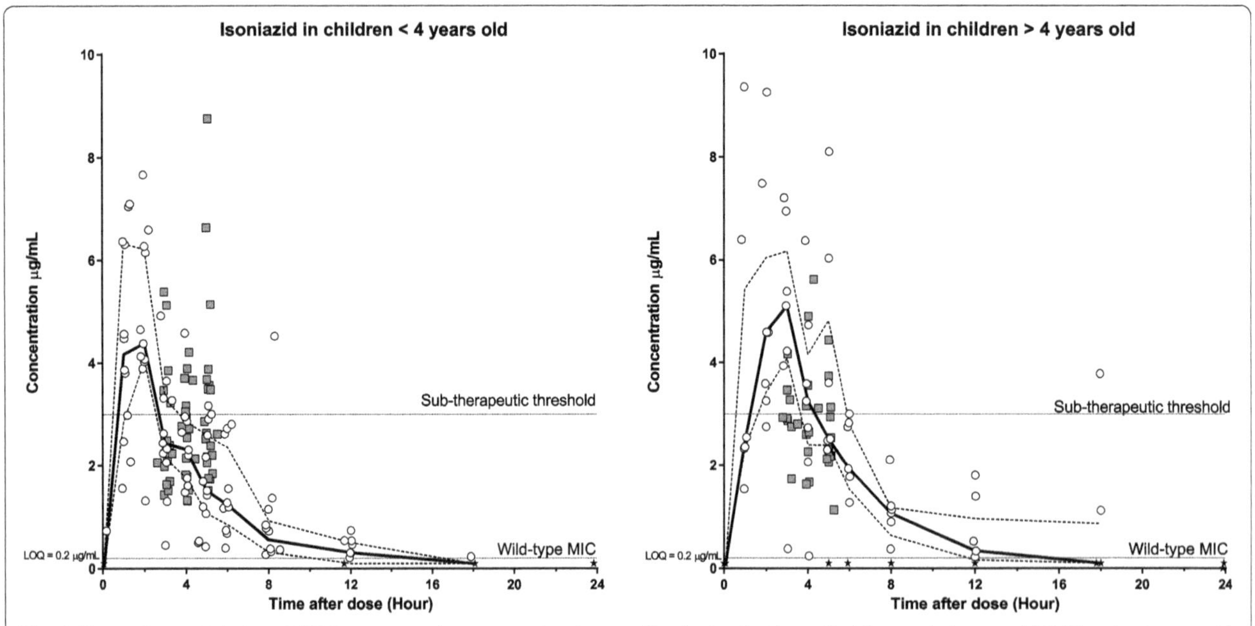

Fig. 2 Plasma (open circles) and CSF (grey squares) concentration-time profiles for isoniazid stratified for age (<4 years old [left] and > 4 years old [right]). Continuous lines represent the median plasma concentration and broken lines represent the plasma upper and lower quartiles. Black stars represent plasma samples with concentrations below LOQ. Sub-therapeutic threshold: 3 µg/mL; Minimum Inhibitory Concentration (MIC) and Limit of Quantification (LOQ): 0.2 µg/mL

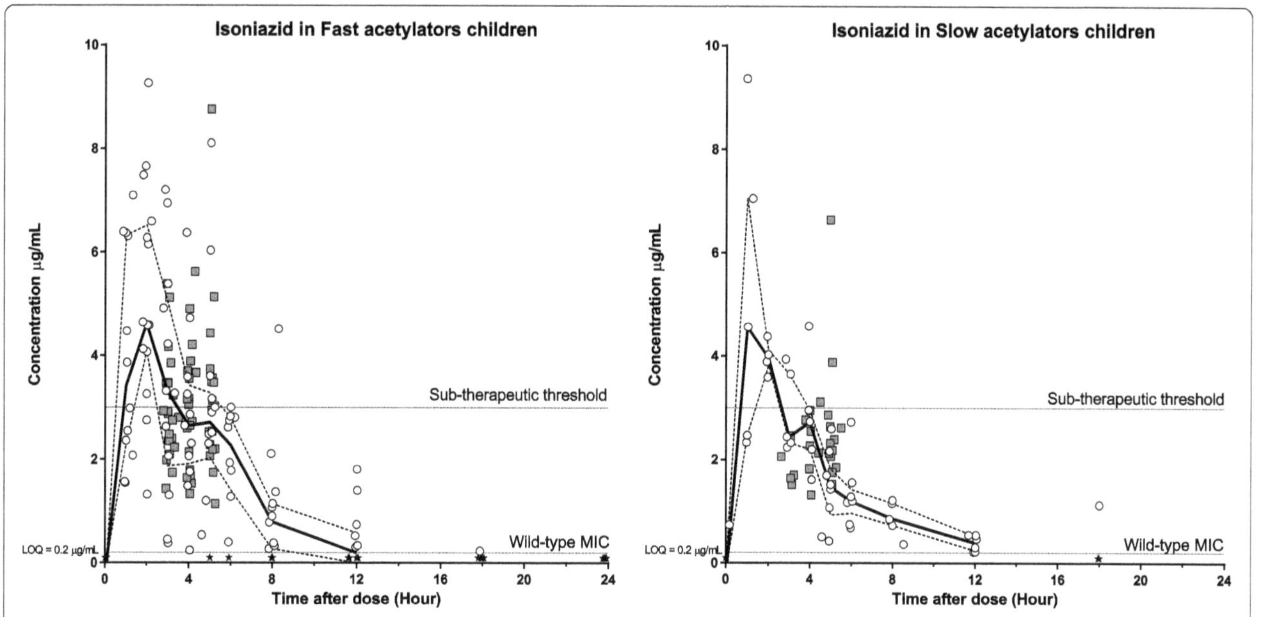

Fig. 3 Plasma (open circles) and CSF (grey squares) concentration-time profiles for isoniazid stratified for Fast acetylators [left] and Slow acetylators [right]. Continuous lines represent the median plasma concentration and broken lines represent the plasma upper and lower quartiles. Black stars represent plasma samples with concentrations below LOQ. Sub-therapeutic threshold: 3 µg/mL; Minimum Inhibitory Concentration (MIC) and Limit of Quantification (LOQ): 0.2 µg/mL

was also seen for body weight-normalized volume of distribution in patients with a slow acetylator phenotype, resulting in a markedly increased terminal elimination half-life (87 %). However, an imbalance in the number of fast and slow acetylators in the two age groups might have confounded these results. Indeed, the ratio was 60 % fast actetylators in the young age group versus 85 % fast actetylators for the over 4 years old (Table 1). Therapeutic plasma concentrations were reached in both groups and there were no observed differences in the distribution into CSF between fast and slow acetylators.

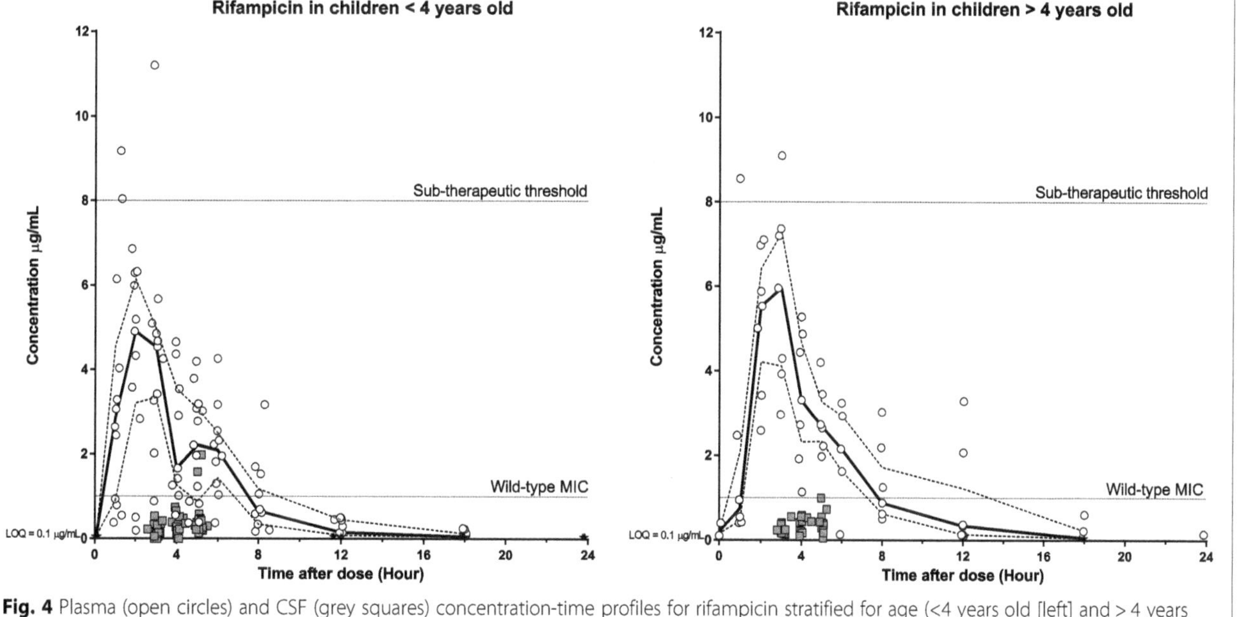

Fig. 4 Plasma (open circles) and CSF (grey squares) concentration-time profiles for rifampicin stratified for age (<4 years old [left] and > 4 years old [right]). Continuous lines represent the median plasma concentration and broken lines represent the plasma upper and lower quartiles. Black stars represent plasma samples with concentrations below LOQ. Sub-therapeutic threshold: 8 µg/mL; Minimum Inhibitory Concentration (MIC): 1.0 µg/mL; Limit of Quantification (LOQ): 0.1 µg/mL

Table 4 Pharmacokinetic non-compartmental results of isoniazid in fast and slow acetylators

Isoniazid	SLOW	FAST	% difference
Number of patients enrolled[a]	28	64	
Body Weight (median kg - range)	10.0 (4.5–26.0)	13.0 (4.4–44.0)	
Age (median months - range)	36 (6–180)	42 (2–180)	
Dosage (mean - % CV)	4.82 (11.7)	4.70 (13.3)	*p*-value: > 0.05[b]
C_{MAX} (ug/mL)	4.56	4.62	−1.3
T_{MAX} (hr)	1	2	−50
CL/F (L/hr)	2.28	2.47	−7.69
CL/F/BW (L/hr/kg)	0.23	0.19	21.1
V/F (L)	12.2	7.05	72.3
V/F/BW (L/kg)	1.21	0.54	124
$T_{1/2}$ (hr)	3.69	1.98	86.4
AUC0-∞ (hr × ug/mL)	21.9	22.8	−3.78
$AUC_{0-\infty}$/dosage (hr × ug/mL/(mg/kg))	4.38	4.95	−11.5
T > MIC (hr)	14.8	11.9	24.7
T > MIC/24 h (%)	61.7	49.4	24.8
$AUC_{0-24\ h}$ > MIC (hr × ug/mL)	17.7	19.8	−10.7

[a]Acetylator genotype was determined in 92 patients. [b]Mann–Whitney T-test. Apart for dosage with mean and % CV, all values are reported as median (range) or as median estimates for pharmacokinetic parameters. C_{MAX} maximum observed plasma concentration after oral administration, T_{MAX} observed time to reach C_{MAX}, *CL/F* oral elimination clearance, *CL/F/BW* elimination clearance corrected by the median body weight, *V/F* apparent volume of distribution, *V/F/BW* apparent volume of distribution corrected by the median body weight, $T_{1/2}$ terminal elimination half-life, $AUC_{0-\infty}$ predicted area under the plasma concentration-time curve after the last dose from zero time to infinity, *T > MIC* time above the minimum inhibitory concentration, *T > MIC/24 h* percentage of the time above the minimum inhibitory concentration over the 24 h dose interval, *AUC > MIC* observed area under the plasma concentration-time curve above the minimum inhibitory concentration. % difference is calculated with the > 4 years group used as the reference

Table 5 Pharmacokinetic non-compartmental results of rifampicin in children above and below 4 years of age

Rifampicin	<4 years old	>4 years old	% difference
Number of patients enrolled	64	36	
Body Weight (median kg - range)	9.0 (4.0–15.0)	19.0 (13.5–43.0)	
Age (median months - range)	12 (2–48)	96 (48–180)	
Dosage (mean - % CV)	9.38 (12.8)	10.2 (9.04)	*p*-value: 0.0002[a]
C_{MAX} (ug/mL)	4.9	5.96	−17.8
T_{MAX} (hr)	2	3	−33.3
CL/F (L/hr)	4.66	7.86	−40.7
CL/F/BW (L/hr/kg)	0.52	0.41	26.8
V/F (L)	15.6	25.5	−38.9
V/F/BW (L/kg)	1.73	1.34	29.1
$T_{1/2}$ (hr)	2.31	2.25	2.67
AUC0-∞ (hr × ug/mL)	21.5	25.4	−15.7
$AUC_{0-\infty}$/dosage (hr × ug/mL/(mg/kg))	2.36	2.6	−9.23
T > MIC (hr)	6.89	6.66	3.45
T > MIC/24 h (%)	28.7	27.8	3.39
$AUC_{0-24\ h}$ > MIC (hr × ug/mL)	11.7	14.7	−20.1

Apart for dosage with mean and % CV, all values are reported as median (range) or as median estimates for pharmacokinetic parameters. C_{MAX} maximum observed plasma concentration after oral administration, T_{MAX} observed time to reach C_{MAX}, *CL/F* oral elimination clearance, *CL/F/BW* elimination clearance corrected by the median body weight, *V/F* apparent volume of distribution, *V/F/BW* apparent volume of distribution corrected by the median body weight, $T_{1/2}$ terminal elimination half-life, $AUC_{0-\infty}$ predicted area under the plasma concentration-time curve after the last dose from zero time to infinity, *T > MIC* time above the minimum inhibitory concentration, *T > MIC/24 h* percentage of the time above the minimum inhibitory concentration over the 24 h dose interval, *AUC > MIC* observed area under the plasma concentration-time curve above the minimum inhibitory concentration. % difference is calculated with the > 4 years group used as the reference. [a]Mann–Whitney T-test

Rifampicin

Overall, rifampicin presented the largest variation in the concentration-time profiles, especially in the younger children (Fig. 4). Pooled pharmacokinetic parameters, stratified for children above and below 4 years of age, are presented in Table 5. Young children, as compared to older children, showed a higher body weight-normalized elimination clearance (25 %) and volume of distribution (29 %), a 18 % lower maximum concentration and a lower total exposure with 16 %. Total exposure, normalized on dosage (mg/kg), showed a less pronounced decrease of only 9 %. Similar times above MIC were observed while the total exposure above MIC was found lower (20 %) in young children compared to older children. Only a few individual concentration measurements and none of the median or interquartile ranges reached the previously defined sub-therapeutic plasma concentration threshold of 8 μg/mL (Fig. 4) [24, 25]. The observed penetration of rifampicin into CSF was very poor with only 2 individual concentration measurements above the wild-type MIC (Fig. 4).

Discussion

The naïve-pooled pharmacokinetic analysis provided a model-independent analysis approach and was graphically proven to represent the central trends and the variability of the measured concentration-time profiles well in both age-groups and for all drugs. Considerable variability was seen in the observed data which might be explained by the relatively large difference in age and body weight of enrolled children. However, although a naïve pooled data approach provides generally fairly accurate PK estimates [32], the observed variability emphasizes the need to evaluate these treatments on a population level and suggests that a nonlinear mixed-effects approach might provide a more mechanistic understanding of the variability and the influence of clinically important covariates. Pharmacokinetic parameter estimates in this study were generally in agreement with previous studies reporting pharmacokinetic properties of this first-line therapy in children with pulmonary TB [31, 33–35] and TBM [4, 36, 37].

All drugs showed a higher body weight-normalized elimination clearance in young children as compared to older children, and a lower drug exposure was observed in the young group. Similar results have been presented in the literature, noticing a lower exposure in children when compared adults, and lower exposure in young children when compared to older children [30, 31, 38, 39]. These observations lead the revision of the pediatric dosing regimen in TB, recommending an increased dosage for all TB drugs in children. This is most likely a consequence of the well-known allometric relationship between body weight and clearance, and emphasizes the need of dose adjustments in young children with a focus on the youngest patients. In order to produce a dosing alternative that provides an equivalent total drug exposure in children of all age, dosing should therefore rather be scaled with, for example, the body surface area or the lean body weight [40, 41] . Large observed variability and a model-independent analysis, as presented in this study, do not provide a reliable tool to suggest new dosing regimens. However, our data support the recent WHO recommendations to increase the doses of anti-tuberculosis drugs in children with TB, and moreover underline the importance of this in TB meningitis. Further studies are needed urgently to evaluate the clinical impact of the new WHO regimen, designed for pulmonary TB, in young children with TBM.

Plasma concentrations of isoniazid and pyrazinamide reached therapeutic levels rapidly after drug administration. However, only a few individual concentration measurements of rifampicin reached a putative therapeutic level of 8 μg/mL, suggesting that rifampicin may still be severely under-dosed with the current dose recommendation of 15 mg/kg. TBM is primarily a disease of the brain and it is therefore crucial that the administered drugs are distributed from blood into the therapeutic site of action in sufficient concentrations to eliminate the bacterium. Only pyrazinamide and isoniazid demonstrated a large distribution from plasma to CSF with approximately equivalent drug concentrations in plasma and CSF.

Pyrazinamide is only active at low pH which makes definition of MIC difficult in the context of TBM [42]. The role of pyrazinamide within the neutral pH environment of the CSF compartment is unclear. It may have a crucial role in clearing persistent metabolically dormant bacilli within tuberculomas. However, although less frequent in children, pyrazinamide is the antituberculous agent most often implicated in the development of drug-induced liver injuries (DILI) and consideration must therefore be given to the risk of DILI with increased doses of pyrazinamide when determining optimal dosage.

Isoniazid is responsible for killing the majority of the bacteria within the first days of treatment in pulmonary TB [43–46]. Achieving adequate drug concentrations in CSF in the treatment of TBM is therefore likely to be crucial in preventing early mortality and morbidity. This emphasizes the importance of dose-optimization of isoniazid since body weight-normalized clearance and volume of distribution were found significantly higher in younger children, resulting in a decreased exposure. This is consistent with previous reports that younger children eliminate isoniazid faster than older children and adults [30, 47]. Patients with fast acetylator status had a modest decreased body weight-normalized clearance of isoniazid as compared to patients with slow acetylator status

(Table 4). These results were unexpected, assuming fast acetylators metabolize isoniazid more rapidly resulting in an increased clearance. However, the results are likely to be confounded by the greater proportion of slow acetylators in the younger age group (40 %) as compared to the older children (15 %). Young children had an overall higher body weight-normalized clearance compared to older children, which may have attenuated the overall difference in isoniazid pharmacokinetics between slow and fast acetylators. Furthermore, Thee et al. previously reported that isoniazid concentrations were not dependent on acetylator status in South African children below 2 years of age [31]. Maturation of the NAT2 enzyme system with age might play an important role in the metabolism of isoniazid and/or there might be ethnic differences in the degree to which NAT2 genotype influences the metabolism of isoniazid. A separate analysis demonstrated an expected 35 % increased body weight-normalized clearance in children with fast acetylator status compared to slow acetylators. It was not deemed reliable to evaluate the fast vs slow phenotype in the older age group considering that only 5 patients of the older children were slow acetylators.

Low concentrations of rifampicin, below the therapeutic threshold, were seen in CSF suggesting higher doses of rifampicin may be more effective in the treatment of childhood TBM. Rifampicin CSF drug concentrations are proportional to dosing and in other forms of TB a dose-related increase in bactericidal activity exists [4, 48] Higher dosages result in increased early bactericidal activity [4, 49] and improved culture conversion rates [50]. A recent Indonesian study showed survival benefit in TBM patients with 13 mg/kg of intravenous rifampicin and additional moxifloxacin for the initial 2 weeks of treatment [7, 51]. These two studies showed the advantage of a higher dosage of rifampicin but here delivered intravenously. An equivalent oral dosage is likely to be between 15 to 25 mg/kg due to the poor and variable bioavailibilty of rifampicin [52, 53]. Children have lower exposure to rifampicin compared to adults, given the same mg/kg dosing. It is likely that dosages of 15–20 mg/kg in children are required to achieve CSF concentration well in excess of the MIC for drug-susceptible strains and higher dosages still (≥20 mg/kg) may be required in very young children [4]. Our findings provide addition support for current and planned studies investigating the use of higher doses for all first-line anti-TB drugs for TBM treatment. The 6-month intensified pediatric regimen used in South Africa with excellent clinical outcomes further supports the hypothesis that higher anti-tuberculosis drug doses, especially of rifampicin, will improve the outcomes of children with TBM [9].

Several limitations of this study deserve comment. First, this was a prospective observational study using an old and no longer recommended regimen. The higher dose regimen recommended by WHO in 2009 was not implemented in Vietnam until 2013. Second, only sparse and small volume CSF sampling was possible and we therefore had to compromise which drugs to analyse. We chose pyrazinamide, isoniazid and rifampicin for a technical reason: ethambutol presents a low molar absorptivity in the UV-visible spectrum and could not be analysed by our LC-UV method. Third, in naïve pooled data analysis, the observations from each individual are grouped or pooled as if it was a single patient. Hence the results from the non-compartmental analysis can only be expressed as group median with no variation. A risk of bias from severe outliers can arise but only with an imbalance of data per individual, which was not the case in this study. Naïve pooled data analysis is a simplistic approach but quickly informative without the need of specialized software and expertise from modelers. However, dedicated population models able to describe the PK/PD of each drug in plasma and CSF of children are on-going. Finally, with few CSF sampling occasions, far from treatment initiation, the relationships between drug exposure, bacterial killing, and clinical outcome are difficult to assess. Most deaths occur rapidly within the first weeks, before any lumbar puncture could be performed giving information on levels of drugs in these patients.

Conclusion

In summary, this study described the pharmacokinetic properties of isoniazid, pyrazinamide and rifampicin in children with TBM and showed the inadequacy of the relatively low-dose regimens, with an emphasis on the youngest patients below 4 years of age. It is crucial that the administered drugs distribute into the CSF in the treatment of TBM. Only isoniazid and pyrazinamide distributed greatly into the CSF of these enrolled children. This study provided a baseline for evaluation of the pharmacokinetic properties of the new WHO pediatric dosage in Vietnam, which was implemented in 2013. It remains to be confirmed if the new dosing regimen is capable of increasing substantially the drug exposure in the CSF and improving clinical outcomes. More data is urgently needed to establish evidence for optimal drug combinations and doses in the treatment of pediatric TBM.

Competing interests

We have read and understood BMC Infectious Diseases policy on declaration of interests and declare that we have no competing interests.

Authors' contributions

TP participated in the study design, validated the quantification method, analysed the clinical samples, performed the non-compartmental analysis and wrote the article. NDB principle investigator of the study, wrote the study protocol, recruited the patients and analysed the clinical data. PVT validated the quantification method and analysed the clinical samples. PNP analysed the clinical samples. NHD recruited the patients, performed the biochemistry tests and processed the PK samples. TND recruited the patients, performed the biochemistry tests and processed the PK samples. MC wrote the study protocol and performed the biochemistry and genotyping tests and analysis. GET co-investigator of the study, head of OUCRU Vietnam brought a significant contribution in the writing of this article. JT head of the clinical pharmacology department at MORU Thailand, assisted in the non-compartmental analysis and helped writing the article. JND co-investigator of the study, designed and wrote the full protocol, funded the clinical investigation through a grant from the Wellcome Trust and assisted in the writing of the article. All authors read and approved the final manuscript.

Acknowledgements
This study was supported by the Wellcome Trust, UK. We are grateful to the Director, the nurses and technicians of the Pham Ngoc Thach Hospital, Ho Chi Minh City for their support, and all the patients who participated in the study for their contribution

Author details
[1]Mahidol-Oxford Tropical Medicine Research Unit, Faculty of Tropical Medicine, Mahidol University, Bangkok, Thailand. [2]Centre for Tropical Medicine and Global Health, Nuffield Department of Medicine, University of Oxford, Oxford, UK. [3]Oxford University Clinical Research Unit, Wellcome Trust Major Overseas Programme, Ho Chi Minh City, Viet Nam. [4]Pham Ngoc Thach Hospital, Ho Chi Minh City, Viet Nam. [5]Liverpool School of Tropical Medicine, Liverpool, UK.

References

1. Farinha NJ, Razali KA, Holzel H, Morgan G, Novelli VM. Tuberculosis of the central nervous system in children: a 20-year survey. J Infect. 2000;41:61–8.
2. Marx GE, Chan ED. Tuberculous meningitis: diagnosis and treatment overview. Tuberc Res Treat. 2011;2011:798764.
3. Peloquin CA, Jaresko GS, Yong C, Keung ACF, Bulpitt AMYE, Jelliffe RW. Population Pharmacokinetic Modeling of Isoniazid, Rifampin, and Pyrazinamide. Antimicrob Agents Chemother. 1997;41:2670–9.
4. Donald PR. Cerebrospinal fluid concentrations of antituberculosis agents in adults and children. Tuberculosis. 2010;90:279–92.
5. Gundert-Remy U, Klett M, Weber E. Concentration of ethambutol in cerebrospinal fluid in man as a function of the non-protein-bound drug fraction in serum. Eur J Clin Pharmacol. 1973;6:133–6.
6. Ellard GA, Humphries M, Gabriel M, Teoh R. Penetration of pyrazinamide into the cerebrospinal fluid in tuberculous meningitis. Br Med J. 1987;294: 284–5.
7. Ruslami R, Ganiem AR, Dian S, et al. Intensified regimen containing rifampicin and moxifloxacin for tuberculous meningitis: an open-label, randomised controlled phase 2 trial. Lancet Infect Dis. 2012;3099:1–9.
8. Heemskerk D, Day J, Chau TTH, et al. Intensified treatment with high dose rifampicin and levofloxacin compared to standard treatment for adult patients with tuberculous meningitis (TBM-IT): protocol for a randomized controlled trial. Trials. 2011;12:1–11.
9. van Toorn R, Schaaf HS, Laubscher J a, van Elsland SL, Donald PR, Schoeman JF. Short intensified treatment in children with drug-susceptible tuberculous meningitis. Pediatr Infect Dis J. 2014;33:248–52.
10. Wolbers M, Heemskerk D, Chau TTH, et al. Sample size requirements for separating out the effects of combination treatments: randomised controlled trials of combination therapy vs. standard treatment compared to factorial designs for patients with tuberculous meningitis. Trials. 2011;12:26.
11. Guidance for national tuberculosis programmes on the management of tuberculosis in children. WHO report 2006. Geneva, World Health Organization, 2006 (WHO/HTM/TB/2006.371 - WHO/FCH/CAH/2006.7).
12. Thwaites GE. Dexamethasone for the treatment of tuberculous meningitis in adolescents and adults. N Engl J Med. 2004;531:1741–51.
13. Brans R, Laizane D, Khan A, Blömeke B. N-acetyltransferase 2 genotyping: an accurate and feasible approach for simultaneous detection of the most common NAT2 alleles. Clin Chem. 2004;50:1264–6.
14. Rihs H-P, John A, Scherenberg M, Seidel A, Brüning T. Concordance between the deduced acetylation status generated by high-speed: real-time PCR based NAT2 genotyping of seven single nucleotide polymorphisms and human NAT2 phenotypes determined by a caffeine assay. Clin Chim acta. 2007;376:240–3.
15. Kilbane a J, Silbart LK, Manis M, Beitins IZ, Weber WW. Human N-acetylation genotype determination with urinary caffeine metabolites. Clin Pharmacol Ther. 1990;47:470–7.
16. Notarianni LJ, Dobrocky P, Godlewski G, Jones RW, Bennett PN. Caffeine as a metabolic probe: NAT2 phenotyping. Br J Clin Pharmacol. 1996;41:169–73.
17. Tiwari G, Tiwari R. Bioanalytical method validation: An updated review. Pharm Methods. 2010;1:25–38.
18. Prahl JB, Johansen IS, Cohen AS, Frimodt-Møller N, Andersen AB. Clinical significance of 2 h plasma concentrations of first-line anti-tuberculosis drugs: a prospective observational study. J Antimicrob Chemother. 2014;69:2841–7.
19. Ruslami R, Nijland HMJ, Alisjahbana B, Parwati I, van Crevel R, Aarnoutse RE. Pharmacokinetics and tolerability of a higher rifampin dose versus the standard dose in pulmonary tuberculosis patients. Antimicrob Agents Chemother. 2007;51:2546–51.
20. Reynolds J, Heysell SK. Understanding pharmacokinetics to improve tuberculosis treatment outcome. Expert Opin Drug Metab Toxicol. 2014;10:1–11.
21. Mugabo P, Hassan MS, Slaughter R. Acute Pharmacokinetics of First Line Anti-tuberculosis Drugs in Patients with Pulmonary Tuberculosis and in Patients with Pulmonary Tuberculosis Co-infected with HIV. J US-China Med Sci. 2011;8:661–6.
22. Mitchison DA, Davies GR. Assessment of the Efficacy of New Anti-Tuberculosis Drugs. Open Infect Dis J. 2008;2:59–76.
23. Ramachandran G, Kumar AK, Swaminathan S. Pharmacokinetics of anti-tuberculosis drugs in children. Indian J Pediatr. 2011;78:435–42.
24. Ramachandran G, Hemanth Kumar AK, Bhavani PK, et al. Age, nutritional status and INH acetylator status affect pharmacokinetics of anti-tuberculosis drugs in children. Int J Tuberc Lung Dis. 2013;17:800–6.
25. Peloquin CA. Therapeutic drug monitoring in the treatment of tuberculosis. Drugs. 2002;62:2169–83.
26. Foster BJ, Platt RW, Zemel BS. Development and validation of a predictive equation for lean body mass in children and adolescents. Ann Hum Biol. 2012;39:171–82.
27. Pouplin T, Phuong PN, Van Toi P, Nguyen Pouplin J, Farrar J. Isoniazid, pyrazinamide and rifampicin content variation in split fixed-dose combination tablets. PLoS One. 2014;9:e102047.
28. Donald PR, Maritz JS, Diacon AH. Pyrazinamide pharmacokinetics and efficacy in adults and children. Tuberculosis. 2012;92:1–8.
29. Rey E, Gendrel D, Treluyer JM, et al. Isoniazid pharmacokinetics in children according to acetylator phenotype. Fundam Clin Pharmacol. 2001;15:355–9.
30. Schaaf HS, Parkin DP, Seifart HI, et al. Isoniazid pharmacokinetics in children treated for respiratory tuberculosis. Arch Dis Child. 2005;90:614–8.
31. Thee S, Seddon JA, Donald PR, et al. Pharmacokinetics of isoniazid, rifampin, and pyrazinamide in children younger than two years of age with tuberculosis: evidence for implementation of revised World Health Organization recommendations. Antimicrob Agents Chemother. 2011;55:5560–7.
32. Mahmood I. Naive pooled-data approach for pharmacokinetic studies in pediatrics with a very small sample size. Am J Ther. 2014;21:269–74.
33. Graham SM, Sismanidis C, Menzies HJ, Marais BJ, Detjen AK, Black RE. Importance of tuberculosis control to address child survival. Lancet. 2014;6736:5–7.
34. Marais BJ, Graham SM. Childhood tuberculosis: a roadmap towards zero deaths. Journal of Paediatrics and Child Health. 2014. doi:10.1111/jpc.12647.
35. Shingadia D. Tuberculosis in childhood. Ther Adv Respir Dis. 2012;6:161–71.
36. van Well GTJ, Paes BF, Terwee CB, et al. Twenty Years of Pediatric Tuberculous Meningitis: A Retrospective Cohort Study in the Western Cape of South Africa. Pediatrics. 2009;123:e1–8.
37. Donald PR. The chemotherapy of tuberculous meningitis in children and adults. Tuberculosis. 2010;90:375–92.
38. Thee S, Detjen A, Wahn U, Magdorf K. Rifampicin serum levels in childhood tuberculosis. Int J Tuberc Lung Dis. 2009;13:1106–11.
39. Graham SM, Bell DJ, Nyirongo S, et al. Low Levels of Pyrazinamide and Ethambutol in Children with Tuberculosis and Impact of Age, Nutritional Status, and Human Immunodeficiency Virus Infection. Antimicrob Agents Chemother. 2006;50:407–13.
40. McLeay SC, Morrish GA, Kirkpatrick CMJ, Green B. The relationship between drug clearance and body size: systematic review and meta-analysis of the literature published from 2000 to 2007. Clin Pharmacokinet. 2012;51:319–30.

41. Holford N. A size standard for pharmacokinetics. Clin Pharmacokinet. 1996; 30:329–32.
42. Zhang Y, Mitchison D. The curious characteristics of pyrazinamide: a review. Int J Tuberc Lung Dis. 2003;7:6–21.
43. Mitchison DA. Role of individual drugs in the chemotherapy of tuberculosis. Int J Tuberc Lung Dis. 2000;4:796–806.
44. Donald PR, Sirgel FA, Venter A, et al. The Influence of Human N-Acetyltransferase Genotype on the Early Bactericidal Activity of Isoniazid. Clin Infect Dis. 2004;39:1425–30.
45. Donald PR, Sirgel FA, Botha FJ, et al. The early bactericidal activity of isoniazid related to its dose size in pulmonary tuberculosis. Am J Respir Crit Care Med. 1997;156:895–900.
46. Jindani A, Aber VR, Edwards EA, Mitchison DA. The early bactericidal activity of drugs in patients with pulmonary tuberculosis. Am Rev Respir Dis. 1980; 121:939–49.
47. McIlleron H, Willemse M, Werely CJ, et al. Isoniazid plasma concentrations in a cohort of South African children with tuberculosis: implications for international pediatric dosing guidelines. Clin Infect Dis. 2009;48:1547–53.
48. Diacon AH, Patientia RF, Venter A, et al. Early bactericidal activity of high-dose rifampin in patients with pulmonary tuberculosis evidenced by positive sputum smears. Antimicrob Agents Chemother. 2007;51:2994–6.
49. Diacon AH, Donald PR. The early bactericidal activity of antituberculosis drugs. Expert Rev Anti Infect Ther. 2014;12:223–37.
50. Steingart KR, Jotblad S, Robsky K, et al. Higher-dose rifampin for the treatment of pulmonary tuberculosis: a systematic review [Review article]. Int J Tuberc Lung Dis. 2011;15:305–16.
51. te Brake L, Dian S, Ganiem AR, et al. Pharmacokinetic/pharmacodynamic analysis of an intensified regimen containing rifampicin and moxifloxacin for tuberculous meningitis. Int J Antimicrob Agents. 2015;45(5):496–503.
52. Mariappan TT, Singh S, Pandey R, Khuller GK. Determination of Absolute Bioavailability of Rifampicin by Varying the Mode of Intravenous Administration and the Time of Sampling. Clin Res Regul Aff. 2005;22:119–28.
53. Koup JR, Williams-Warren J, Viswanathan CT, Weber A, Smith AL. Pharmacokinetics of rifampin in children. II. Oral bioavailability. Ther Drug Monit. 1986;8:17–22.

Permissions

All chapters in this book were first published in ID, by BioMed Central; hereby published with permission under the Creative Commons Attribution License or equivalent. Every chapter published in this book has been scrutinized by our experts. Their significance has been extensively debated. The topics covered herein carry significant findings which will fuel the growth of the discipline. They may even be implemented as practical applications or may be referred to as a beginning point for another development.

The contributors of this book come from diverse backgrounds, making this book a truly international effort. This book will bring forth new frontiers with its revolutionizing research information and detailed analysis of the nascent developments around the world.

We would like to thank all the contributing authors for lending their expertise to make the book truly unique. They have played a crucial role in the development of this book. Without their invaluable contributions this book wouldn't have been possible. They have made vital efforts to compile up to date information on the varied aspects of this subject to make this book a valuable addition to the collection of many professionals and students.

This book was conceptualized with the vision of imparting up-to-date information and advanced data in this field. To ensure the same, a matchless editorial board was set up. Every individual on the board went through rigorous rounds of assessment to prove their worth. After which they invested a large part of their time researching and compiling the most relevant data for our readers.

The editorial board has been involved in producing this book since its inception. They have spent rigorous hours researching and exploring the diverse topics which have resulted in the successful publishing of this book. They have passed on their knowledge of decades through this book. To expedite this challenging task, the publisher supported the team at every step. A small team of assistant editors was also appointed to further simplify the editing procedure and attain best results for the readers.

Apart from the editorial board, the designing team has also invested a significant amount of their time in understanding the subject and creating the most relevant covers. They scrutinized every image to scout for the most suitable representation of the subject and create an appropriate cover for the book.

The publishing team has been an ardent support to the editorial, designing and production team. Their endless efforts to recruit the best for this project, has resulted in the accomplishment of this book. They are a veteran in the field of academics and their pool of knowledge is as vast as their experience in printing. Their expertise and guidance has proved useful at every step. Their uncompromising quality standards have made this book an exceptional effort. Their encouragement from time to time has been an inspiration for everyone.

The publisher and the editorial board hope that this book will prove to be a valuable piece of knowledge for researchers, students, practitioners and scholars across the globe.

List of Contributors

Mireille Prince-David and Mounerou Salou
Centre de Biologie Moléculaire et d'Immunologie, Université de Lomé, BP 101, Lomé, Togo
Service de Microbiologie, Centre Hospitalier Universitaire Sylvanus Olympio, Tokoin Hôpital, BP 57, Lomé, Togo

Corinne Marois-Créhan
Agence nationale de sécurité sanitaire de l'alimentation, de l'environnement et du travail, 22440 Ploufragan, France
Université Bretagne Loire, 22440 Ploufragan, France

Komi Assogba and Koffi A. Balogou
Service de Neurologie, Centre Hospitalier Universitaire Campus, BP 30284, Lomé, Togo

Céline Plainvert
Service de Bactériologie, Hôpitaux Universitaires Paris Centre, site Cochin, 75679 Paris cedex 14, France
Centre National de Référence des Streptocoques, Hôpital Cochin, 75679 Paris cedex 14, France

Claire Poyart and Asmaa Tazi
Service de Bactériologie, Hôpitaux Universitaires Paris Centre, site Cochin, 75679 Paris cedex 14, France
Centre National de Référence des Streptocoques, Hôpital Cochin, 75679 Paris cedex 14, France
Université Paris Descartes, 75006 Paris, France

Xiong Xiao, Yang Zhang, Liwei Zhang, Peng Kang and Nan Ji
Department of Neurosurgery/China National Clinical Research Center for Neurological Diseases, Beijing Tiantan Hospital, Capital Medical University, 6 Tian Tan Xi Li, Beijing 100050, China

Thai Thanh Truc
Oxford University Clinical Research Unit, Wellcome Trust Major Overseas Programme, 764 Vo Van Kiet, Quan 5, Ho Chi Minh City, Vietnam

Nguyen Duc Bang and Dang Thi Minh Ha
Oxford University Clinical Research Unit, Wellcome Trust Major Overseas Programme, 764 Vo Van Kiet, Quan 5, Ho Chi Minh City, Vietnam
Pham Ngoc Thach Hospital, 120 Hung Vuong, Quan 5, Ho Chi Minh City, Vietnam

Thomas Pouplin
Oxford University Clinical Research Unit, Wellcome Trust Major Overseas Programme, 764 Vo Van Kiet, Quan 5, Ho Chi Minh City, Vietnam
Centre for Tropical Medicine and Global Health, Nuffield Department of Medicine Research Building, University of Oxford, Old Road campus, Roosevelt Drive, Oxford, UK
Mahidol-Oxford Tropical Medicine Research Unit, Faculty of Tropical Medicine, 420/6 Ratchawithi Rd., Bangkok, Thailand

Tran Ngoc Duong and Nguyen Huy Dung
Pham Ngoc Thach Hospital, 120 Hung Vuong, Quan 5, Ho Chi Minh City, Vietnam

Maxine Caws
Oxford University Clinical Research Unit, Wellcome Trust Major Overseas Programme, 764 Vo Van Kiet, Quan 5, Ho Chi Minh City, Vietnam
Department of Clinical Sciences, Liverpool School of Tropical Medicine, Pembroke Place, L3 5QA Liverpool, UK
Centre for Tropical Medicine and Global Health, Nuffield Department of Medicine Research Building, University of Oxford, Old Road campus, Roosevelt Drive, Oxford, UK

Guy E. Thwaites, Doortje Heemskerk, Laura Merson, Pham Van Toi, Jeremy J. Farrar, Marcel Wolbers and Jeremy N. Day
Oxford University Clinical Research Unit, Wellcome Trust Major Overseas Programme, 764 Vo Van Kiet, Quan 5, Ho Chi Minh City, Vietnam
Centre for Tropical Medicine and Global Health, Nuffield Department of Medicine Research Building, University of Oxford, Old Road campus, Roosevelt Drive, Oxford, UK

Joel Tarning
Centre for Tropical Medicine and Global Health, Nuffield Department of Medicine Research Building, University of Oxford, Old Road campus, Roosevelt Drive, Oxford, UK
Mahidol-Oxford Tropical Medicine Research Unit, Faculty of Tropical Medicine, 420/6 Ratchawithi Rd., Bangkok, Thailand

S. Majeed and S. Sharma
Department of Biochemistry, Postgraduate Institute of Medical Education & Research, Chandigarh 160012, India

P. Singh
Department of Neurology, Postgraduate Institute of Medical Education & Research, Chandigarh 160012, India

N. Sharma
Department of Internal Medicine, Postgraduate Institute of Medical Education & Research, Chandigarh 160012, India

Anurag Kumar Singh, Hardeep Singh Malhotra, Ravindra Kumar Garg, Neeraj Kumar, Rajesh Verma and Praveen Kumar Sharma
Department of Neurology, King George Medical University, Uttar Pradesh, Lucknow, India

Amita Jain
Department of Microbiology, King George Medical University, Uttar Pradesh, Lucknow, India

Neera Kohli
Department of Radiodiagnosis, King George Medical University, Uttar Pradesh, Lucknow, India

Lei Shen
Department of Thoracic Intensive Care Units, Shanghai Pulmonary Hospital, Shanghai, China

Jianming Zheng, Mengqi Zhu, Haoxiang Zhu, Qi Cheng and Qian Li
Department of Infectious Diseases, Huashan Hospital, Fudan University, Shanghai, China

Yan Wang
Central Laboratory, Huashan Hospital, Fudan University, Shanghai, China

Aniruddha More, Ravindra Kumar Garg, Hardeep Singh Malhotra, Neeraj Kumar and Ravi Uniyal
Department of Neurology, King George Medical University, Lucknow PIN-226003, Uttar Pradesh, India

Junyan Qu, Taoyou Zhou, Cejun Zhong, Rong Deng and Xiaoju Lü
Center of Infectious Disease, West China Hospital, Sichuan University, 37 Guoxue Lane, Chengdu 610041, China

Peng Wang, Meng Xiao and Yingchun Xu
Department of Clinical Laboratory, Peking Union Medical College Hospital, Chinese Academy of Medical Sciences, Beijing 100730, People's Republic of China

Menglan Zhou
Department of Clinical Laboratory, Peking Union Medical College Hospital, Chinese Academy of Medical Sciences, Beijing 100730, People's Republic of China
Graduate School, Peking Union Medical College, Chinese Academy of Medical Sciences, Beijing, China

Sharon Chen and Fanrong Kong
Centre for Infectious Diseases and Microbiology Laboratory Services, Pathology West, Westmead Hospital, University of Sydney Darcy Road, Westmead, New South Wales 2145, Australia

Bin Du
Department of Medical Intensive Care Unit, Peking Union Medical College Hospital, Chinese Academy of Medical Sciences, Beijing, China

Jinlong Du
Department of Clinical Laboratory, Fu Xing Hospital, Capital Medical University, Beijing, China

Fengdan Wang
Department of Radiology, Peking Union Medical College Hospital, Chinese Academy of Medical Sciences, Beijing, China

Shayne Mason and Carolus J. Reinecke
Centre for Human Metabolomics, Faculty of Natural Sciences, North-West University (Potchefstroom Campus), Potchefstroom 2531, South Africa

Willem Kulik and Arno van Cruchten
Laboratory Genetic Metabolic Diseases, Department of Clinical Chemistry, Academic Medical Center, University of Amsterdam, Amsterdam, The Netherlands

Regan Solomons
Department of Paediatrics and Child Health, Faculty of Medicine and Health Sciences, Stellenbosch University, Tygerberg 7505, South Africa

A. Marceline Tutu van Furth
Department of Paediatric Infectious Diseases–Immunology and Rheumatology, Vrije Universiteit Medical Centre, De Boelelaan 1117, 1081HV Amsterdam, The Netherlands

Jaya George
Department of Chemical Pathology, University of Witwatersrand and National Health Laboratory Service, Johannesburg, South Africa

Adriano Dusé
Department of Clinical Microbiology and Infectious Diseases, University of Witwatersrand and National Health Laboratory Service, Johannesburg, South Africa

Pieter Ekermans
Department of Chemical Pathology, University of Witwatersrand and National Health Laboratory Service, Johannesburg, South Africa
Department of Chemical Pathology and Department of Clinical Microbiology and Infectious Diseases, School of Pathology, Faculty of Health Sciences, University of Witwatersrand and National Health Laboratory Service, 7 York Road, Johannesburg, South Africa

Brenda Anna Kwambana-Adams, Ebenezer Foster-Nyarko, Archibald Kwame Worwui, Catherine Okoi, Madikay Senghore, Jacob Kweku Otu and Chinelo Ebruke
Vaccines and Immunity Theme, The Medical Research Council Unit The Gambia, Banjul, Fajara, The Gambia

Franklin Asiedu-Bekoe, Badu Sarkodie, Kwame Amponsa-Achiano and Ebenezer Appiah-Denkyira
Ghana Health Service, Accra, Ghana

Osei Kuffour Afreh, Richard Bannerman and Timothy Letsa
Brong Ahafo Regional Health Directorate, Sunyani, Brong Ahafo, Ghana

George Khumalo Kuma
Regional Hospital Sunyani, Sunyani, Brong Ahafo Region, Ghana

Godfred Owusu-Okyere and David Opare
National Public Health Reference Laboratory, Ghana Health Service, Accra, Ghana

Sally-Ann Ohene, Charles Okot and Owen Kaluwa
WHO Country Office Ghana, Accra, Ghana

Gemma Kay and Mark J. Pallen
Microbiology and Infection Unit, Warwick Medical School, Warwick, UK

Victor Bampoe
Ministry of Health, Accra, Ghana

Syed M. A. Zaman
Disease Control and Elimination Theme, Medical Research Council Unit The Gambia, Fajara, The Gambia
London School of Hygiene and Tropical Medicine, London, UK

Martin Antonio
Vaccines and Immunity Theme, The Medical Research Council Unit The Gambia, Banjul, Fajara, The Gambia
Microbiology and Infection Unit, Warwick Medical School, Warwick, UK
London School of Hygiene and Tropical Medicine, London, UK

Umberto D'Alessandro
Disease Control and Elimination Theme, Medical Research Council Unit The Gambia, Fajara, The Gambia
London School of Hygiene and Tropical Medicine, London, UK
Institute of Tropical Medicine, Antwerp, Belgium

Jason M. Mwenda
WHO Regional Office for Africa, Brazzaville, Republic of Congo

Heng Gee Lee and Jayaram Menon
Department of Medicine, The Infectious Disease Unit, Queen Elizabeth Hospital, Kota Kinabalu, Sabah, Malaysia

Timothy William
Department of Medicine, The Infectious Disease Unit, Queen Elizabeth Hospital, Kota Kinabalu, Sabah, Malaysia
Jesselton Medical Centre, Kota Kinabalu, Sabah, Malaysia

Anna P. Ralph
Menzies School of Health Research, Darwin, Australia

Eng Eong Ooi, Yan'an Hou and October Sessions
Program in Emerging Infectious Diseases, Duke-NUS Graduate Medical School, Singapore, Singapore

Tsin Wen Yeo
Menzies School of Health Research, Darwin, Australia
Lee Kong Chian School of Medicine, Nanyang Technological University, Singapore, Singapore
Communicable Disease Centre, Institute of Infectious Diseases and Epidemiology, Tan Tock Seng Hospital, Singapore, Singapore

Lin-lin Liu, Tian-ming Chen, Shao-ying Li and Gang Liu
Department of Infectious Diseases, Beijing Children's Hospital, Capital Medical University, Beijing, China

Ling-yun Guo
Department of Infectious Diseases, Beijing Children's Hospital, Capital Medical University, Beijing, China
Key Laboratory of Major Diseases in Children and National Key Discipline of Pediatrics (Capital Medical University), Ministry of Education, National Clinical Research Centre for Respiratory Diseases, Beijing Key Laboratory of Pediatric Respiratory Infection Diseases, Beijing Pediatric Research Institute, Beijing Children's Hospital, Capital Medical University, Beijing, China

Yong-hong Yang
Key Laboratory of Major Diseases in Children and National Key Discipline of Pediatrics (Capital Medical University), Ministry of Education, National Clinical Research Centre for Respiratory Diseases, Beijing Key Laboratory of Pediatric Respiratory Infection Diseases, Beijing Pediatric Research Institute, Beijing Children's Hospital, Capital Medical University, Beijing, China

Yue Liu
Department of Radiology, Beijing Children's Hospital, Capital Medical University, Beijing, China

Michael Dalager-Pedersen
Department of Infectious Diseases, Aalborg University Hospital, Mølleparkvej 4, 9100 Aalborg, Denmark

Jacob Bodilsen
Department of Infectious Diseases, Aalborg University Hospital, Mølleparkvej 4, 9100 Aalborg, Denmark
Department of Medicine, Vendsyssel Hospital, Hjørring, Denmark

Henrik Carl Schønheyder
Department of Clinical Microbiology, Aalborg University Hospital, Aalborg, Denmark
Department of Clinical Medicine, Aalborg University, Aalborg, Denmark

Henrik Nielsen
Department of Infectious Diseases, Aalborg University Hospital, Mølleparkvej 4, 9100 Aalborg, Denmark
Department of Clinical Medicine, Aalborg University, Aalborg, Denmark

Anu Ramachandran and Maunank Shah
Johns Hopkins University School of Medicine, 725 N. Wolfe St. PCTB building-224, Baltimore, MD 21205, USA

Yukari Manabe
Johns Hopkins University School of Medicine, 725 N. Wolfe St. PCTB building-224, Baltimore, MD 21205, USA
Infectious Diseases Institute, Makerere University College of Health Sciences, Kampala, Uganda

Radha Rajasingham
Division of Infectious Diseases and International Medicine, Department of Medicine, University of Minnesota, Minneapolis, MN, USA

Hua-Zhen Zhao, Rui-Ying Wang, Xuan Wang, Ying-Kui Jiang, Ling-Hong Zhou, Jia-Hui Cheng, Li-Ping Huang and Li-Ping Zhu
Department of Infectious Diseases, Huashan Hospital, Fudan University, 12 Central Urumqi Road, Shanghai, China

Thomas Stephen Harrison
Institute of Infection and Immunity, St George's, University of London, London SW17, 0RE, UK

Yu He
Department of Clinical Laboratory, First Affiliated Hospital of Guangxi Medical University, Nanning, China
Department of Epidemiology, Affiliated Tumor Hospital of Guangxi Medical University, 71#, Hedi Road, Nanning 530021, China

Chao Han
Department of Geriatrics, Shandong Mental Health Center, Jinan, China

Kai-Feng Chang
Department of Infection Prevention, Pingyi Center for Disease Control and Prevention, Pingyi, China

Mao-Shui Wang
Department of Lab Medicine, Shandong Provincial Chest Hospital, Jinan, China

Tian-Ren Huang
Department of Epidemiology, Affiliated Tumor Hospital of Guangxi Medical University, 71#, Hedi Road, Nanning 530021, China

Shigeo Iijima
Department of Pediatrics, Hamamatsu University School of Medicine, Hamamatsu, Japan

Newton Kalata
Malawi-Liverpool-Wellcome Trust Clinical Research Programme, College of Medicine, Chichiri, Blantyre, Malawi

Jayne P. Ellis
Malawi-Liverpool-Wellcome Trust Clinical Research Programme, College of Medicine, Chichiri, Blantyre, Malawi
Hospital for Tropical Diseases, University College London Hospitals NHS Foundation Trust, London, UK

Elizabeth C. Joekes
Department of Radiology, The Royal Liverpool University Hospitals NHS Trust, Liverpool, UK

Samuel Kampondeni
Blantyre Malaria Project, Blantyre, Malawi

Laura A. Benjamin
Brain Infections Group, Walton Centre NHS Foundation Trust and Institute of Infection and Global Health, University of Liverpool, Liverpool, UK

Thomas S. Harrison
Institute for Infection and Immunity, St George's, University of London, London, UK

David G. Lalloo
Department of Clinical Sciences, Liverpool School of Tropical Medicine, Liverpool, UK

Robert S. Heyderman
Malawi-Liverpool-Wellcome Trust Clinical Research Programme, College of Medicine, Chichiri, Blantyre, Malawi
Division of Infection and Immunity, University College London, London, UK

Nguyen Thi Cam Huong, Nguyen My Hoa, Le Anh Tuan and Pham Thi Le Hoa
Department of Infectious Diseases, University of Medicine and Pharmacy at Ho Chi Minh City, Ho Chi Minh city, Vietnam
The Hospital for Tropical Diseases, Ho Chi Minh City, Vietnam

Ahmed M. A. Altibi
Faculty of Medicine, University of Jordan, Amman, Jordan

Samar Salman
Dermatology and Venereology Department, Tanta University Hospital, Tanta, Egypt

Sara Morsy
Biochemistry Department, Faculty of Medicine, Tanta University, Tanta, Egypt

Nguyen Thi Bich Lien
Ho Chi Minh City Hospital of Dermatology-Venereology, Ho Chi Minh City, Vietnam

Nguyen Thanh Truong
The Hospital for Tropical Diseases, Ho Chi Minh City, Vietnam

Van The Trung
Department of Dermatology, University of Medicine and Pharmacy at Ho Chi Minh City, Ho Chi Minh City, Vietnam

Nguyen Thi Hoang Mai
Oxford University Clinical Research Unit, Ho Chi Minh City, Vietnam

Nguyen Ba Thang
Department of Neurology, University of Medicine and Pharmacy at Ho Chi Minh City, Ho Chi Minh City, Vietnam

Siri Laura Feruglio
Division for Infection Control and Environmental Health, Norwegian Institute of Public Health, Oslo, Norway

Guro K. Bårnes and Dominique A. Caugant
Division for Infection Control and Environmental Health, Norwegian Institute of Public Health, Oslo, Norway
Faculty of Medicine, University of Oslo, Oslo, Norway

Esayas Kebede Gudina, Melkamu Berhane, Alemseged Abdissa and Getnet Tesfaw
Institute of Health, Jimma University, Jimma, Ethiopia

Hannah Joan Jørgensen
Division for Infection Control and Environmental Health, Norwegian Institute of Public Health, Oslo, Norway
Norwegian Veterinary Institute, Oslo, Norway

Gemeda Abebe
Institute of Health, Jimma University, Jimma, Ethiopia
Mycobacteriology Research Center, Jimma University, Jimma, Ethiopia

Eveline Pipolo Milan, Jéssica Jacinto Salviano de Almeida, Tatiane Uetti Gomes Fernandes and André Luciano de Araújo Prudente
Departamento de Infectologia, Universidade Federal do Rio Grande do Norte, Natal, Rio Grande do Norte, Brazil

Walicyranison Plinio Silva-Rocha, Matheus Firmino de Azevedo and Guilherme Maranhão Chaves
Centro de Ciências da Saúde, Laboratório de Micologia Médica e Molecular, Departamento de Análises Clínicas e Toxicológicas, Universidade Federal do Rio Grande do Norte, Rua Gal. Gustavo Cordeiro de Faria S/N, Petrópolis, Natal, Rio Grande do Norte, Brazil

Elaine Cristina Francisco, Analy Salles de Azevedo Melo and Arnaldo Lopes Colombo
Laboratório Especial de Micologia, Disciplina de Infectologia, Universidade Federal de São Paulo, São Paulo, Brazil

Béla Kocsis and Dóra Szabó
Semmelweis University, Institute of Medical Microbiology, Budapest, Hungary

Zoltán Tiszlavicz and Gabriella Jakab
SYNLAB Székesfehérvár Microbiology Laboratory, Székesfehérvár, Hungary
Réka Brassay, Márton Orbán and Ágnes Sárkány
"Szent György" University Teaching Hospital, Székesfehérvár, Hungary

Basil Benduri Kaburi, Ernest Kenu, Kofi Mensah Nyarko, Samuel Oko Sackey and Edwin Andrew Afari
Field Epidemiology and Laboratory Training Programme, Department of Epidemiology and Disease Control, School of Public Health, College of Health Sciences, University of Ghana, Legon, Accra, Ghana

Chrysantus Kubio
Field Epidemiology and Laboratory Training Programme, Department of Epidemiology and Disease Control, School of Public Health, College of Health Sciences, University of Ghana, Legon, Accra, Ghana
Ghana Health Service, West Gonja District Health Directorate, Damongo, Ghana

Jacob Yakubu Mahama
Ghana Health Service, Northern Regional Health Directorate, Tamale, Ghana

Heidi Smuts, Stephen Korsman and Diana Hardie
Division of Medical Virology, Department of Pathology, Faculty of Health Sciences, University of Cape Town, South Africa and the National Health Laboratory Service, Anzio Road, Observatory, Cape Town 7925, South Africa

Sarah Cronje
Life Bay View Private Hospital, Ryk Tulbach Street & Alhof Drive, De Nova, Mossel Bay 6506, South Africa

Juno Thomas
Centre for Enteric Diseases, National Institute for Communicable Diseases, 1 Modderfontein Road, Sandringham, Johannesburg 2130, South Africa

Delene Brink
PathCare George Laboratory, 1 Gloucester Avenue, George 6529, South Africa

Thomas Pouplin and Joel Tarning
Mahidol-Oxford Tropical Medicine Research Unit, Faculty of Tropical Medicine, Mahidol University, Bangkok, Thailand
Centre for Tropical Medicine and Global Health, Nuffield Department of Medicine, University of Oxford, Oxford, UK

Guy E. Thwaites and Jeremy N. Day
Centre for Tropical Medicine and Global Health, Nuffield Department of Medicine, University of Oxford, Oxford, UK
Oxford University Clinical Research Unit, Wellcome Trust Major Overseas Programme, Ho Chi Minh City, Viet Nam

Nguyen Duc Bang
Oxford University Clinical Research Unit, Wellcome Trust Major Overseas Programme, Ho Chi Minh City, Viet Nam
Pham Ngoc Thach Hospital, Ho Chi Minh City, Viet Nam

Pham Van Toi and Pham Nguyen Phuong
Oxford University Clinical Research Unit, Wellcome Trust Major Overseas Programme, Ho Chi Minh City, Viet Nam

Nguyen Huy Dung and Tran Ngoc Duong
Pham Ngoc Thach Hospital, Ho Chi Minh City, Viet Nam

Maxine Caws
Centre for Tropical Medicine and Global Health, Nuffield Department of Medicine, University of Oxford, Oxford, UK
Oxford University Clinical Research Unit, Wellcome Trust Major Overseas Programme, Ho Chi Minh City, Viet Nam
Liverpool School of Tropical Medicine, Liverpool, UK

Index

Lightning Source UK Ltd.
Milton Keynes UK
UKHW021141030622
403936UK00002B/20

9 781639 273034